Clinical Examples in Pediatric Rheumatology

Christian Huemer · Hermann Girschick

(Editors)

Clinical Examples in Pediatric Rheumatology

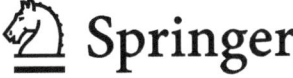 Springer

Editors
Christian Huemer
Landeskrankenhaus Bregenz
Bregenz, Austria

Hermann Girschick
Klinik für Kinder und Jugendmedizin
Vivantes Netzwerk f. Gesundheit GmbH
Berlin, Germany

ISBN 978-3-662-68731-4   ISBN 978-3-662-68732-1   (eBook)
https://doi.org/10.1007/978-3-662-68732-1

Translation from the German language edition: "Klinische Beispiele Pädiatrische Rheumatologie" by Christian Huemer and Hermann Girschick, © Der/die Herausgeber bzw. der/die Autor(en), exklusiv lizenziert an Springer-Verlag GmbH, DE, ein Teil von Springer Nature 2023. Published by Springer Berlin Heidelberg. All Rights Reserved

This book is a translation of the original German edition "Klinische Beispiele Pädiatrische Rheumatologie" by Huemer, Christian, published by Springer-Verlag GmbH, DE in 2023. The translation was done with the help of an artificial intelligence machine translation tool. A subsequent human revision was done primarily in terms of content, so that the book will read stylistically differently from a conventional translation. Springer Nature works continuously to further the development of tools for the production of books and on the related technologies to support the authors.

This Springer imprint is published by the registered company Springer-Verlag GmbH, DE, part of Springer Nature.
The registered company address is: Heidelberger Platz 3, 14197 Berlin, Germany

Paper in this product is recyclable.

Preface

Dear readers,

Complaints about the musculoskeletal system can have a variety of differential diagnostic causes, ranging from traumatology to oncology. Inflammatory changes from the field of rheumatology are assigned to "classic" disease entities, although the existing symptoms of the patient do not always immediately allow such an assignment. Therefore, the pattern recognition of a symptom complex is a crucial task in training and in daily routine in consultation and inpatient care. The "proving" symptoms are often missing in pediatric and adolescent rheumatology. Therefore, the mentioned symptoms are assessed within classification systems, and ultimately they are then assigned to a disease. This assignment is not necessarily synonymous with a clear diagnosis. It may even be possible to assign within several classifications. Laboratory values, including autoantibody patterns or even genetic analyses, can be helpful in clinical practice for the assignment. All of this ultimately forms the basis for a drug therapy decision. Recently, attempts have been made to standardize procedures nationally and internationally through targeted therapy strategies (Treat-to-Target protocols). Modern biologics are available here alongside proven conventional anti-inflammatory drugs and basic therapeutics.

The editors and co-authors of this book have endeavored to provide a wide range of clinical pictures for the practicing pediatrician and also for the training assistant for the additional designation of pediatric rheumatology. The approach within a rheumatological clinic, starting with anamnesis, clinical examination findings and symptom recognition, further diagnostics and then determination of the therapy strategy based on the above-mentioned algorithms, we try to explain in detail in this present case collection using impressive examples, in order to show you decision-making paths and procedures.

We hope that you find joy in reading!

Christian Huemer
Bregenz, Austria

Hermann Girschick
Berlin, Germany

Contents

List of Contributors

Prof. Dr. med. Hermann Girschick Klinik für Kinder- und Jugendmedizin, Vivantes Netzwerk für Gesundheit GmbH, Klinikum im Friedrichshain, Berlin, Germany; Kinderklinik und Poliklinik, Universitätsklinikum Würzburg, Würzburg, Germany

Dr. med. Annette Holl-Wieden Kinderklinik und Poliklinik, Universitätsklinikum Würzburg, Würzburg, Germany

Prim. Univ. Prof. Dr. med. Christian Huemer Ostschweizer Kinderspital, St.Gallen, Switzerland; Abt. für Kinder- und Jugendheilkunde, Landeskrankenhaus Bregenz, Akademisches Lehrkrankenhaus der Universitäten Wien, Innsbruck & Graz, Bregenz, Austria

Dr. med. Ae-Rie Im-Schipolowski Klinik für Kinder- und Jugendmedizin, Vivantes Netzwerk für Gesundheit GmbH, Klinikum im Friedrichshain, Berlin, Germany

Dr. med. Moritz Klaas Klinik für Kinder- und Jugendmedizin, Vivantes Netzwerk für Gesundheit GmbH, Klinikum im Friedrichshain, Berlin, Germany

PD Dr. med. Henner Morbach Kinderklinik und Poliklinik, Universitätsklinikum Würzburg, Würzburg, Germany

Dr. med. Christiane Reiser Abt. für Kinder- und Jugendheilkunde, Landeskrankenhaus Bregenz, Akademisches Lehrkrankenhaus der Universitäten Wien, Innsbruck & Graz, Bregenz, Austria; Abt. für Kinderrheumatologie, Klinik für Kinderheilkunde und Jugendmedizin, Universitätsklinikum Tübingen, Tübingen, Germany

A Tired Toddler Who Wants to be Carried, and a Teenage Athlete with a Swollen Knee

Christiane Reiser

Contents

© The Author(s), under exclusive license to Springer-Verlag GmbH, DE, part of Springer Nature 2024
C. Huemer and H. Girschick (eds.), *Clinical Examples in Pediatric Rheumatology*,
https://doi.org/10.1007/978-3-662-68732-1_1

1

1.1 Medical History

■■ Mila

The referral of the just over 2-year-old patient was initially to neuropediatrics due to suspected gait disorder. Accompanying the uncertain gait, the patient had been showing swellings in the area of the wrists for several months, as well as a **morning stiffness** with pain. The stiffness significantly improved over the course of the day. The mother had noticed a **general fatigue** in the child, and the general well-being of the child had changed according to the mother, the child was listless and grumpy.

The child had already been seen by an orthopedist, and the X-ray of both hip joints showed a normal finding appropriate for her age. Since no pathologies could be detected in neuropediatrics, the patient was referred to pediatric rheumatology. Family history: Maternal grandmother: Crohn's disease; Father: Restless Legs Syndrome. Vaccination status complete, previous development age-appropriate.

■■ Ebru

The 15-year-old patient, who was passionate about playing football, was initially referred by his general practitioner to the colleagues in trauma surgery, as he had been experiencing **knee joint pain** on the right side with effusion for months. The joint puncture performed there gave no indications of an infectious event. No trauma was remembered, however, the patient had to give up playing football due to the joint complaints, which he suffered greatly from. After an MRI examination, there was suspicion of a disease from the rheumatic spectrum, and he was referred to pediatric rheumatology. The medical history revealed no significant new aspects, the patient reported occasional pain now also in the left knee joint. The family history was bland, a tick bite was not remembered.

1.2 Examination Findings

■■ Mila

26-month-old toddler in good general condition and slim nutritional status. Weight 10 kg (Third percentile), length Fiftieth percentile. No abnormalities in pediatric internal medicine.

The musculoskeletal status revealed the presence of a **polyarthritis** involving multiple large and small joints. Hands, elbows, knees, and ankle joints were significantly swollen and painful on movement. Also, MCP and PIP joints (right hand emphasized) were swollen.

■■ Ebru

15-year-old patient in good general and nutritional condition, very athletic, muscular. **Knee joint arthritis** on the right with significant effusion, limited flexion and extension. Left knee joint unremarkable.

1.3 Laboratory Values and Imaging

1.3.1 Laboratory Values

■■ Mila

Inflammatory markers: **ESR 32 mm/h**, CRP 4.2 mg/dl (normal value < 0.5). **ANA titer 1:640,** rheumatoid factor negative. HLA-B27 negative. Borrelia serology negative. Blood count: leukocytes 16,700/μl, Hb 11.1 g/dl (norm 10.7–13.9), MCV 71.9 (norm 73–91), otherwise unremarkable. Serological findings, especially regarding bone metabolism and cell turnover, were unremarkable. Coagulation analysis: unremarkable overview parameters.

■■ Ebru

Inflammatory markers: ESR 13 mm/h, CRP 0.6 mg/dl (normal value < 0.5). Borrelia serology negative. HLA-B27 negative. ANA negative. Rheumatoid factor negative. Blood count and serological findings, especially regarding bone metabolism and cell turnover, were unremarkable. Uric acid 7.2 mg/dl (borderline normal). Coagulation analysis: unremarkable overview parameters.

1.3.2 Imaging

■■ Mila

Due to the multitude of inflamed joints and the sonographic evidence of **polyarthritis**, a whole-body MRI with i.v. contrast was performed for accurate assessment and differential diagnostic delineation, which revealed the following findings: symmetrical, synovial changes of the small and large joints of the upper and lower extremities with effusion and synovial enhancement: including the glenohumeral joint, carpus and the MCP joints on both sides with right-sided emphasis, upper ankle joint on both sides, in the area of the tarsus and the metatarsophalangeal joints on both sides.

■■ Ebru

Conventional X-ray of the left knee joint: soft tissue swelling, otherwise unremarkable. Sonography: pronounced effusion, synovitis with significant thickening and proliferation. MRI of the left knee joint: extensive joint effusion with soft tissue and bone edema in the attachment area of the quadriceps, popliteal and lateral femoral condyle consistent with **oligoarthritis**.

1.4 Educational Questions

1. What tentative diagnosis should be considered based on the symptoms? What is the most likely diagnosis?
2. How useful would it be to perform a conventional X-ray in this situation?
3. What options exist for patient education and training?
4. What is the prognosis of JIA, especially with regard to the mental health of children and adolescents?

1.5 Further Course

■■ Mila

The patient is diagnosed with **ANA-positive, seronegative polyarthritis**. Initially, a whole-body MRI was performed, which showed a symmetrical involvement of large and small joints with effusion formations of varying degrees. The examination had to be performed under anesthesia due to the patient's age. The **intra-articular steroid injection** was performed in the same sedation in the hands, knees, and ankle joints on both sides. After receiving negative results for Hepatitis B, C, and Tuberculosis (intradermal tuberculin test), we started immunosuppressive therapy with **Methotrexate** (dosage 10–15 mg/m^2 BSA) once a week per os. Folic acid 2.5 mg is given 24 hours after MTX intake in patients under approx. 20 kg body weight (5 mg from 20 kg body weight). The patient receives anti-inflammatory ibuprofen 30 mg/kg body weight in 3 single doses per day. At the first presentation after 4 weeks and also in the further course, a very rapid excellent response to the therapy was shown. Only the hand and elbow joints were still slightly painful and swollen after 8 weeks. The medications were well tolerated. The therapy with ibuprofen was discontinued in the meantime.

■■ Ebru

The adolescent is diagnosed with **ANA-negative, limited oligoarthritis**. After receiving negative Lyme serology, intra-articular steroid injection was performed under sedation and accompanying anti-inflammatory therapy with ibuprofen. Although there was

1

a rapid and significant improvement in arthritis within 3 weeks, there was no complete remission, so therapy with MTX was started 4 weeks later. At this time, there was also arthritis of the left big toe joint. In the further course, the patient's mother repeatedly reported that Ebru was "depressed" because the situation was not improving and he still could not play football, so measures for disease coping were necessary. Conversations with a psychologist resulted in a stabilization of the situation. From the side of the underlying disease, there was an exacerbation of the pain 12 weeks after the start of MTX, which required hospital admission. The repeated MRI examination revealed arthritic changes in the left midfoot. Immediate improvement of the pain under oral steroids for 4 weeks (tapering), start with Adalimumab in addition to Methotrexate as extended immunosuppressive therapy. Rapid achievement of a sustained remission under this.

Ophthalmological examinations to exclude uveitis were performed in both children according to the recommendation of the guideline (German Ophthalmological Society e.V. 2021), without any inflammatory changes being seen.

1.6 Educational Answers

- 1. **What presumptive diagnosis should be considered based on the symptoms? What is the most likely diagnosis?**

In the case of oligoarticular progression, a number of differential diagnoses should be considered depending on the medical history and examination findings. For detailed explanations, we refer to the textbooks of pediatric rheumatology. After excluding acute causes such as trauma, septic arthritis/osteomyelitis (including tuberculous) and Lyme arthritis, reactive arthritides and arthritides that occur in the context of rheumatic diseases are found, with juvenile idiopathic arthritis (JIA) being the most common rheumatic disease in childhood. **Lyme arthritis**, as the most common differential diagnosis, typically presents with oligoarthritis of the lower extremity. The diagnosis is usually made serologically. The eubacterial PCR from the joint aspirate can also be indicative. In the case of oligoarticular progression, Borrelia diagnostics are mandatory. In addition, there are rarer diseases such as chronic non-bacterial osteomyelitis (CNO) or pigmented villonodular synovitis (this rare diagnosis should be particularly considered in the case of [mono-] arthritis of the knee joint), which should be included in the differential diagnostic considerations depending on the clinic, imaging and course. In particular, celiac serology should also be performed in younger children, as this autoimmune disease can manifest with the first symptom of arthritis.

Since the findings and the course in Ebru were well compatible with the presence of JIA, the corresponding therapy was initiated. According to the ILAR classification criteria (Petty et al. 2004), Ebru has oligoarthritis, "persistent"/limited form.

In Mila, the diagnosis of polyarticular JIA is quickly made (◘ Fig. 1.1), with a distinction being made here between the rheumatoid factor (RF) positive and negative form. The RF-positive JIA only accounts for about 1–4% of our JIA cases, it corresponds among other things to genetically predisposing factors, laboratory parameters and course most likely to adult rheumatoid arthritis and occurs more often in older/adolescent patients. The much more common **"seronegative" polyarthritis (RF and ACPA negative)** is defined by joint involvement ≥ 5 joints and the exclusion of other causes (◘ Fig. 1.2 shows the clinical findings of a boy as an example). After the clinic, laboratory findings and course in the patient made JIA appear as the most likely diagnosis, therapy was quickly initiated. An

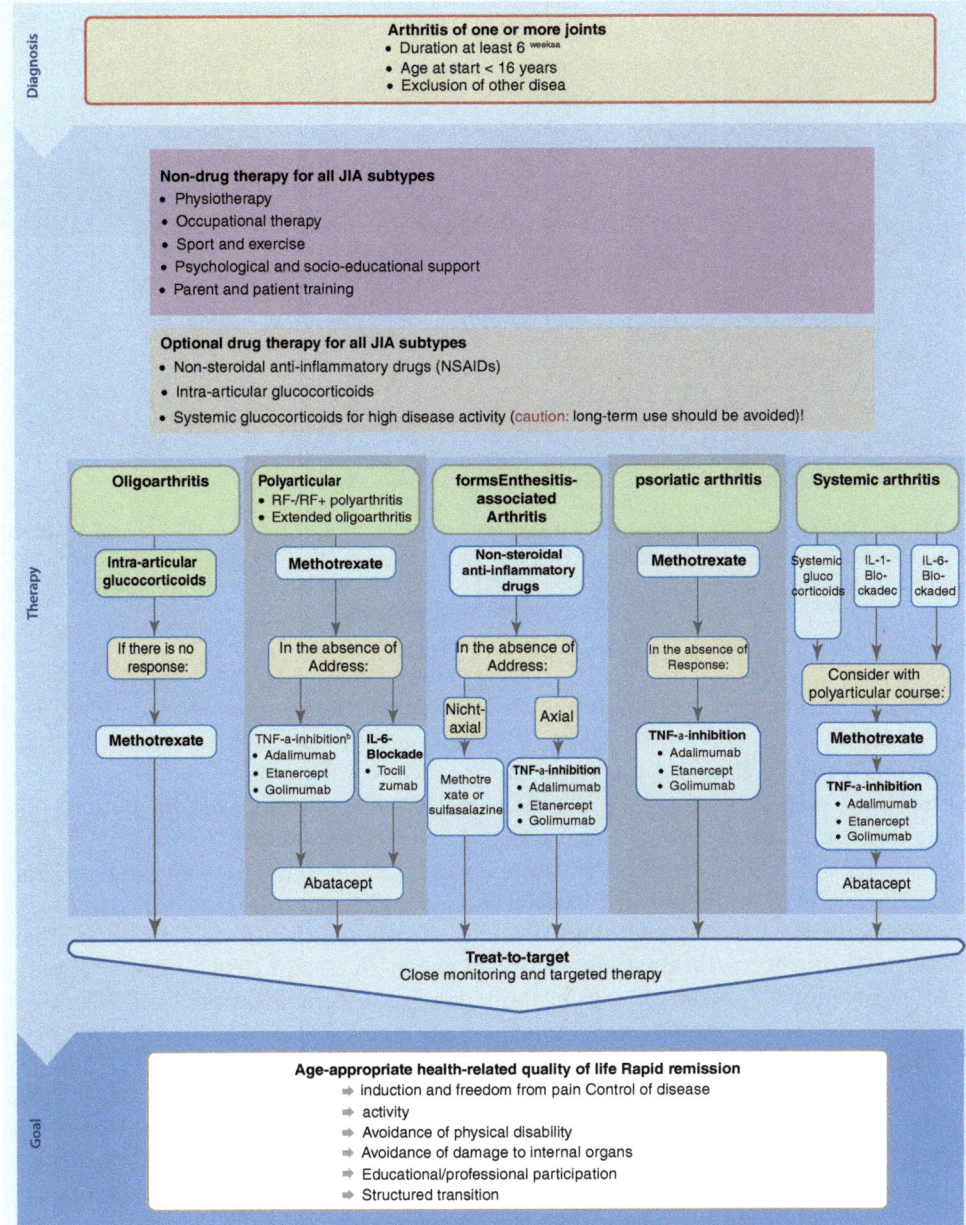

☐ **Fig. 1.1** **Recommendations for diagnostic and therapeutic approach in different subtypes of juvenile idiopathic arthritis.** From: Oommen 2020, recommendation for action according to the S2k guideline therapy of juvenile idiopathic arthritis (▶ https://doi.org/10.1007/s00112-020-00982-0)

1

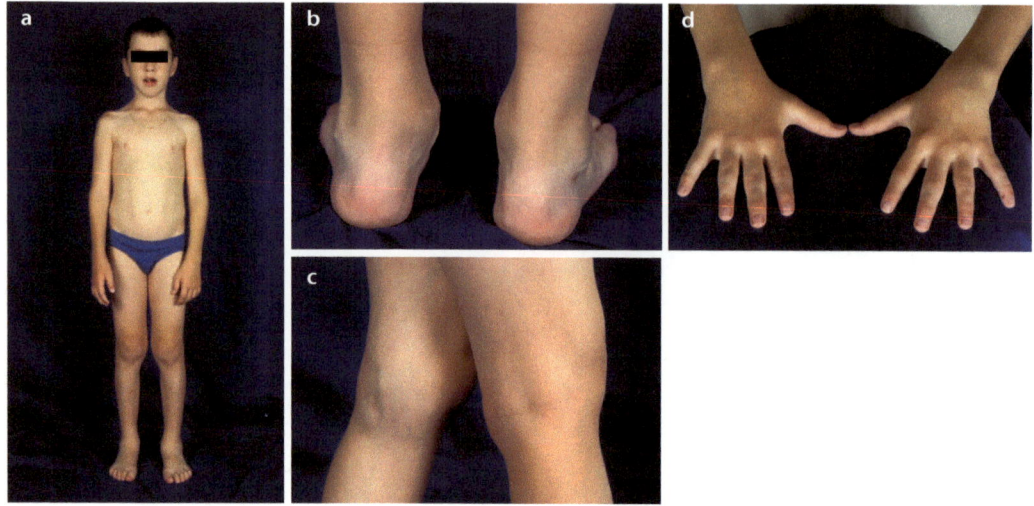

◘ Fig. 1.2 a–d RF-negative polyarthritis, clinical picture. 7-year-old boy with complaints for 3 years; affected by arthritis: both knees, wrists, finger joints, OSG, USG, cervical spine, shoulders with significant restriction of joint mobility, fortunately no bony destructions. Laboratory chemistry shows slight signs of inflammation, RF negative, ANA negative, HLA-B27 negative. No eye involvement in the course

overview of the therapy strategies is shown in ◘ Fig. 1.1.

Depending on the duration and type of complaints, as well as particularly the accompanying symptoms, there are a number of differential diagnostic considerations in polyarthritis, here we would like to refer to textbooks of pediatric rheumatology. Behind polyarthritis/polyarthralgia, in addition to an oncological diagnosis, e.g. in the sense of leukemia, a symptom of a collagen disease such as systemic lupus erythematosus (SLE) can also be hidden. Therefore, the initial laboratory diagnostics are of great importance, which should include all relevant organ systems, especially bone metabolism and extended autoimmunology.

■ **2. How useful would it be to perform a conventional X-ray in this situation?**

Especially for differential diagnostic clarification, a conventional X-ray of at least one joint/region can be useful. Erosive changes are to be expected especially in psoriasis ar-

thritis and seropositive polyarthritis, as well as in protracted or untreated courses.

■ **3. What options exist for patient education and training?**

Improved disease understanding and knowledge enhances therapy adherence. Training is offered, for example, by the Rheuma League or rheumatism clinics. Digital offers are also increasingly available (▶ www.my-rheumatism-is-growing-up.com; ▶ www.children-rheumatism-info.com) and their effectiveness has been reviewed (Reiser et al. 2021). For older teenagers and young adults, transition training exists, for example, in the context of camps (▶ www.rheumatism-camp.org). The aim is, among other things, to address the emotional burden of the patient, as impressively existing in Ebru.

■ **4. What is the prognosis of JIA, especially with regard to the mental health of children and adolescents?**

Special attention should be paid to comorbidities, the presence of which can worsen the outcome (Favier et al. 2018). Mental illnesses, especially **depression**, are associated with increased pain and limited joint function (Lipstein et al. 2016). This should be taken into account at any age by the treating physicians and, if necessary, therapeutic measures should be initiated. The presence of untreated mental illnesses is defined as a risk factor for the failure of the **transition to adult medicine** (Society for Transition Medicine 2021).

1.7 Summary

1.7.1 Definition

JIA is defined as arthritis of one or more joints, with the following characteristics:
- Onset before the Sixteenth birthday
- Duration of arthritis ≥ 6 weeks
- Unclear etiology
- Exclusion of other causes

The disease is classified based on clinical and laboratory findings within the first 6 months and divided into the corresponding subtypes (see textbooks of pediatric rheumatology).

1.7.2 Pathogenesis/Clinic

In oligoarthritis, arthritis often begins insidiously in early childhood—often of the knee joint—which often manifests less through pain than through **behavioral changes** (child does not want to run anymore). Other typical findings are morning stiffness, start-up pain after inactivity, and possibly the protective posture of the affected limb. Some parents report that the child is less active or more tired than before.

Seronegative polyarthritis often manifests with symmetrical involvement of small and large joints. In the case of small joints, the MCP and PIP joints are often affected, in the case of large joints initially the knee, ankle, hand, and elbow joints, although in principle all joints can be affected. The temporomandibular joint is also particularly worth mentioning, which is often only noticed by facial asymmetry or pain when chewing, which gives great importance to history and careful examination. General symptoms of polyarthritis can be fatigue, subfebrile temperatures, or developmental stagnation.

1.7.3 Diagnosis

- *Laboratory* (also individually expandable with regard to differential diagnostic considerations):
  ESR, CRP, blood count, differential blood count; liver and kidney function parameters, uric acid, LDH; ANA (if positive, including dsDNA, ENA), HLA-B27; rheumatoid factors or anti-CCP-AB; Lyme serology (possibly also serologies in relation to streptococci, Yersinia, salmonella, shigella, campylobacter, chlamydia, mycoplasma); possibly complement C3, C4 and CH50; urine status
- *Sonography:*
  Established diagnostic tool in the consultation, excellent for follow-up controls.
- *Radiological:*
  Conventional X-ray of individual joints for differential diagnostic clarification and assessment of existing complications (erosions, joint space narrowing, especially in polyarthritis: periarticular osteoporosis); MRI especially in axial involvement, involvement of the temporomandibular joints and differential diagnostic considerations

1.7.4 Therapy

An overview of the therapeutic options is given in ◘ Fig. 1.1 from the S2k guideline for JIA (Oommen 2020). Intra-articular

1

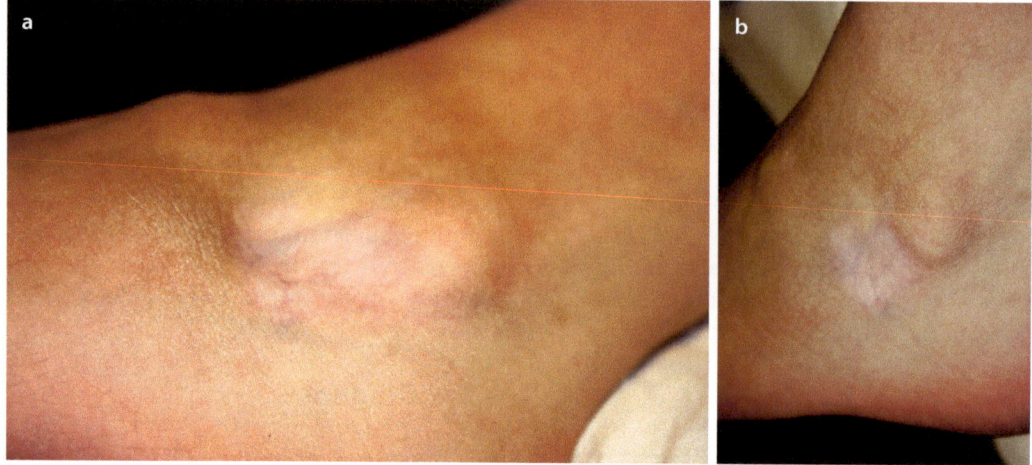

◘ Fig. 1.3   a,b Joint status after intra-articular steroid application. Lipoatrophy and depigmentation after therapeutic puncture with triamcinolone hexacetonide of the lower left ankle joint

steroid injection still plays an important role, which should always be performed under sedation/anesthesia in the pediatric setting to avoid traumatization. Side effects that can occur here include bacterial joint infections, joint bleeding, and lipoatrophy after instillation of triamcinolone hexacetonide (◘ Fig. 1.3).

1.7.5 Diagnosis

The diagnosis is an exclusion diagnosis, which can be made based on the mentioned clinical and laboratory findings as well as the anamnestic and differential diagnostic considerations.

1.7.6 Prognosis

In about half of the patients, a remission (long-term without further drug therapy) is achieved therapeutically, although the individual courses are very different. Early start of effective therapy forms (Treat-to-Target) appear to be of decisive importance

for the prognosis. To achieve good therapy adherence, educational measures are important.

> **Conclusion**
>
> The diagnosis of JIA requires careful work-up of the differential diagnoses. Nowadays, a variety of effective medications are available that can enable children and adolescents to participate as unimpaired as possible, especially when used early.

References

Deutsche Ophthalmologische Gesellschaft e.V. (2021) S2k Leitlinie: Diagnostik und antientzündliche Therapie der Uveitis bei juveniler idiopathischer Arthritis. AWMF-Leitlinie

Favier LA, Taylor J, Loiselle Rich K et al (2018) Barriers to adherence in juvenile idiopathic arthritis: a multicenter collaborative experience and preliminary results. J Rheumatol 45:690–696. ► https://doi.org/10.3899/jrheum.171087

Gesellschaft für Transitionsmedizin (2021) S3-Leitlinie: Von der Pädiatrie in die Erwachsenenmedizin

Lipstein EA, Lovell DJ, Denson LA et al (2016) Parents' information needs and influential factors when making decisions about TNF-α inhibitors. Pediatr Rheumatol Online J 14:53. ► https://doi.org/10.1186/s12969-016-0113-5

Oommen PT (2020) Handlungsempfehlung nach der S2k-Leitlinie Therapie der juvenilen idiopathischen Arthritis. Monatsschr Kinderheilkd 168:947–949. ► https://doi.org/10.1007/s00112-020-00982-0

Petty RE, Southwood TR, Manners P et al (2004) International League of Associations for Rheumatology classification of juvenile idiopathic arthritis: second revision, Edmonton, 2001. J Rheumatol 31:390–392

Reiser C, Zeltner NA, Rettenbacher B et al (2021) Explaining juvenile idiopathic arthritis to paediatric patients using illustrations and easy-to-read texts: improvement of disease knowledge and adherence to treatment. Pediatr Rheumatol Online J 19:158. ► https://doi.org/10.1186/s12969-021-00644-9

A 14-Year-Old Boy with Spinal Pain and Heel Pain

Christian Huemer

Contents

2.1 Medical History

Moritz, at the age of 15, is presented at the rheumatology clinic for further investigation of complaints in the spinal area and bilateral heel pain that have been present for 8 weeks. The symptoms began a year ago, gradually with pain in the entire spine at rest, but especially during school sports; initially, the family doctor referred him to an orthopedist. An X-ray of the spine was taken, but no specific diagnosis was made. Physiotherapy was initially prescribed and showed little improvement. Regarding the bilateral heel pain that has occurred in recent months, there was initially suspicion of growing pains. No further specific therapy was suggested. Now, at the insistence of his mother, who herself has sacroiliitis, he is referred to the rheumatology clinic for further investigation.

2.2 Examination Findings

15-year-old boy in good general and nutritional condition.

Musculoskeletal status shows no signs of palpable synovitis in the joints, active and passive mobility in all peripheral joints is inconspicuous. There is tenderness to pressure in the area of the Achilles tendon attachments. Examination of the spine with slight **paravertebral tenderness to pressure**, especially in the sacroiliac region, modified Schober test 18 cm (thus slightly restricted).

Internal status (auscultation findings, cardiopulmonary, abdomen, ENT findings) inconspicuous. Skin findings inconspicuous except for mild facial acne.

2.3 Laboratory Values and Imaging

2.3.1 Laboratory Values

Blood count, CRP inconspicuous. ESR inconspicuous. Rheumatoid factor negative.

Antinuclear antibodies negative. C3, C4 complement negative. Anti-CCP negative. **HLA-B27 positive**.

2.3.2 Imaging

MRI examination of the ileosacral region (◘ Fig. 2.1) showed symmetrical bone marrow edema adjacent to the SI joint space on both sides. No joint effusion, no signs of erosive changes. In summary, findings consistent with **bilateral sacroiliitis**.

2.4 Educational Questions

1. What suspected diagnosis should be considered based on the symptom of back pain, and what is the most likely diagnosis?
2. How useful would additional laboratory or imaging diagnostics be in this situation?
3. What questions would you add to the family history?

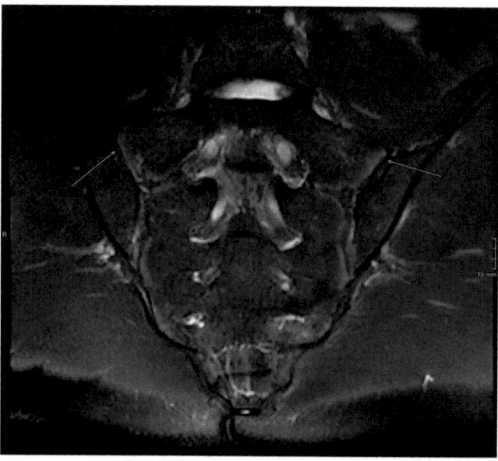

◘ **Fig. 2.1 MRI of the sacroiliac region.** Bilateral symmetrical sacroiliitis without evidence of erosive changes, significant edema (T2 weighting). (With kind permission from Prim. Dr. A. Schuster, Radiology Department LKH Bregenz)

2.5 Differential Diagnostic Considerations

Back pain in adolescents is a common symptom and requires an economical, graduated differential diagnostic clarification. In addition to ruling out a non-inflammatory diagnosis (juvenile scoliosis, osteodystrophies of the adolescent, e.g. Scheuermann's disease), differential diagnoses should also consider conditions with radiating back pain: kidney diseases or gastrointestinal diseases are common. Further diagnostics using laboratory and imaging diagnostics are indicated primarily in cases of suspected inflammatory spinal diseases.

Acute or chronic inflammatory diseases of the vertebral bodies (osteomyelitis) and the joint structures of the spine and sacroiliac region must be ruled out. A positive family history of rheumatic diseases or diseases with HLA-B27 positivity in family members can be an important indication of an autoimmune/inflammatory process in the adolescent: however, HLA-B27 positivity alone is not proof of this disease.

2.6 Further Progress

The patient, with clear indications of an inflammatory process in imaging diagnostics (**bilateral sacroiliitis**) and in the clinical picture (pressure tenderness and functional restriction in the sacroiliac region, **enthesitis** of the heel region on both sides), initially received non-steroidal anti-inflammatory therapy (NSAID) and physiotherapy. This did not show lasting success—a therapeutic trial with **sulfasalazine** (2 times 2 g p.o./day) was carried out for 3 months. The patient then reported partial improvement in back mobility and was able to regularly participate in recreational sports again. After a few months, an intolerance to sulfasalazine developed, and a switch to a basic thera-

peutic agent (methotrexate 15 mg/m^2 BSA/week s.c.) was suggested. Current findings: complete clinical improvement under this therapy, the patient currently without restrictions in his everyday life (studies, recreational sports).

2.7 Educative Answers

- **1. What suspected diagnosis should be considered based on the symptom of back pain, what is the most likely diagnosis?**

Given the chronic symptoms, there is a high suspicion of a rheumatological diagnosis in the adolescent, and further diagnostics should be planned accordingly.

- **2. How useful would additional laboratory or imaging diagnostics be in this situation?**

To further narrow down the process, a native X-ray of the spine and especially an MRI examination should be planned. The autoimmune laboratory (ANA, rheumatoid factor, complement, HLA-B27) complements this diagnostics.

- **What questions would you add to the family history?**

Rheumatological diseases involving the axial skeleton often have a positive family history for HLA-B27-associated diseases (Ankylosing spondylitis, **chronic inflammatory bowel disease**, Psoriasis). Therefore, a detailed family history is very useful.

2.8 Summary

The 15-year-old Moritz was diagnosed with juvenile idiopathic arthritis. Based on the clinical picture and the laboratory and imaging findings, there was an enthesitis-associated arthritis (EAA).

2.8.1 Classification

Due to its clinical characteristics and genetic background, EAA belongs to the family of spondyloarthritides (SpA). This includes ankylosing spondylitis, axial SpA, reactive arthritis, psoriatic arthritis, enteropathic arthritis, and the seronegative enthesiopathy and arthropathy syndrome (SEA) (Girschick et al. 2022). Patients with these diseases tend to have **arthritis**, preferably of the large joints of the lower extremities, involvement of the sacroiliac joints and spine, **enthesitis**, **dactylitis**, acute anterior uveitis as well as inflammatory lesions of bone, intestine, and neck. They often have a positive family history for these diseases and HLA-B27 positivity.

> **ILAR Classification: Enthesitis-associated Arthritis (Petty et al. 1998, 2004)**
> ━ **Arthritis and Enthesitis,**
> *or*
> ━ **Arthritis or Enthesitis** with two or more of the following criteria:
> – Sacroiliac joint complaints/lumbosacral pain
> – HLA-B27 positivity
> – Positive family history for HLA-B27-associated diseases (ankylosing spondylitis, EAA, chronic inflammatory bowel diseases, reactive arthritis, acute anterior uveitis)
> – Acute symptomatic anterior uveitis
> – Onset of arthritis in a male patient > 6 years of age

2.8.2 Etiology

A specific singular etiology of EAA is not known. In most cohorts, there is a strong presence of HLA-B27 up to almost 70%.

2.8.3 Clinic

Initially, arthritis occurs in the context of an EAA at one or more peripheral joints (Cassidy and Petty 2001). In addition, there is enthesitis at one or more sites, most commonly in the knee or foot area. Back pain is usually absent at the time of manifestation, only about 24% of children also report pain in the lumbosacral and sacroiliac region.

2.8.4 Diagnosis

The diagnosis of EAA is a clinical diagnosis. Clues are provided by the family history and the typical clinical manifestations. Although the ILAR classification criteria are not diagnostic criteria, they are often used:

Compared to the ILAR classification of 1998, there are competing classifications that describe almost the same group of patients but weigh different things differently. For example, the so-called New York criteria for the diagnosis of ankylosing spondylitis essentially refer to the inflammatory involvement of the spine (Bennett 1968). The criteria established by Armor in 1990 group a set of diseases under the name Spondylarthropathies (Amor et al. 1990): the inflammation of joints and the axial skeleton, the inflammation of tendon, ligament and capsule attachments to the bone. Arthritis in the context of inflammatory bowel diseases, reactive arthritis, including Reiter's syndrome, and psoriasis arthritis were also included here. Already in the early 1980s, Petty (Rosenberg and Petty 1982) had described a similar group of diseases as SEA syndrome (seronegative enthesiopathy and arthropathy), which referred to patients under the age of 17. The aim of the ILAR classification was to define as homogeneous and well describable study populations as possible, which largely exclude each other and thus enable international comparisons. This resulted in the broader juvenile spondylarthropathy being classified in everyday life within the ILAR classification into the groups EAA, psoriatic arthritis and also undifferentiated arthritis. A new proposal for the classification of JIA attempts to take into account both the predominant picture of peripheral SpA in adolescence and the classification of SpA in adulthood (by including imaging and adopting the definition of inflammatory back pain) (Martini et al. 2019).

PRINTO-JIA Criteria of EAA (Martini et al. 2019)
- **Peripheral Arthritis** and **Enthesitis** or:
- Arthritis **or** Enthesitis **plus** > 3 months of inflammatory back pain and radiological sacroiliitis or:
- Arthritis **or** Enthesitis **plus** 2 of the following parameters:
  a) Pressure pain over the sacroiliac joints
  b) Inflammatory back pain
  c) Acute anterior uveitis
  d) Evidence of HLA B27
  e) Positive family history for a SpA in a first-degree relative

---

2.8.5 Therapy

The goal of therapy is to achieve inactive disease and, if possible, to maintain all desired athletic activities. The use of medication depends on the clinical severity of the inflammation. In the case of rapidly developing (poly-)arthritis and pronounced enthesitis, the use of locally or systemically administered glucocorticoids should be considered. If only a few joints are affected, an intra-articular steroid injection may be useful. A steroid injection into the sacroiliac joint can be a therapeutic option. If

there is insufficient response to these therapies, basic therapy with sulfasalazine (20–50 mg/kg body weight p.o.) should be indicated (Brooks 2001; Varbanova and Dyankov 1999). Alternatively, therapy with methotrexate (10–15 mg/m^2 BSA/week p.o. or s.c.) could be discussed. However, there are insufficient study data on methotrexate and EAA in children and adolescents. Corresponding data from adult patients show no effect for MTX (and also for sulfasalazine) in axial disease and only limited efficacy in peripheral arthritis. As a third option, TNF-α-blocking biologics are available (Henrickson and Reiff 2004; Hospach et al. 2022). Explicitly approved for the treatment of children and adolescents with EAA are adalimumab from the age of 6 and etanercept from the age of 12 (Foeldvari et al. 2019; Horneff et al. 2015).

2.8.6 Prognosis

EAA has—in addition to systemic JIA and rheumatoid factor-positive JIA—among the subgroups of JIA a significantly worse prognosis. In a study published in 2002, 56% of patients still had disease activity of their EAA 16 years after diagnosis. This underlines the enormous importance of individualized treat-to-target therapy for this group of patients.

Conclusion

The investigation of back pain in adolescents requires a step-by-step approach to exclude important non-inflammatory and other non-rheumatic differential diagnoses.

The diagnosis of EAA should be defined quickly, as a clear individual treatment concept must be established promptly in order to influence the already unfavorable prognosis.

References

Amor B, Dougados M, Mijiyawa M (1990) Criteria of the classifcation of spondylarothpathies. Rev Rheum Mal Osteoartic 57:85–89

Bennett W (1968) Population studies of the rheumatic disease. Excerpta Medica, New York, pp 4–6

Brooks CD (2001) Sulfasalazine for the management of juvenile rheumatoid arthritis. J Rheumatol 28:845–853

Cassidy JT, Petty RE (2001) Juvenile ankylosing spondylitis. In: Cassidy JT, Petty RE (Eds) Textbook of pediatric rheumatology. Saunders, Philadelphia, pp 323–345

Foeldvari I, Constantin T, Vojinović J, Horneff G, Chasnyk V, Dehoorne J, Panaviene V, Sušić G, Stanevicha V, Kobusinska K, Zuber Z, Dobrzyniecka B, Nikishina I, Bader-Meunier B, Breda L, Doležalová P, Job-Deslandre C, Rumba-Rozenfelde I, Wulffraat N, Pedersen RD, Bukowski JF, Vlahos B, Martini A, Ruperto N, Paediatric Rheumatology International Trials Organisation (PRINTO) (2019) Etanercept treatment for extended oligoarticular juvenile idiopathic arthritis, enthesitis-related arthritis, or psoriatic arthritis: 6-year efficacy and safety data from an open-label trial. Arthritis Res Ther 21(1):125. ▶ https://doi.org/10.1186/s13075-019-1916-9

Girschick H, Hospach T, Minden K (2022) Enthesitis-assoziierte Arthritis bei Kindern und Jugendlichen. In: Wagner N, Dannecker G, Kallinich T (Hrsg) Pädiatrische Rheumatologie. Springer, Berlin/Heidelberg, S 393–402

Henrickson M, Reiff A (2004) Prolonged efficacy of etanercept in refractory enthesitis-related arthritis. J Rheumatol 31:2055–2061

Horneff G, Foeldvari I, Minden K, Trauzeddel R, Kümmerle-Deschner JB, Tenbrock K, Ganser G, Huppertz HI (2015) Efficacy and safety of etanercept in patients with the enthesitis-related arthritis category of juvenile idiopathic arthritis: results from a phase III randomized, double-blind study. Arthritis Rheumatol 67(8):2240–2249. ▶ https://doi.org/10.1002/art.39145

Hospach T, Horneff G, Poddubnyy D (2022) Spondyloarthritis in childhood and adulthood. Z Rheumatol 81(1):14–21. ▶ https://doi.org/10.1007/s00393-021-01135-8

Martini A, Ravelli A, Avcin T, Beresford MW, Burgos-Vargas R, Cuttica R, Ilowite NT, Khubchandani R, Laxer RM, Lovell DJ, Petty RE, Wallace CA, Wulffraat NM, Pistorio A, Ruperto N, Pediatric Rheumatology International Trials Organization (PRINTO) (2019) Toward new classification criteria for juvenile idiopathic arthritis: first steps, Pediatric Rheumatology International Trials Organization International Consensus. J Rheumatol 46(2):190–197. ▶ https://doi.org/10.3899/jrheum.180168

Petty RE, Southwood TR, Baum J, Bhettay E, Glass DN, Manners P, Maldonado-Cocco J, Suarez-Almazor M, Orozco-Alcala J, Prieur AM (1998) Revision of the proposed classification criteria for juvenile idiopathic arthritis: Durban, 1997. J Rheumatol 25(10):1991–1994

Petty RE, Southwood TR, Manners P et al (2004) International League of Associations for Rheumatology classification of juvenile idiopathic arthritis, Second revision. Edmonton J Rheumatol 31:390–392

Rosenberg AM, Petty RE (1982) A syndrome of seronegative enthesiopathy and arthropathy in children. Arthritis Rheum 25:1041–1047

Varbanova BB, Dyankov ED (1999) Sulphasalazine. An alternative drug for second-line treatment of juvenile idiopathic arthritis. J Rheumatol 38:2482–2487

A 16-Year-Old Girl with Swelling of 3 Fingers for Several Months: What's Going On?

Christian Huemer

Contents

© The Author(s), under exclusive license to Springer-Verlag GmbH, DE, part of Springer Nature 2024
C. Huemer and H. Girschick (eds.), *Clinical Examples in Pediatric Rheumatology*,
https://doi.org/10.1007/978-3-662-68732-1_3

3.1 Medical History

The 16-year-old patient presented herself at the rheumatology clinic with a swelling in the area of the Second, Third, and Fourth fingers of the right hand that had been present for about 8 months. She had previously seen an orthopedist, who had suspected a sports injury—the girl occasionally played volleyball—and initially recommended a 3-month therapy with a nonsteroidal anti-inflammatory drug. Over time, the symptoms increased, involving also the thumb and possibly the Third ray of the right hand and the Second ray of the right hand. No other complaints. Only in the area of the elbow joints on both sides, there was recurrent dry skin with slight skin redness. No other previous illnesses known. Family history positive for psoriasis in the father of the child, otherwise unremarkable family history.

3.2 Examination Findings

16-year-old girl in the best general and nutritional condition, no abnormalities in the internal status. Skin findings show slightly reddened, scaly-eczematous skin in the area of the elbow extensor sides on both sides.

Joint status shows swelling at the left knee joint, swelling of the thumb base joint, and a swelling of the Second-Fourth fingers of the right hand in the sense of dactylitis. Functionally, there is an end-stage flexion deficit in the affected fingers, there is slight pressure tenderness over the proximal interphalangeal joints of the affected fingers.

3.3 Laboratory Values and Imaging

3.3.1 Laboratory Values

Unremarkable blood count, CRP negative, ESR slightly elevated (28 mm/h), antinu-clear antibodies, ANCA, rheumatoid factor, complement C3, C4, anti-CCP antibodies each negative, **HLA-B27 positive**.

Liver and kidney function parameters unremarkable, thyroid parameters unremarkable. Gliadin IgG antibodies and transglutaminase IgA antibodies negative.

3.3.2 Imaging

Plain radiograph of the right hand (◘ Fig. 3.1): In the Fourth digit of the right hand, there are arthritic changes in the distal and proximal interphalangeal joint with erosive changes. Clearly visible soft tissue swelling of the Third and Fourth digits in the sense of dactylitis.

3.4 Educational Questions

1. What differential diagnoses do you consider with this described symptomatology?
2. What significance do the consistently negative findings of the "rheumatism laboratory" have for further diagnostic and also therapeutic planning?
3. What strategic therapeutic considerations need to be taken into account, especially including a target-defined therapy?

3.5 Educational Answers

- **1. What differential diagnoses do you consider with this described symptomatology?**

The swelling of initially one finger and subsequently other finger joints that has been present for several months primarily suggests a high suspicion of a rheumatic process. A post-traumatic lesion with this clinical picture or an infectious process would be extremely unlikely after 8 months of disease duration.

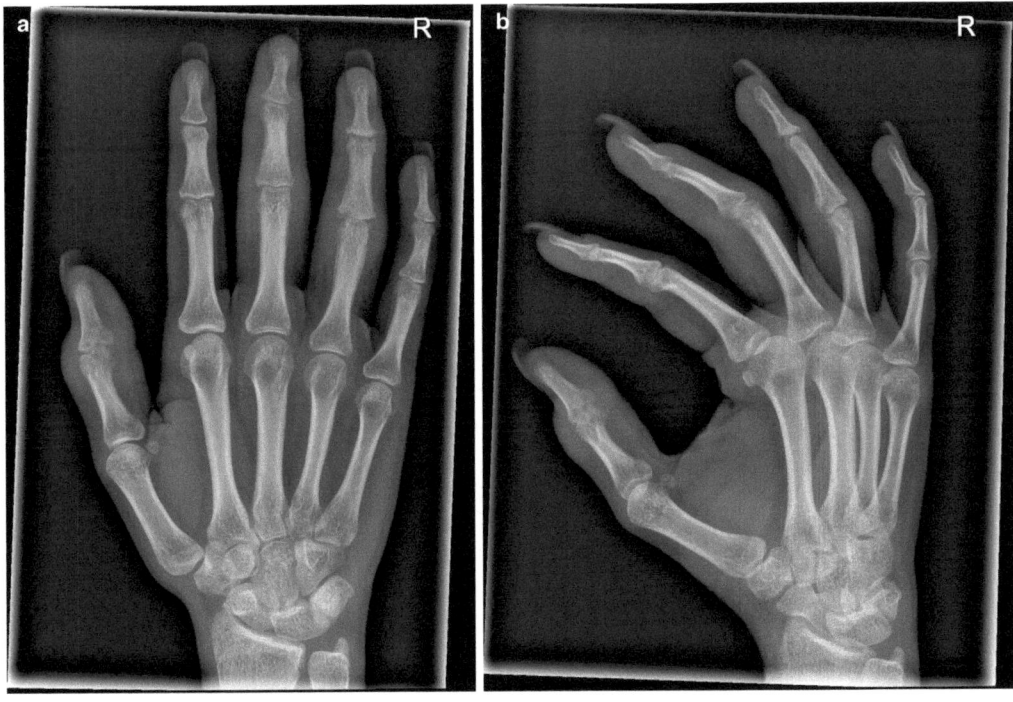

☐ **Fig. 3.1** X-ray of the right hand in psoriatic arthritis. In the Fourth digit of the right hand, there are arthritic changes in the distal and proximal interphalangeal joint with erosive changes. Clearly visible soft tissue swelling of the Third and Fourth digits in the sense of dactylitis. (With kind permission from Dr. A. Schuster, Department of Radiology, LKH Bregenz)

- **2. What significance do the consistently negative findings of the rheumatism laboratory have for further diagnostic and also therapeutic planning?**

The negative autoimmune findings help on the one hand to exclude specific subgroups of juvenile idiopathic arthritis, interesting of course is the **HLA-B27 positivity** of the child—this points to a genetic predisposition of her clinical picture.

- **3. What strategic therapeutic considerations need to be taken into account, especially including a target-defined therapy?**

In the context of a treat-to-target concept, it should be particularly considered at the time of diagnosis which rheumatological entities are particularly unfavorably classified in terms of their prognosis. These entities demand a significantly more aggressive therapy concept.

3.6 Further Course

In the 16-year-old girl, based on the clinical findings on joints and skin, the **diagnosis of juvenile psoriasis arthritis (JPsA)** was defined and immediately a basic therapy with methotrexate (15 mg/m^2 BSA/week s.c.) was started; as supportive therapy folic acid (5 mg p.o./week on the day after the MTX injection) and an NSAID therapy. Concurrently, occupational therapy with night splints was initiated. After 6 months of therapy, there was still insufficient remission (both in terms of joint status and skin findings, hence additional biologic therapy with adalimumab (1-time 40 mg s.c. every

2 weeks). Even with this combined therapy, the set goal of clinical remission was not achieved after another 12 months. Currently, initiation of therapy with an interleukin-17A blocking antibody secukinumab (1-time 300 mg s.c. every 4 weeks)).

3.7 Summary

3.7.1 Classification

Juvenile psoriasis arthritis (JPsA) is defined according to the ILAR classification as arthritis of unknown cause in a child < 16 years when psoriasis is also present (Petty et al. 1998, 2004). However, skin and joint symptoms do not have to start at the same time, joint symptoms can precede the dermatological symptoms in many cases, making the recognition of psoriasis arthritis often difficult. Patients with psoriasis arthritis can also be identified without psoriasis based on certain features such as dactylitis, nail changes (pitting, cracks, thickening, color changes) or positive family history for psoriasis (◘ Tab. 3.1).

3.7.2 Etiology and Frequency

The cause of psoriatic arthritis is still unclear. The connection between the simultaneous or consecutive development of **arthritis** and **psoriasis** is also unclear. Approximately 30–35% of all psoriasis cases manifest before the age of 20. In Germany, about 1–2% of children and adolescents have psoriasis, the proportion of patients

◘ **Tab. 3.1**   Diagnostic or classification criteria for juvenile psoriasis arthritis

Vancouver criteria (Petty et al. 1998)[a]	ILAR criteria (Petty et al. 2004)
Arthritis and psoriasis or:	Arthritis and psoriasis or:
Arthritis with at least 3 of the following secondary criteria:	Arthritis and at least 2 of the following secondary criteria:
– Dactylitis	– Dactylitis
– Nail pitting	– Nail pitting or onycholysis
– Family history of psoriasis (First and Second degree relatives)	– Family history of psoriasis (1st degree relatives)
– Psoriasis-like skin lesion	Exclusion criteria:
	– Positive rheumatoid factor
	– Arthritis in a HLA-B27 positive boy after the 6th birthday
	– Ankylosing spondylitis
	– Enthesitis-associated arthritis
	– Sacroiliitis in inflammatory bowel disease
	– Reiter's syndrome, acute anterior uveitis (anamnestic or current) in a first-degree relative
	Signs of systemic arthritis

[a] Definitive juvenile psoriasis arthritis; possible juvenile psoriasis arthritis: Arthritis with 2 of the 4 secondary criteria

with additional symptoms is lower. The prevalence of juvenile psoriatic arthritis is estimated at about 10–15 per 100,000 with an annual incidence rate between 2 and 3 per 100,000 (Consolaro et al. 2019).

3.7.3 Clinic

Within the first 6 months of the disease, juvenile psoriatic arthritis usually manifests as arthritis of a few joints (oligoarthritis), only in a few cases does juvenile psoriatic arthritis manifest as symmetrical polyarthritis at the onset of the disease (Huemer et al. 2022). The joint most commonly affected by juvenile psoriatic arthritis is the knee joint, but there is also a clear predilection for small joints in the hands and feet. The isolated swelling of a single small joint, especially a single toe, is highly pathognomonic for juvenile psoriatic arthritis, see ◗ Fig. 3.2.

Inflammation of **distal interphalangeal joints** occurs in up to 30% of cases, dactylitis in up to 49% of psoriatic arthritis patients. Inflammatory changes in the area of the bony insertion sites of tendons, ligaments or joint capsules lead to localized redness, swelling and pressure pain, this **enthesopathy** is defined as a significant clinical sign in psoriatic arthritis. The typical dermatological symptoms in children consist of well-demarcated, erythematous and desquamative skin lesions in the area of the extensor sides of the elbow, knee and interphalangeal joints (Stoll et al. 2006). Psoriasis vulgaris, the classic form of psoriasis, is found in more than 80% of children with arthritis and psoriasis. The diagnostically helpful Auspitz phenomenon can contribute to the diagnosis of psoriasis: after careful rubbing with a wooden spatula, there is a whitish-opaque discoloration of the scales: "candle wax phenomenon" (Reece et al. 1999). With further rubbing, there is minimal pinpoint skin bleeding: "bloody dew".

A number of changes in finger and toenails are found in psoriasis, the most common sign is **nail pitting,** it is found in about a third of patients: smallest round depressions in the area of the nails, 0.5–1 mm in diameter associated with slightly reduced light reflection of the otherwise shiny nail surface.

The diagnosis of juvenile psoriasis is made clinically, there are no pathognomonic laboratory parameters.

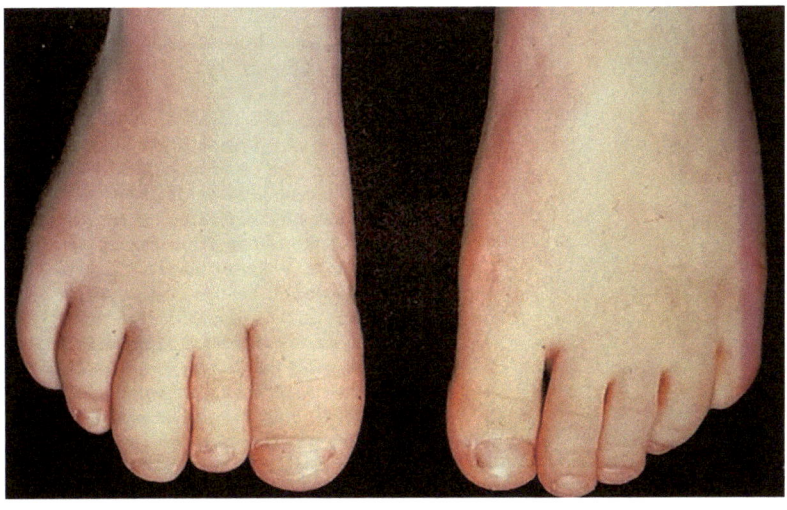

◗ **Fig. 3.2**   Child with dactylitis of the third toe on the right due to psoriasis. (From Huemer and Minden 2022)

3.7.4 Therapy

The recommendations for the treatment of juvenile psoriatic arthritis are based on study results for juvenile idiopathic arthritis and adult psoriatic arthritis. Randomized controlled therapy studies for juvenile psoriatic arthritis are not yet available. Thus, nonsteroidal anti-rheumatic drugs are established in the initial therapy, depending on the clinical picture followed by disease-modifying therapies such as methotrexate (Reece et al. 1999) or sulfasalazine (Acosta Felquer et al. 2014). Within the group of biologics, the most extensive clinical data is available for the treatment of psoriatic arthritis with TNF-α inhibitors (etanercept, infliximab, adalimumab, golimumab) (Acosta Felquer 2014; Li et al. 2019).

3.7.5 Prognosis

Compared to other forms of arthritis in childhood, the prognosis of psoriatic arthritis is considered unfavorable. In a study with 63 JPsA patients who were examined for more than 5 years, more than 70% of cases still showed signs of active arthritis at the end of the study period.

Conclusion

The diagnosis of JPsA is of relevance, as a more aggressive basic therapy should be established very early for this form of childhood arthritis. The diagnosis of JPsA is based on the clinical picture of psoriasis and simultaneous chronic arthritis. In the quite common case of not yet clear skin findings, further clinical symptoms (family history, dactylitis and nail pitting) can facilitate the diagnosis.

References

Acosta Felquer ML, Coates LC, Soriano ER (2014) Drug therapies for peripheral joint disease in psoriatic arthritis: a systematic review. J Rheumatol 41:2277–2285

Consolaro A, Giancane G, Alongi A (2019) Paediatric Rheumatology International Trials Organisation. Phenotypic variability and disparities in treatment and outcomes of childhood arthritis throughout the world: an observational cohort study. Lancet Child Adolesc Health 3(4):255–263

Huemer C, Minden K (2022) Juvenile Psoriasis-Arthritis. In: Wagner N, Dannecker G, Kallinich T (Hrsg) Pädiatrische Rheumatologie. Springer, Berlin/Heidelberg, pp 403–412

Li SJ, Perez-Chada LM, Merola JF (2019) TNF inhibitor-induced psoriasis: proposed algorithm for treatment and management. J Psoriasis Psoriatic Arthritis 4(2):70–80

Petty RE, Southwood TR, Baum J (1998) Revision of the proposed classification criteria for juvenile idiopathic arthritis: Durban 1997. J Rheumatol 25:10

Petty RE, Southwood TR, Manners P (2004) International league of associations for rheumatology classification of juvenile idiopathic arthritis: second revision Edmonton 2001. J Rheumatol 31:2

Reece RJ, Canete JD, Parsons WJ (1999) Distinct vascular patterns of early synovitis in psoriatic, reactive and rheumatoid arthritis. Arthritis Rheum 42:1481–1484

Stoll ML, Zurakowski D, Nigrovic LR, Nichols DP (2006) Patients with juvenile psoriatic arthritis comprise two distinct populations. Arthritis Rheum 54:3564–3572

Fever, Rash, and Joint Pain—Just an Infection?

Annette Holl-Wieden

Contents

4.1 Medical History

Maja, 13 years old, had been experiencing **sore throat, fever,** a **skin rash,** and **pain in her wrists and ankles** for 2 weeks. She was admitted to an external children's hospital for further clarification. The inflammation values were elevated, but the blood cultures were negative. Tonsillopharyngitis was suspected and antibiotic treatment with cefuroxime was started. A microbiological examination of a throat swab and an antistreptolysin (ASL) titer were inconspicuous. Due to the unclear symptoms, she was transferred to our clinic.

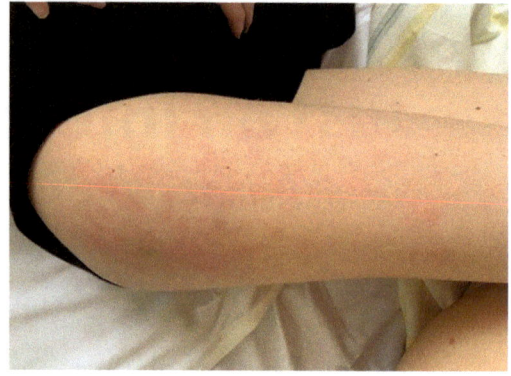

◘ **Fig. 4.1** Maja, 13 years old, with macular exanthema during fever increase

4.2 Examination Findings

Maja was tired and "weak" and had **fever.** There was a slight cervical **lymph node swelling,** the rest of the lymph node status was inconspicuous. She had **arthritis** of the knee joints, the left ankle, the wrists, and the metacarpophalangeal (MCP) joints of both index and middle fingers. The affected joints were swollen and the movement was painfully restricted. Close observation of the fever course showed 2 fever spikes per day. The fever dropped spontaneously. Close observation showed that a **fine-spotted exanthema** appeared on the limbs and trunk during the fever increase (◘ Fig. 4.1).

4.3 Laboratory Values and Imaging

4.3.1 Laboratory Values

The blood count with manual differential blood count showed leukocytosis, neutrophilia, normochromic, normocytic anemia, and thrombocytosis (**leukocytes 16,590/ μl** [normal value 4500–13,000], **neutrophils** 87.3% [normal value 40–61.5], **Hb 9.7 g/dl** [normal value 12–16], **platelets 773,000/μl** [normal value 150,000–450,000]). The inflammation parameters were significantly elevated (**ESR 73 mm/h, CRP 20.4 mg/ dl** [normal value 0–0.5], **ferritin 1519 μg/l** [9.3–59], **S100 A8/A9-proteins 28,400 ng/ml** [normal value<2900]). The overview laboratory values (including liver and kidney values) were inconspicuous. The complement factors (C3 and C4) were within the normal range. The blood culture and the urine examination showed no conspicuous findings. ANA, anti-dsDNA-AB and ENA as well as ANCA and RF were negative. The calprotectin in the stool was within the normal range. Serologically, there was no indication of an HIV, hepatitis B, hepatitis C, EBV, CMV, and mycoplasma infection.

4.3.2 Imaging

The echocardiography showed a small **pericardial effusion,** the heart function was not restricted. The ECG was inconspicuous. The sonography of the pleura revealed a small **pleural effusion.** An abdominal sonography, a chest X-ray, and a bone marrow puncture were inconspicuous.

4.4 Educational Questions

1. What differential diagnoses should be considered based on the medical history of 2-week fever, exanthema, arthritis, and high inflammation values?
2. What diagnosis should be made?
3. What therapy should be administered?

4.5 Differential Diagnostic Considerations

In the case of a 2-week fever, rash, arthritis, and high inflammation markers, the presence of an **infectious disease** should be considered. Tonsillopharyngitis with streptococci, rheumatic fever, and sepsis have already been ruled out elsewhere. Serological tests for various bacterial and especially viral pathogens were negative. Ultimately, there was no indication of an infectious disease. It is important to rule out a **malignant disease** such as leukemia or lymphoma. The differential blood count, a bone marrow puncture, a chest X-ray, and an ultrasound of the abdomen provided no indication of these diseases. Furthermore, rheumatic diseases such as **collagenoses**, e.g., lupus erythematosus, but also **systemic vasculitides** must be ruled out. In particular, the **Kawasaki syndrome**, known as "mucocutaneous lymph node syndrome," is an important differential diagnosis. However, the clinical and immunological criteria for these diseases were not met. There was also no indication of a **chronic inflammatory bowel disease**. Therefore, the presence of an autoinflammatory disease had to be primarily considered. Maja had no previous similar disease episodes, the family history was empty, the presence of a **hereditary autoinflammatory disease**, a so-called hereditary periodic fever syndrome, was therefore rather unlikely. Corresponding genetic tests were therefore not carried out. The triad of fever, rash, and arthritis,

as well as the slight lymphadenopathy, the small pericardial effusion, and pleural effusion, suggested a systemic **juvenile idiopathic arthritis (sJIA)**. Typical for the disease was the fever course with 2 fever peaks per day, the spontaneous drop in fever, and the fine-spotted rash during the fever increase. The high inflammation values, especially the high ferritin and the high S100A8/A9 proteins, also supported the diagnosis. The diagnosis of SJIA could be made. In adult patients with Still's disease (AOSD), sore throat often occurs as an additional symptom. In our patient, the sore throat occurred as part of the SJIA. Consideration should also be given to a **macrophage activation syndrome (MAS)**. This can occur as a severe complication of sJIA, but can also be the result of another disease, such as an infectious disease. The laboratory findings typical for MAS (see below) were not present.

4.6 Further Course

After the diagnosis of sJIA, therapy with **Anakinra** (2 mg/kg BW/day, corresponding to 100 mg/day) was started. Anakinra is an IL-1 receptor antagonist that is administered subcutaneously once a day. On the Third day of therapy, the fever subsided. Maja was discharged. On the Eleventh day of therapy, she developed a fever again. The inflammation values increased again. An **oral glucocorticoid therapy** (prednisolone 0.7 mg/kg BW/day) was started, and the therapy with Anakinra was continued. This led to the subsidence of the fever and a decrease in inflammation values. The general condition and the arthritis improved quickly. In the course, the glucocorticoid therapy was reduced. After 4 weeks, Maja developed a fear of injections. The therapy with Anakinra was switched to **Canakinumab**, an anti-IL-1β antibody. Canakinumab (150 mg s.c.) was administered subcutaneously every

4 weeks. The medication with predniso-lone was stopped after 6 weeks. The girl re-mained symptom-free in the course, the in-flammation values were not elevated. The therapy with Canakinumab was stopped af-ter 5 months (◨ Fig. 4.2). Maja has been in remission for 1 year. We assume that she had a monophasic course of the disease.

4.7 Educational Answers

■ **1. What differential diagnoses should be considered based on the medical history of 2-week fever, rash, arthritis, and high inflammation values?**
The following differential diagnoses should be considered: infections, malignant diseases, collagenoses, systemic vasculitides, hereditary periodic "fever" syndromes, macrophage ac-tivation syndrome.

■ **2. What diagnosis should be made?**
The diagnosis of systemic juvenile idio-pathic arthritis (sJIA) should be made. This is indicated by the triad of fever, rash, ar-thritis, and especially the course of fever and the typical rash. The high inflamma-tion values, especially the high **ferritin** and the high S100A8/A9 proteins, also point to sJIA. The above-mentioned differential di-agnoses could be excluded.

■ **3. What therapy should be administered?**
After diagnosing sJIA, there are various ther-apy options: In addition to a general fever-re-ducing NSAID therapy, treatment with glu-cocorticoids is possible. Approved is the ther-apy with an interleukin-1 blocker, namely Anakinra or Canakinumab, or a therapy with an interleukin-6 blocker, i.e., Tocilizumab.

4.8 Summary

4.8.1 Background/Pathogenesis

sJIA is often still referred to as **Morbus Still** after its first describer Georg Frederic

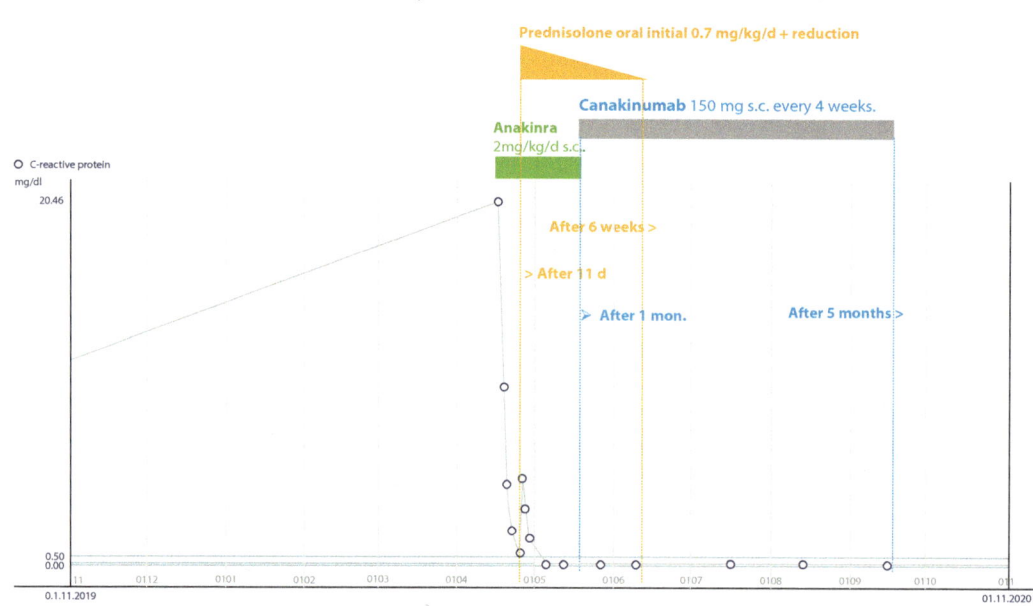

◨ **Fig. 4.2** Maja's disease course based on the CRP value in relation to the chosen therapy

Still. If the disease occurs in adults, it is referred to as **AOSD (Adult-onset Still's Disease)** (De Benedetti and Schneider 2016). According to the ILAR classification criteria, sJIA is classified as one of the 7 subgroups of juvenile idiopathic arthritis (JIA). However, the disease differs significantly in pathogenesis and clinic from the other forms of JIA. SJIA is primarily considered an autoinflammatory disease in the initial phase (De Benedetti and Schneider 2016).

4.8.2 Clinic

Characteristic for sJIA is the triad: fever, rash, arthritis. There can also be organ manifestations, such as splenomegaly, hepatomegaly, pericarditis, pleuritis, lymph node swellings. Typical are 1-2 fever peaks per day with spontaneous defervescence. During the fever rise, a fine-spotted, fleeting, usually salmon-colored rash is found. This rash must be specifically searched for. The diagnosis is currently made according to the ILAR classification criteria (De Benedetti and Schneider 2016). According to this, the presence of arthritis is required for the diagnosis. However, some children with sJIA do not have arthritis in the early phase of the disease, so the diagnosis is often significantly delayed. This is addressed by a newly proposed classification according to PRINTO (Martini et al. 2019). According to this, the diagnosis could also be made without the presence of arthritis. However, the criteria have not yet been validated and are therefore not generally valid.

sJIA is considered a biphasic disease. In the beginning, autoinflammation with overactivation of the innate immunity dominates. This leads to an increased release of proinflammatory cytokines (including IL-1, IL-6). The patients have systemic signs, i.e., fever, a rash, and high inflammation signs. If the disease is not effectively treated

in this phase, it transitions into another phase of the disease. Here, there is primarily a dysregulation of the acquired immunity. The patients have a persistent severe destructive polyarthritis. It is assumed that there is a time window ("window of opportunity") at the beginning of the disease in which treatment e.g., with IL-1 blockade can have a particularly positive effect. This early biologic therapy seems to be able to prevent the transition into a chronic destructive arthritis. In the phase of persistent severe destructive polyarthritis, on the other hand, the patients usually show a poor response to any therapy (Foll et al. 2020; Nigrovic 2014). A life-threatening complication of sJIA is a macrophage activation syndrome (MAS). This leads to a strong activation of macrophages and T lymphocytes with the result of a cytokine storm. Clinical signs of MAS are continuous high fever, bleeding, purpura, enlargements of lymph nodes, liver and spleen, a liver dysfunction with jaundice, also liver failure, a CNS involvement and ultimately multiorgan failure. Typical laboratory findings are a drop in ESR, leukocytes and platelets, an increase in ferritin, liver values, LDH, triglycerides, a drop in fibrinogen and increased D-dimers, a prolonged prothrombin time and partial thromboplastin time as well as hemophagocytosis in the bone marrow (De Benedetti and Schneider 2016). Especially ferritin and the soluble interleukin-2 receptor are important parameters for activity assessment. For MAS in SJIA, there are EULAR/ACR classification criteria (Ravelli et al. 2016).

4.8.3 Diagnosis

The diagnosis of sJIA is made clinically and confirmed by typical laboratory findings. Moreover, sJIA is a diagnosis of exclusion (De Benedetti and Schneider 2016). In sJIA, the inflammation parameters are elevated. There is an increase in ESR and CRP, leukocytosis with granulocytosis as well as thrombocytosis and often anemia. Ferritin, S100A8/A9 proteins, and interleukin-18 are elevated. The latter are considered diagnostically helpful biomarkers (Nirmala et al. 2014).

4.8.4 Therapy

In the past, only a few drugs were available for therapy. Glucocorticoids were usually given in high doses and for a long time. Most children developed severe side effects such as pronounced **Cushing's symptoms** or osseous structure deficits. Today, targeted therapy approaches are available, drugs for interleukin-1 blockade such as Anakinra or Canakinumab, and Tocilizumab for interleukin-6 blockade. Studies have well documented the effectiveness of these drugs and led to their approval (De Benedetti et al. 2012; Quartier et al. 2011; Ruperto et al. 2012). There are also some new therapeutic approaches: Studies are being conducted on JAK inhibitors, a recombinant IL-18-binding protein (IL-18BP), and a monoclonal anti-interferon(IFN)-γ antibody (Foll et al. 2020). Overall, the therapy of sJIA is still very inconsistent. There are too few clinical studies and therefore no evidence-based guidelines. The CARRA initiative of North American pediatric rheumatologists and the Pro-Child initiative of the German Society of Pediatric and Adolescent Rheumatology (GKJR) have formulated consensus-based treatment plans for the first 9 or 12 months of the disease (DeWitt et al. 2012; Hinze et al. 2018). They serve to harmonize and optimize therapy in the long term. Various therapy options are presented, in the recommendations of the Pro-Child initiative the therapy with glucocorticoids, Anakinra, Canakinumab or Tocilizumab. Treatment goals are formulated, if not achieved, a change in therapy should be discussed with the patient and parents (Treat-to-Target therapy). The aim is to achieve the fastest possible remission with the most limited use of glucocorticoids (Hinze et al. 2018).

> **Conclusion**
>
> In sJIA, early diagnosis and therapy are crucial. In the "window of opportunity", targeted therapy with cytokine blockade drugs (e.g., IL-1 or IL-6 blockade) can be effective and even lead to remission.

References

De Benedetti F, Schneider R (2016) Systemic juvenile idiopathic arthritis. In: Petty RE, Laxer RM, Lindsley CB, Wedderburn LR (Eds) Textbook of pediatric rheumatology, 7. edn. Elsevier, Philadelphia, pp 205–216

De Benedetti F, Brunner HI, Ruperto N, Kenwright A, Wright S, Calvo I, Cuttica R, Ravelli A, Schneider R, Woo P, Wouters C, Xavier R, Zemel L, Baildam E, Burgos-Vargas R, Dolezalova P, Garay SM, Merino R, Joos R, Grom A, Wulffraat N, Zuber Z, Zulian F, Lovell D, Martini A, Printo P (2012) Randomized trial of tocilizumab in systemic juvenile idiopathic arthritis. N Engl J Med 367(25):2385–2395. ▶ https://doi.org/10.1056/NEJMoa1112802

DeWitt EM, Kimura Y, Beukelman T, Nigrovic PA, Onel K, Prahalad S, Schneider R, Stoll ML, Angeles-Han S, Milojevic D, Schikler KN, Vehe RK, Weiss JE, Weiss P, Ilowite NT, Wallace CA, Juvenile Idiopathic Arthritis Disease-specific Research Committee of Childhood Arthritis R, Research A (2012) Consensus treatment plans for new-onset systemic juvenile idiopathic arthritis. Arthritis Care Res (Hoboken) 64(7):1001–1010. ▶ https://doi.org/10.1002/acr.21625

Foll D, Wittkowski H, Hinze C (2020) [Still's disease as biphasic disorder: current knowledge on pathogenesis and novel treatment approaches]. Z Rheumatol 79(7):639-648. ▶ https://doi.org/10.1007/s00393-020-00779-2

Hinze CH, Holzinger D, Lainka E, Haas JP, Speth F, Kallinich T, Rieber N, Hufnagel M, Jansson AF, Hedrich C, Winowski H, Berger T, Foeldvari I, Ganser G, Hospach A, Huppertz HI, Monkemoller K, Neudorf U, Weissbarth-Riedel E, Wittkowski H, Horneff G, Foell D, collaborators P-KSp (2018) Practice and consensus-based strategies in diagnosing and managing systemic juvenile idiopathic arthritis in Germany. Pediatr Rheumatol Online J 16(1):7. ▶ https://doi.org/10.1186/s12969-018-0224-2

Martini A, Ravelli A, Avcin T, Beresford MW, Burgos-Vargas R, Cuttica R, Ilowite NT, Khubchandani R, Laxer RM, Lovell DJ, Petty RE, Wallace CA, Wulffraat NM, Pistorio A, Ruperto N, Pediatric Rheumatology International Trials O (2019) Toward new classification criteria for juvenile idiopathic arthritis: first steps, Pediatric Rheumatology International Trials Organization International Consensus. J Rheumatol 46(2):190–197. ▶ https://doi.org/10.3899/jrheum.180168

Nigrovic PA (2014) Review: is there a window of opportunity for treatment of systemic juvenile idiopathic arthritis? Arthritis Rheumatol 66(6):1405–1413. ▶ https://doi.org/10.1002/art.38615

Nirmala N, Grom A, Gram H (2014) Biomarkers in systemic juvenile idiopathic arthritis: a comparison with biomarkers in cryopyrin-associated periodic syndromes. Curr Opin Rheumatol 26(5):543–552. ▶ https://doi.org/10.1097/BOR.0000000000000098

Quartier P, Allantaz F, Cimaz R, Pillet P, Messiaen C, Bardin C, Bossuyt X, Boutten A, Bienvenu J, Duquesne A, Richer O, Chaussabel D, Mogenet A, Banchereau J, Treluyer JM, Landais P, Pascual V (2011) A multicentre, randomised, double-blind, placebo-controlled trial with the interleukin-1 receptor antagonist anakinra in patients with systemic-onset juvenile idiopathic arthritis (ANAJIS trial). Ann Rheum Dis 70(5):747–754. ▶ https://doi.org/10.1136/ard.2010.134254

Ravelli A, Minoia F, Davi S, Horne A, Bovis F, Pistorio A, Arico M, Avcin T, Behrens EM, De Benedetti F, Filipovic L, Grom AA, Henter JI, Ilowite NT, Jordan MB, Khubchandani R, Kitoh T, Lehmberg K, Lovell DJ, Miettunen P, Nichols KE, Ozen S, Pachlopnik Schmid J, Ramanan AV, Russo R, Schneider R, Sterba G, Uziel Y, Wallace C, Wouters C, Wulffraat N, Demirkaya E, Brunner HI, Martini A, Ruperto N, Cron RQ, Paediatric Rheumatology International Trials O, Childhood A, Rheumatology Research A, Pediatric Rheumatology Collaborative Study G, Histiocyte S (2016) 2016 Classification criteria for macrophage activation syndrome complicating systemic juvenile idiopathic arthritis: a European League Against Rheumatism/American College of Rheumatology/Paediatric Rheumatology International Trials Organisation Collaborative Initiative. Arthritis Rheumatol 68(3):566–576. ▶ https://doi.org/10.1002/art.39332

Ruperto N, Brunner HI, Quartier P, Constantin T, Wulffraat N, Horneff G, Brik R, McCann L, Kasapcopur O, Rutkowska-Sak L, Schneider R, Berkun Y, Calvo I, Erguven M, Goffin L, Hofer M, Kallinich T, Oliveira SK, Uziel Y, Viola S, Nistala K, Wouters C, Cimaz R, Ferrandiz MA, Flato B, Gamir ML, Kone-Paut I, Grom A, Magnusson B, Ozen S, Sztajnbok F, Lheritier K, Abrams K, Kim D, Martini A, Lovell DJ, Printo P (2012) Two randomized trials of canakinumab in systemic juvenile idiopathic arthritis. N Engl J Med 367(25):2396–2406. ▶ https://doi.org/10.1056/NEJMoa1205099

What to do When the Immune System Goes into a Storm?

Henner Morbach

Contents

5.1 Medical History

A $4^1/_2$ year old boy developed a febrile infection with rhinitis and tonsillopharyngitis as well as mild, dry cough in December. The emergency medical service prescribed an antibiotic therapy with Cefaclor©. The fever persisted over the next 3 weeks with daily 1–2 fever spikes. Due to the long-standing fever of unknown origin, the boy was admitted to the hospital.

The boy is the second of three children of consanguineous parents. So far, the child had not suffered from any severe infections, nor was there a clustering of infections. The family history is empty regarding recurrent or severe infections as well as fever spikes. The boy has a known Beta-Thalassaemia minor, which does not require treatment.

5.2 Examination Findings

Upon hospital admission, the boy was in a compromised general condition. There was tachypnea, coarse crackles could be auscultated ubiquitously, some of them transmitted. The tonsils were hyperplastic, sporadically with whitish-gray deposits. The spleen was palpable 2 cm below the rib arch, otherwise the abdominal examination was unremarkable. There was no lymphadenopathy. Nor was there any exanthema.

5.3 Laboratory Values and Imaging

5.3.1 Laboratory Values

The blood count showed a **lymphocytosis** with 21,300 leukocytes/ul and 54% lymphocytes, microscopically increased numbers of reactive lymphocytes were detectable. The hemoglobin content had dropped by 2 points compared to the previous values, now at 7.6 g/dl (Anemia), there was also a **thrombocytopenia** (98,000/ul). The inflammation values were significantly increased (CRP 6.3 mg/dl; Procalcitonin 9.6 ng/ml). Notably, there was also a significantly increased **ferritin (12,188 μg/l)**. In addition, increased **D-dimers** (22.9 mg/l) and low **fibrinogen** (1.8 g/l) indicated signs of **hyperfibrinolysis**. There was also a **hepatopathy** (GOT 420 U/l; GPT 136 U/l, GGT 109 U/l, alkaline phosphatase 627 U/l) and signs of increased cell breakdown (LDH 2110 U/l). The **triglycerides** in the serum were elevated despite the absence of food intake (309 mg/dl).

5.3.2 Imaging

In the chest X-ray, small patchy parahilar opacities were noticeable in both lungs. Sonographically, the spleen was enlarged (8.7 cm length, splenomegaly), and mesenteric lymphadenopathy was also noticeable.

5.4 Educational Questions

1. How can the striking laboratory constellation be interpreted in view of the fever that has been present for 3 weeks?
2. What triggers could have caused the current disease picture and what diagnostic steps should be taken to clarify this?
3. Are further examinations relevant in view of the current disease picture with regard to a possible underlying disease?
4. What therapeutic steps could be considered?

5.5 Differential Diagnostic Considerations

The initial symptoms of rhinitis, tonsillopharyngitis, and cough suggest a viral respiratory infection as the trigger for the current disease picture. The concurrent splenomegaly and the noticeable lymphocytosis in the blood count, with microscopically detectable reactive lymphocytes, would be consistent with an infection by Epstein-Barr virus (EBV). The child's disease picture would be classified under the clinical picture of an **infectious mononucleosis**, in the context of which hepatitis often occurs. In principle, other viral pathogens (e.g., CMV, adenovirus) could also explain the child's initial symptoms.

However, the long fever course of over 3 weeks seems to indicate an uncontrolled (virus) infection and/or an initially infection-related and now detached excessive inflammatory response. This would also be consistent with the significantly elevated inflammatory parameters detected in the blood test. The very high ferritin levels ("**hyperferritinemia**"), the **(pan)cytopenia** as well as the signs of hyperfibrinolysis with low fibrinogen levels are almost pathognomonic in the situation of an unclear, prolonged fever for a hemophagocytic lymphohistiocytosis (HLH) or a **macrophage activation syndrome** (MAS) (Henter et al. 2007; Ravelli et al. 2016). This disease picture can be triggered by various causes. Viruses, and especially EBV, are typical triggering factors of HLH, with varying degrees of genetic predisposition existing in the affected individuals. This should be included in the differential diagnostic considerations for a possibly existing underlying disease. In addition to EBV, other viruses, but also non-viral infectious agents, can trigger HLH (Crayne et al. 2019). It is worth highlighting **Leishmania**, whose infection can occur under the laboratory constellation of HLH.

In addition to infections as triggers of HLH, this excessive inflammatory constellation can also occur on the basis of rheumatic diseases and malignancies. In this case, the term MAS is often used. The most common rheumatic diseases in which MAS develops as a complication are the systemic form of JIA and the collagenoses. The clinical examination did not provide any indicative hint of the existence of a collagenosis in the patient. However, the cytopenia could be autoimmune-mediated and exist within the context of a **systemic lupus erythematosus**. The prolonged fever and the laboratory constellation would in principle be compatible with sJIA, although no rash had occurred in the patient so far and there were no arthralgias or signs of arthritis. A malignant disease, especially with involvement of the bone marrow, is possible in the patient and should always be included in the differential diagnosis given the clinical symptoms and laboratory constellation.

5.6 Further Course

Due to the typical laboratory constellation with cytopenia, hyperferritinemia, hyperfibrinolysis, and increased transaminases, a suspicion of HLH was raised. In the infectious disease diagnostics, an **EBV infection** could be detected both in the direct pathogen diagnostics in the blood by PCR and serologically (DNA copy number $1.6 * 10^3$/ ml; EBV-VCA-IgM and IgG antibodies positive). Other respiratory or hepatotropic viruses could not be detected. The examination of the bone marrow showed no evidence of a malignant hematological disease, occasional **hemophagocytosis** was detectable (◘ Fig. 5.1). The molecular genetic examination of the bone marrow gave no indication of visceral leishmaniasis. Autoantibodies (ANA, ENA) were not detectable. To investigate a possible CNS involvement in the context of the infection or HLH, a cerebrospinal fluid examination was performed, which showed a slight **pleocytosis** (leukocyte count 34/µl with 92% lymphocytes), and EBV-DNA was weakly detectable at the edge of the detection limit. The cranial MRI showed an unremarkable finding.

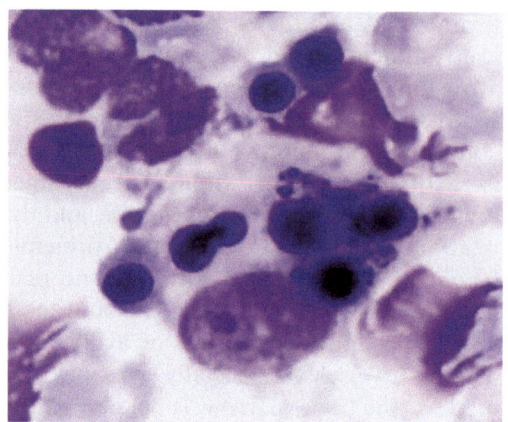

Fig. 5.1 Bone marrow cytology in HLH/MAS. Representation of a hyperactive bone marrow macrophage with hemophagocytosis

The serum immunoglobulin levels G, A, M were within the normal range. In the more specialized immunological diagnostics, the picture of a significant **T-cell activation** was shown (HLA-DR expression on 78% of the CD8$^+$ T cells, **soluble IL-2 receptor** (sCD25) in the serum significantly increased to 7480 U/ml). As EBV-associated HLH often underlies an inherited immune system disease, further diagnostic efforts were made in this regard. A typical finding that can indicate a genetically caused HLH/MAS is the **reduced function of NK cells**, which was demonstrated in the patient by a significantly **reduced degranulation of the NK cells** in vitro. The investigations regarding a specific defect showed a lack of expression of XIAP in T and NK cells and a hemizygous deletion of exon 3 in the XIAP gene. Consequently, the diagnosis of HLH/MAS based on a **XIAP deficiency** (X-linked inhibitor of apoptosis protein) was made.

The immunosuppressive therapy of HLH was initially carried out with a combination of dexamethasone and high-dose immunoglobulin administration. Under this, there was a very rapid significant de-crease in the inflammatory parameters and the patient became fever-free. An intensification of the therapy (e.g., by adding specific cytokine-blocking drugs or cytostatics such as etoposide) was initially held back due to the good response and was not necessary due to the positive course under reduction of dexamethasone.

5.7 Educative Responses

■ **1. How can the striking laboratory constellation be interpreted in view of the fever that has been present for 3 weeks?**
Noteworthy in the laboratory constellation is the significantly increased ferritin, which in the context of an unclear and prolonged fever can indicate an excessive and uncontrolled inflammatory response as part of one of the "Hyperferritinemia syndromes". Another specific characteristic of this pathological inflammatory response is the reduced or relatively **low** (but still within normal range) **fibrinogen**. This is due to hyperfibrinolysis. HLH and MAS are the typical hyperinflammation syndromes associated with this laboratory constellation. These are not specific diseases, rather HLH and MAS are pathological inflammatory responses that occur with a specific inflammation pattern and can occur in etiologically different constellations (Crayne and Cron 2019). The term HLH is mainly used in the context of (virus) infections as a trigger for hyperinflammation. HLH mainly occurs in genetically determined immune defects associated with a **defect in perforin-**/granzyme-mediated cytotoxicity, and is referred to as **familial and primary HLH**. The defects in cytotoxicity are associated with increased activation and **cytokine production** due to insufficient control of the triggering pathogen, with **interferon(IFN)-γ** playing a key role. As a result of strong immunological activation of the immune system, which

can be caused by a severe or persistent infection, secondary HLH can also occur in the absence of strong or missing genetic predisposition. In the patient, the **diagnostic criteria for HLH were met** solely based on the clinical symptoms (fever, splenomegaly) and easily determinable laboratory parameters (blood count, ferritin, fibrinogen, triglycerides) (Henter et al. 2007) (see overview). The abnormalities in the more specific immunological diagnostics (increased sCD25 and impaired NK cell function) confirmed the suspected diagnosis.

Diagnostic criteria for hemophago-cytic lymphohistiocytosis (Henter et al. 2007)

Five of the following eight criteria should be met:
- Fever
- Splenomegaly
- Cytopenia ≥ 2 cell lines
- Hypertriglyceridemia and/or hypofibrinogenemia
- Increased ferritin (>500 µg/l)
- Elevated soluble IL-2 receptor (sCD25) (>2400 U/ml)
- NK cell activity reduced or not detectable
- Hemophagocytosis in bone marrow, cerebrospinal fluid or lymph nodes

Secondary HLH can also develop on the basis of a malignant disease. For the diagnosis of HLH, **diagnostic criteria** have been developed that, in addition to ferritin, signs of hyperfibrinolysis and cytopenia, also include the molecular genetic constellation and the examination of NK cell function (Henter et al. 2007). The occurrence of **MAS** has been observed mainly in the context of certain rheumatic diseases (sJIA, collagenoses) and is predominantly used in this context in terms of terminology. MAS seems to be mainly caused by an increased activity of certain cytokines and especially **IL-18 and IFN-γ**. Classification criteria have also been developed for MAS in the context of rheumatic diseases (sJIA) (Ravelli et al. 2016). In particular, an increase in ferritin together with an increased activity of transaminases and falling (but possibly still normal) cell counts in the blood count indicates MAS in sJIA. Ultimately, the two hyperferritinemia syndromes (HLH and MAS) do not seem to be clearly distinguishable from each other and converge pathophysiologically at the level of overactivation of parts of T-cell function with excessive secretion of specific cytokines.

- **2. What triggers could have caused the current disease pattern and what diagnostic steps need to be taken to clarify this?**

When diagnosing HLH or MAS, the **triggering factor** of the excessive inflammatory response needs to be identified. First and foremost, it is necessary to define infectious agents as a possible trigger. This primarily includes viruses, but also bacteria and, rarely, fungi and parasites (Leishmania). The EBV infection is a typical trigger of primary HLH due to specific immune defects. In some patients, the specific antibody production is disturbed, so a **direct examination of the pathogen**, e.g., by PCR, should always be carried out in diagnostics. The preceding tonsillopharyngitis and the laboratory chemical signs of hepatitis already suggested infectious mononucleosis in the context of an EBV infection in the patient. In addition to infections, the presence of a malignant or rheumatic disease should be considered. For differential diagnosis regarding the presence of a **collagenosis**, autoantibody diagnostics (ANA, ENA) can be helpful, which yielded inconspicuous findings in the patient. A characteristic rash and arthralgia/arthritis can indicate sJIA.

5

- **3. Are further examinations regarding a possible underlying disease relevant due to the current disease pattern?**

In addition to the above-mentioned causes as a trigger of HLH, the question arises of a genetically caused underlying disease. In particular, the EBV infection as a triggering trigger of HLH is a warning sign for this. The first functional screening is an **NK cell degranulation test**, which is offered in specific immunological laboratories. In parallel, a flow cytometric examination of individual proteins can be carried out, in which changes are associated with primary HLH (e.g., **Perforin, SAP** [Signaling lymphocytic activation molecule associated protein], **XIAP, CD27**). The confirmatory diagnostics or extended examination is usually carried out by means of molecular genetic examinations as part of a **panel sequencing or exome sequencing** and subsequent focused bioinformatic analysis. The clinically phenotypically based classification of congenital diseases of the immune system, which is regularly updated by the International Union of Immunological Societies (IUIS), is helpful for selecting the genes to be examined.

In the further observation period of about 2 years, the patient did not experience any further occurrences of prolonged fever episodes. Recurrent bouts with the development of HLH/MAS can be possible in patients with XIAP deficiency (Latour and Aguilar 2015; Pachlopnik Schmid et al. 2011). In addition, the disease carries a high risk of developing chronic inflammatory bowel disease, which resembles Crohn's disease and often runs therapy-resistant. Since a significantly increased calprotectin was detectable in the stool of the patient once during the course, an endoscopic examination was carried out, but no inflammation could be detected in either the upper or lower gastrointestinal tract. XIAP deficiency is not associated with the risk of lymphoma development, which is possible with other genetically caused diseases with disturbed EBV immunity (Pachlopnik Schmid et al. 2011).

- **4. What therapeutic steps could be considered?**

The therapy for HLH or MAS is based on the extent of the manifestation, the triggering factors, and underlying diseases (Wegehaupt et al. 2020). An important therapeutic goal is to eliminate the triggering trigger if possible. For the treatment of the excessive inflammation, **glucocorticoids** (dexamethasone), possibly supplemented with **cyclosporin A** or high-dose, intravenously administered immunoglobulins (IVIG) are usually used in HLH. In very severely affected patients, especially in the context of primary HLH or lack of response to initial therapy, treatment is usually carried out within the framework of the HLH protocol with etoposide. In primary HLH, an allogeneic stem cell transplantation is usually aimed for. Specific cytokine blockades (e.g., JAK inhibitor ruxolitinib; IFN-γ antibody emapalumab; recombinant IL-18 binding protein tadekinig alfa) represent a promising therapy option, but are currently still being tested or not approved in Europe for this indication. Also for MAS in rheumatic diseases, **glucocorticoids** (prednisone) in combination with **cyclosporin A** are often used drugs in the initial therapy. In addition, an **IL-1 blockade by anakinra** is also an option here.

In the patient, the excessive inflammation in the context of HLH could be successfully and permanently controlled by treatment with dexamethasone and IVIG, so that no escalation of the immunosuppressive therapy by e.g., etoposide was necessary. The EBV infection also came under control; in the case of persistent infection, a treatment attempt by depletion of the virus-infected B cells with rituximab would have been considered. Due to the so far further inflammation-free course, no long-term therapy in the sense of an anti-inflammatory basic therapy was necessary. In the special case of XIAP deficiency, an allogeneic stem cell transplantation can be considered in severe courses. However, this is not always successful, which can also be explained by the expression of XIAP in non-hematopoietic cells.

5.8 Summary

5.8.1 Etiology

HLH or MAS can have changes especially in genes that are important for cytotoxicity.

5.8.2 Pathogenesis/Clinic

Functional restrictions of cytotoxicity and an excessive T-cell activation with the production of certain cytokines (IFN-γ, IL-18) are among others responsible for the development of HLH/MAS.

5.8.3 Diagnosis

The determination of simple laboratory parameters (blood count, ferritin, fibrinogen, transaminases, triglycerides) can provide a clue to the presence of HLH or MAS. In particular, the significantly increased **ferritin** is a diagnostic key.

5.8.4 Therapy

Corticosteroids are used in the initial therapy and are partly supplemented with cyclosporin A and/or IVIG. Etoposide is used in severe courses. Specific cytokine blockades (IFN-γ) or JAK inhibitors are gaining in importance. In particular, in the case of

MAS in the context of sJIA, an IL-1 blockade is carried out. In the case of a strong genetic basis of HLH, an allogeneic stem cell transplantation is aimed for/considered.

5.8.5 Diagnosis

The diagnosis of HLH and MAS is based on medical history, clinical symptoms, and laboratory parameters and is supplemented by specific diagnostics regarding the trigger and a possible underlying congenital disease.

> **Conclusion**
>
> In the case of prolonged fever and inflammation, the presence of HLH or MAS should be included in the differential diagnostic considerations. In particular, the easily determinable ferritin can serve as a diagnostic key for these hyperferritinemia syndromes.

References

Crayne C, Cron RQ (2019) Pediatric macrophage activation syndrome, recognizing the tip of the iceberg. Eur J Rheumatol:1–8. ► https://doi.org/10.5152/eurjrheum.2019.19150

Crayne CB, Albeituni S, Nichols KE, Cron RQ (2019) The immunology of macrophage activation syndrome. Front Immunol 10:119. ► https://doi.org/10.3389/fimmu.2019.00119

Henter JI, Horne A, Arico M, Egeler RM, Filipovich AH, Imashuku S, Ladisch S, McClain K, Webb D, Winiarski J, Janka G (2007) HLH-2004: diagnostic and therapeutic guidelines for hemophagocytic lymphohistiocytosis. Pediatr Blood Cancer 48(2):124–131. ► https://doi.org/10.1002/pbc.21039

Latour S, Aguilar C (2015) XIAP deficiency syndrome in humans. Semin Cell Dev Biol 39:115–123. ► https://doi.org/10.1016/j.semcdb.2015.01.015

Pachlopnik Schmid J, Canioni D, Moshous D, Touzot F, Mahlaoui N, Hauck F, Kanegane H, Lopez-Granados E, Mejstrikova E, Pellier I, Galicier L, Galambrun C, Barlogis V, Bordigoni P, Fourmaintraux A, Hamidou M, Dabadie A, Le

Deist F, Haerynck F, Ouachee-Chardin M, Rohrlich P, Stephan JL, Lenoir C, Rigaud S, Lambert N, Milili M, Schiff C, Chapel H, Picard C, de Saint BG, Blanche S, Fischer A, Latour S (2011) Clinical similarities and differences of patients with X-linked lymphoproliferative syndrome type 1 (XLP-1/SAP deficiency) versus type 2 (XLP-2/XIAP deficiency). Blood 117(5):1522–1529. ▶ https://doi.org/10.1182/blood-2010-07-298372

Ravelli A, Minoia F, Davi S, Horne A, Bovis F, Pistorio A, Arico M, Avcin T, Behrens EM, De Benedetti F, Filipovic L, Grom AA, Henter JI, Ilowite NT, Jordan MB, Khubchandani R, Kitoh T, Lehmberg K, Lovell DJ, Miettunen P, Nichols KE, Ozen S, Pachlopnik Schmid J, Ramanan AV, Russo R, Schneider R, Sterba G, Uziel Y, Wallace C, Wouters C, Wulffraat N, Demirkaya E, Brunner HI, Martini A, Ruperto N, Cron RQ, Paediatric Rheumatology International Trials O, Childhood A, Rheumatology Research A, Pediatric Rheumatology Collaborative Study G, Histiocyte S (2016) 2016 Classification criteria for macrophage activation syndrome complicating systemic juvenile idiopathic arthritis: a European League Against Rheumatism/American College of Rheumatology/Paediatric Rheumatology International Trials Organisation Collaborative Initiative. Ann Rheum Dis 75(3):481–489. ▶ https://doi.org/10.1136/annrheumdis-2015-208982

Wegehaupt O, Wustrau K, Lehmberg K, Ehl S (2020) Cell versus cytokine—directed therapies for hemophagocytic lymphohistiocytosis (HLH) in inborn errors of immunity. Front Immunol 11:808. ▶ https://doi.org/10.3389/fimmu.2020.00808

A 10-Year-Old Girl with Visual Impairment

Christian Huemer

Contents

6.1 Medical History

The 10-year-old girl was presented at our rheumatology clinic with a referral diagnosis of **Uveitis** on both sides for rheumatological examination. The girl was presented at the eye clinic 4 weeks earlier due to a subjectively perceived impairment of vision, no further specific ocular symptoms or additional symptoms were described. The girl had been presented to the ophthalmologist at the request of the school, there was the impression of a slight impairment of vision in class—a surprising finding for the parents. There was no indication of musculoskeletal symptoms. At the eye clinic, the diagnosis of **Uveitis intermedia** on both sides with **Iridocyclitis** and also vitreous opacity in the left eye was made. General medical history was unremarkable except for several preceding episodes of tonsillopharyngitis. An adenotomy had already been performed a few months before the child was presented. Family history was unremarkable regarding chronic inflammatory diseases.

6.2 Examination Findings

Right Eye: Visual acuity 80%, tension 15 mmHg. Anterior eye segment: Conjunctiva injected 1+, cornea with superior temporal fine small foreign body, inferior fine endothelial coating. Anterior chamber cells 2+. Tyndall 2+.

Fundus: Vitreous with vitreous cells 1+. Vitreous haze 1+. Optic disc sharply defined, vital. Macula dry. Peripapillary snowball, vessels without evidence of vascular incision. Retina circularly attached.

Left Eye: Visual acuity 100%, tension 17 mmHg. Anterior eye segment: Conjunctiva irritation-free, cornea clear, smooth, reflective, anterior chamber deep, optically empty, pupil round, lens clear.

Fundus: Optic disc sharply defined, vital, macula dry. Vitreous haze 1+. Nasal inferior suspicion of vitreous opacity, DD Snowball.

Musculoskeletal status completely unremarkable without evidence of arthritis or enthesitis. Internal status completely unremarkable, good general and nutritional status. No focal signs of inflammation. No cardiopulmonary, gastrointestinal or dermal symptoms. ENT findings unremarkable (no ulcerous or aphthous mucosal lesions).

6.3 Laboratory Values

Blood count, routine serum chemistry findings (electrolytes, liver, kidney function parameters, iron status, CRP, ESR) and infection serological findings (streptococci, toxoplasmosis, Lyme disease, toxocara, HSV, VZV, CMV) unremarkable; Tuberculosis test (Quantiferon) negative; Autoimmunology (ANA, ENA, dsDNA, complement factors, ANCA, rheumatoid factor, ACE) unremarkable.

6.4 Educational Questions

1. What differential diagnostic considerations should be discussed in the diagnosis of uveitis in this patient?
2. What further diagnostic procedures result from this?
3. What treatment recommendations need to be coordinated with the eye clinic?
4. What associated diseases should be considered?

6.5 Further Course

The further course in this child with already initially significant bilateral uveitis is protracted. After initial systemic and topical steroid therapy, an immunomodulatory therapy with Methotrexate (15 mg/m^{2}BSA/week p.o.) was started 8 weeks after diagnosis, after another 6 months, due to insufficient improvement of the eye findings, an additional biologic therapy with Adalimumab (1-time 40 mg s.c. every 2 weeks) had to be indicated. This therapy achieved sustained remission for the first time; since then, there has been a significantly improved eye finding. At no time were there additional complications or any other e.g. musculoskeletal symptoms. The uveitis of our patient is therefore to be considered as isolated **idiopathic uveitis**.

6.6 Educational Answers

- **1. What differential diagnostic considerations should be discussed in the diagnosis of uveitis in this patient?**

When first presenting a child with the diagnosis of uveitis, a number of infections must be clinically excluded (◙ Tab. 6.1) and in the laboratory, depending on the anatomical form of uveitis. This diagnostic is naturally important *before* initiating a long-term anti-inflammatory and immunomodulatory therapy that is generally planned for uveitis.

- **2. What further diagnostics result from this?**

See the laboratory findings obtained in our patient. If there are clinical indications of organ-specific symptoms (TBC, nephritis), additional radiological examinations result.

- **3. What therapy recommendations need to be coordinated with the ophthalmology clinic?**

The therapy of pediatric uveitis is published in recent guidelines (Heiligenhaus et al. 2019, 2022). See also ▶ Sect. 6.7.4.

- **4. What associated diseases should be considered?**

Uveitis is often associated with one of the subforms of juvenile idiopathic arthritis, and can also be part of the underlying disease in the context of collagenoses, periodic fever/autoinflammatory syndromes, or systemic vasculitides.

6.7 Summary

Pediatric uveitis can occur in various forms (iritis, cyclitis, iridocyclitis, retinitis, vitritis) either isolated as an autoimmune reaction or as part of various infectious or non-infectious inflammatory-rheumatic diseases (Heiligenhaus et al. 2022). In childhood, the associated systemic underlying diseases include juvenile idiopathic arthritis (JIA), juvenile sarcoidosis, chronic inflammatory bowel diseases, or Behcet's disease. Pediatric uveitis is a severe eye disease that can lead to permanent visual impairment despite all advances in diagnostics and therapy, especially if it is detected too late or inadequately treated.

◙ **Tab. 6.1** Typical infections in the different anatomical forms of uveitis. (After Heiligenhaus et al. 2022)

Form of Uveitis	Characteristics
Anterior Uveitis	Herpes simplex virus (HSV), Varicella-Zoster virus (VZV), Lyme disease, Syphilis, Tuberculosis
Intermediate Uveitis	Lyme disease, Syphilis, Tuberculosis
Posterior Uveitis	Toxoplasmosis, Toxocariasis, HSV, VZV, Cytomegalovirus (CMV), HIV, Syphilis

6.7.1 Etiology

In the absence of an associated infectious or inflammatory-rheumatic disease, uveitis is referred to as "idiopathic". In the different anatomical forms of uveitis, very different infectious diseases must be considered differentially (e.g., herpetic anterior uveitis, retinochoroiditis in toxoplasmosis, etc.). In about 80% of pediatric uveitis cases, an oligoarticular form of JIA is found simultaneously. The cumulative incidence of uveitis with the basic diagnosis of JIA is 8.3% of the affected children (Carvounis et al. 2006).

6.7.2 Clinic

Uveitis is detected in most JIA children between the ages of 5 and 7. In up to 10% of cases, uveitis manifests before arthritis, in 50% uveitis is detected simultaneously with or in the first 6 months after the diagnosis of arthritis (Kotaniemi et al. 1999). Uveitis in children typically progresses with an externally inconspicuous eye. A typical example is JIA-associated uveitis in young children with an **oligoarthritis**, especially when considering the "early childhood oligoarthritis". This form of childhood rheumatism, typically classified in the 1990s, was then included in the ILAR classification in the "overgroup" oligoarthritis. Occasionally, the children are only noticed when they have very poor vision. In children with enthesitis-associated arthritis, uveitis can (typically) impress with redness of the eyes, tearing, photophobia, pain, and visual impairment.

6.7.3 Diagnosis

A decisive factor for the diagnosis of uveitis is an ophthalmological examination using a slit lamp. The severity of the inflammation is determined by the number of cells in the anterior chamber and in the vitreous body. A high Tyndall effect (protein content) in the anterior chamber correlates with the risk of inflammation-related complications in the eye: In the case of chronic uveitis, **band keratopathies** can develop in the eyelid gap. It is also common for **posterior synechiae** to form, which pose a risk for subsequent cataract formation (◘ Fig. 6.1). A severe complication of uveitis in childhood is **glaucoma**, usually due to excessively high intraocular pressure.

6.7.4 Therapy

The goal of treating pediatric uveitis is to avoid vision-limiting complications and

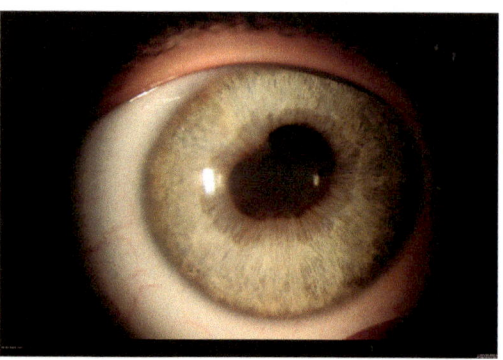

◘ **Fig. 6.1** Posterior synechiae in a JIA patient with anterior uveitis. (From Heiligenhaus et al. 2022)

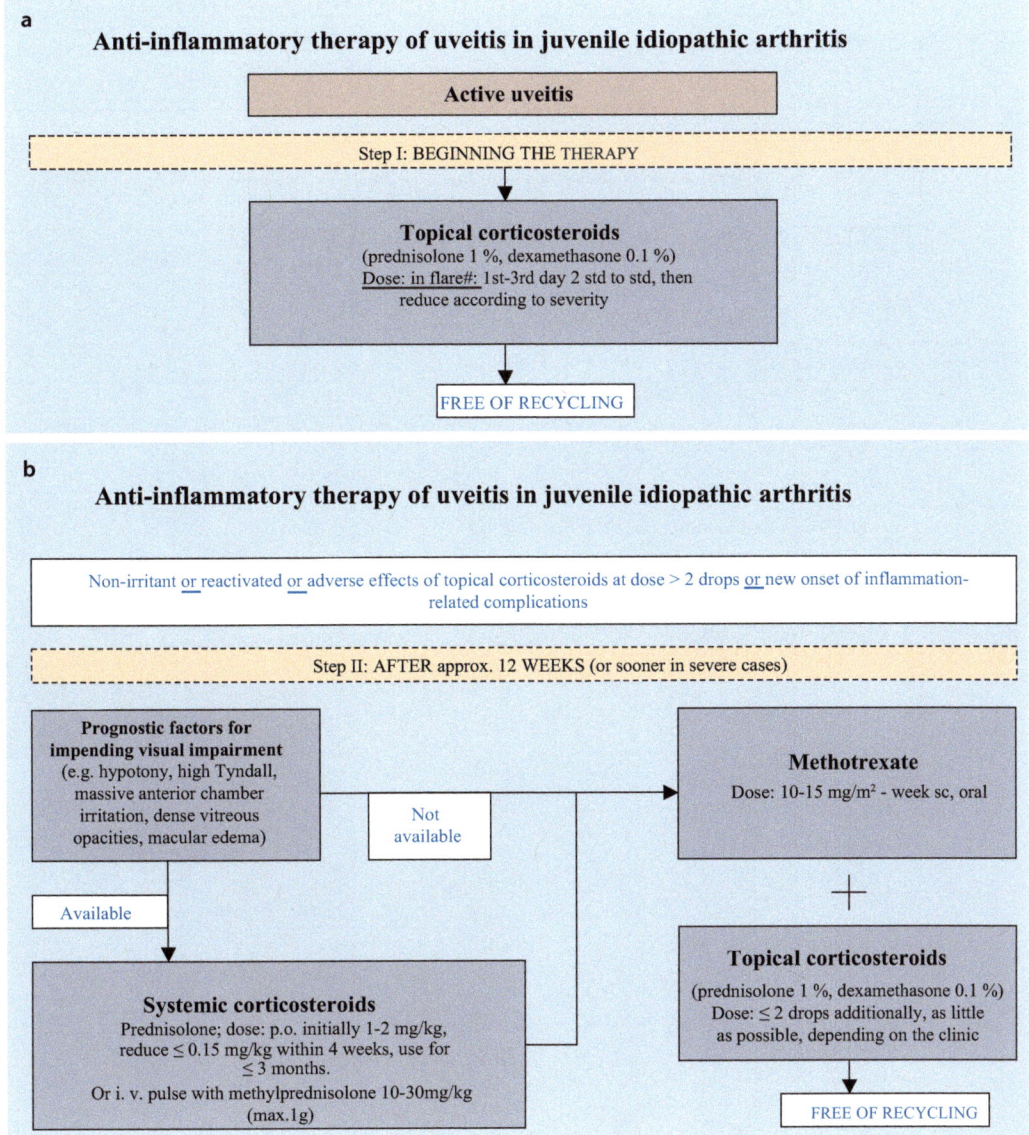

a

Anti-inflammatory therapy of uveitis in juvenile idiopathic arthritis

Active uveitis

Step I: BEGINNING THE THERAPY

Topical corticosteroids
(prednisolone 1 %, dexamethasone 0.1 %)
Dose: in flare#: 1st-3rd day 2 std to std, then
reduce according to severity

FREE OF RECYCLING

b

Anti-inflammatory therapy of uveitis in juvenile idiopathic arthritis

Non-irritant or reactivated or adverse effects of topical corticosteroids at dose > 2 drops or new onset of inflammation-related complications

Step II: AFTER approx. 12 WEEKS (or sooner in severe cases)

Prognostic factors for impending visual impairment
(e.g. hypotony, high Tyndall, massive anterior chamber irritation, dense vitreous opacities, macular edema)

Not available

Methotrexate
Dose: 10-15 mg/m² - week sc, oral

Available

Systemic corticosteroids
Prednisolone; dose: p.o. initially 1-2 mg/kg, reduce ≤ 0.15 mg/kg within 4 weeks, use for ≤ 3 months.
Or i. v. pulse with methylprednisolone 10-30mg/kg (max.1g)

Topical corticosteroids
(prednisolone 1 %, dexamethasone 0.1 %)
Dose: ≤ 2 drops additionally, as little as possible, depending on the clinic

FREE OF RECYCLING

Fig. 6.2 **a–d** Anti-inflammatory step therapy of JIA-associated anterior uveitis. (From Heiligenhaus et al. 2022)

to preserve vision. AWMF guidelines are available for this purpose (Heiligenhaus et al. 2019), which propose the anti-inflammatory therapy of JIA-associated uveitis according to a step-by-step scheme (■ Fig. 6.2a–c). Here, topical and systemic steroid therapy are the initial treatment options (Thorne et al. 2010; Kothari et al. 2015) and in the further course also the basic therapy with methotrexate is the therapy of choice (Beukelman et al. 2012). If these therapies do not respond adequately, the in-

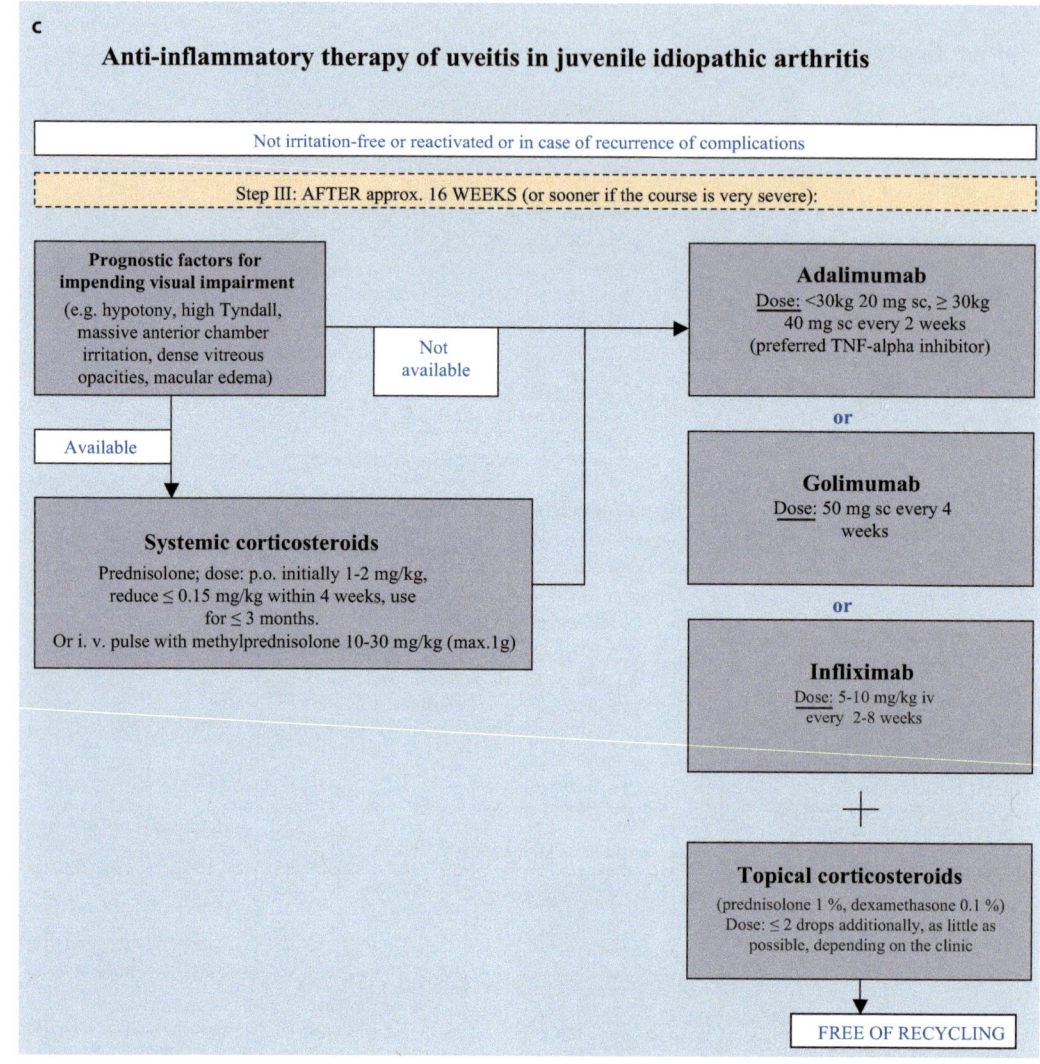

. Fig. 6.2   (continued)

dication for the start of additional biologic therapy (Ramanan et al. 2017; Simonini et al. 2011, 2013) may be given.

6.7.5 Uveitis Screening

The aim of ophthalmological screening examinations is to detect uveitis as early as possible and before complications develop. The uveitis screening intervals in JIA patients are based on the expected uveitis symptoms and incidence in the various arthritis subgroups. These intervals are suggested at closer intervals (every 3 to 6 months) at the beginning of JIA, and then every 6 to 12 months in the further course.

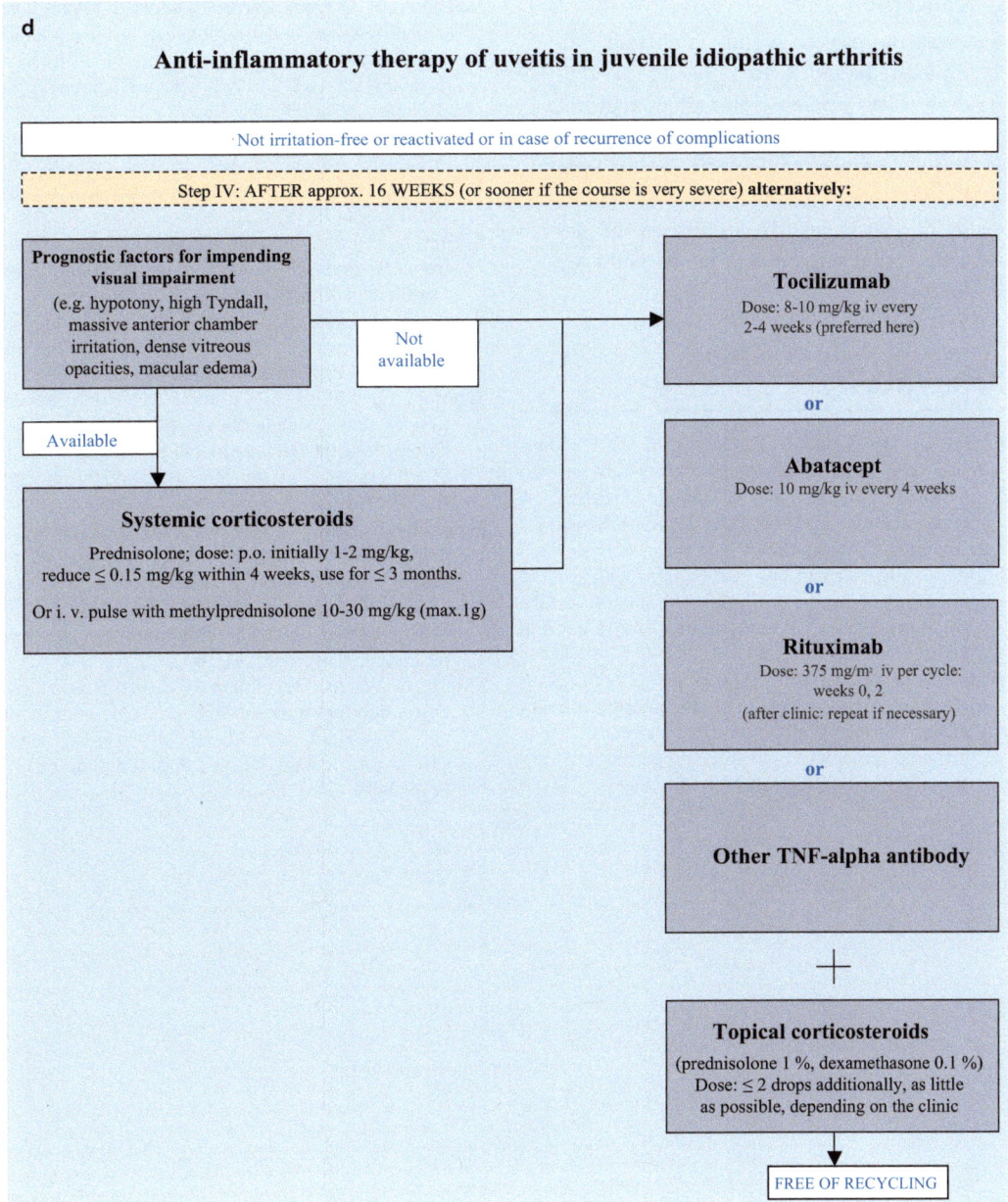

. Fig. 6.2 (continued)

Conclusion

Pediatric uveitis is an important additional diagnosis to consider in children with juvenile idiopathic arthritis, but it can also occur as isolated uveitis. Early detection and referral to an ophthalmologist at the initial diagnosis of oligoarticular JIA or in case of unclear visual impairment in the child are important.

References

Beukelman T, Ringold S, Davis TE (2012) Disease-modifying antirheumatic drug use in the treatment of juvenile idiopathic arthritis. A cross-sectional analysis of the CARRA Registry. J Rheumatol 39:1867–1874

Carvounis PR, Herman DC et al (2006) Incidence and outcomes of uveitis in juvenile rheumatoid arthritis, a synthesis of the literature. Arch Clin Exp Ophthalmol 244:281–290

Heiligenhaus A, Minden K, Tappeiner C et al (2019) Update of the evidence based, interdisciplinary guideline for anti-inflammatory treatment of uveitis associated with juvenile idiopathic arthritis. Semin Arthritis Rheum 49:43–55

Heiligenhaus A, Tappeiner C, Neudorf U (2022) Uveitis bei Kindern und Jugendlichen mit juveniler idiopathischer Arthritis. In: Wagner N, Dannecker G, Kallinich T (Eds) Pädiatrische Rheumatologie. Springer, Berlin/Heidelberg, pp 413–427

Kotaniemi K, Kaipiainen-Seppanen O, Savolainen A, Karma A (1999) A population-based study on uveitis in juvenile rheumatoid arthritis. Clin Exp Rheumatol 17:119–122

Kothari S, Foster CS, Pistilli M (2015) The risk of intraocular pressure elevation in pediatric non-infectious uveitis. Ophthalmology 122:1987–2001

Ramanan AV, Dick AD, Jones AP (2017) Adalimumab plus methotrexate for uveitis in juvenile idiopathic arthritis. N Engl J Med 376:1637–1646

Simonini G, Taddio A, Cattalini M (2011) Prevention of flare recurrences in childhood refractory chronic uveitis: an open-label comparative study of adalimumab versus infliximab. Arthritis Care Res 63:612–618

Simonini G, Taddio A, Cattalini M (2013) Superior efficacy of adalimumab in treating childhood refractory chronic uveitis when used as first biologic modifier drug: adalimumab as starting anti-TNF-alpha therapy in childhood chronic uveitis. Pediatr Rheumatol 11:16

Thorne JE, Woreta FA, Dunn JP (2010) Risk of cataract development among children with juvenile idiopathic arthritis-related uveitis treated with topical corticosteroids. Ophthalmology 117: 1436–1441

6

Cold and Arthritis—Do They Go Together?

Christian Huemer

© The Author(s), under exclusive license to Springer-Verlag GmbH, DE, part of Springer Nature 2024
C. Huemer and H. Girschick (eds.), *Clinical Examples in Pediatric Rheumatology*,
https://doi.org/10.1007/978-3-662-68732-1_7

7.1 Medical History

The 4-year-old girl was presented to the emergency outpatient clinic due to severe pain in the left groin region and abdomen. The child was referred from the general practitioner's office with the suspicion of a trapped inguinal hernia. The child had been experiencing severe pain for a day, which the parents had difficulty localizing. They were not sure whether the child had abdominal pain or leg pain. The child refused to walk, curled up her legs. Specific gastrointestinal symptoms could not be confirmed, nor was there any fever. Therefore, she was presented to the general practitioner on the same day, who made the suspected diagnosis of a trapped inguinal hernia and referred the child to the emergency outpatient clinic of the children's hospital. General medical history so far completely unremarkable. Family medical history unremarkable.

7.2 Examination Findings

4-year-old girl in slightly reduced general condition (pain) and good nutritional status. Under somewhat difficult examination conditions, there is the impression of primarily musculoskeletal symptoms with pain mainly in the area of the right hip joint. This can only be passively flexed to a limited extent, and rotation in the right hip joint is also significantly limited due to pain. Auscultation findings unremarkable. Abdomen palpably soft, regular peristalsis, no tenderness on pressure. No evidence of inguinal hernia. ENT findings without focal signs of inflammation.

7.3 Laboratory Values and Imaging

7.3.1 Laboratory Values

Blood count, CRP, sedimentation rate, liver and kidney function parameters, electrolytes unremarkable.

7.3.2 Imaging

An ultrasound of the abdomen and pelvic region shows an unremarkable finding, especially of the hernial orifices, the kidneys and urinary tract. The same sonographic finding shows an **effusion in the area of the right hip joint** (❏ Fig. 7.1). The effusion appears echo-poor, the synovia somewhat widened.

7.4 Educational Questions

1. What differential diagnoses should be discussed for acute hip pain with sonographically confirmed joint effusion?
2. What additional diagnostics would still be indicated?
3. What therapy would you suggest for this child?

7.5 Differential Diagnostic Considerations and Educative Responses

The presenting symptoms in the toddler with acute, very severe pain in the area of a hip joint necessitates a rapid *differential di-*

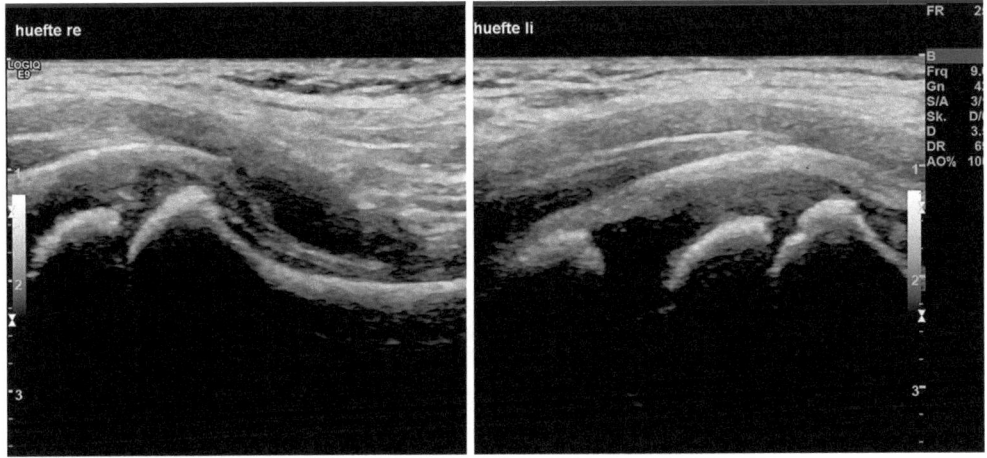

◘ Fig. 7.1 The joint sonography of the hip joints shows a clear echo-poor effusion in the right hip joint and widened synovia, left unremarkable finding

agnosis regarding infectious and non-infectious causes. Although the child did not have a fever, there were clear clinical indications of an inflammatory issue in the area of the hip joint. In such case scenarios, it should always be assessed whether, in addition to sonography, further *imaging diagnostics* (native radiological examination or MRI examination) are indicated. A native radiological examination would be indicated to rule out a primary osseous process (e.g., trauma, neoplastic process, malformations), but not in the early stage of an inflammatory process. Here, there would be a clear indication for performing an MRI. An echogenic sonographic joint finding could provide indications of a primary infectious event and quickly guide the diagnostics in relation to performing a diagnostic joint puncture and an MRI examination. A very important differential diagnosis in this 4-year-old girl is also a diagnosis from the spectrum of osteodystrophies. Foremost among these would be the aseptic necrosis of the femoral head (Perthes disease). This would be a diagnosis that could be made very precisely by MRI

early in the course of the disease after ruling out infectious processes and malignant processes (◘ Fig. 7.2, as an example). Nevertheless, sonography would also be a suitable means of displaying the hip epiphysis in 2 planes, an integral part of hip sonography when searching for effusion and arthritis.

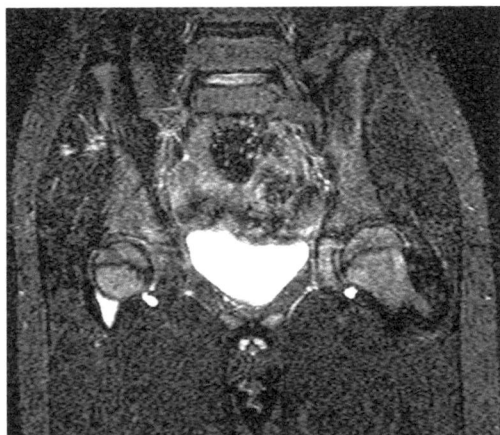

◘ Fig. 7.2 Monoarthritis of the right hip in MRI (TIRM sequence with fat saturation): Arthritis in the right hip 2 weeks after a viral respiratory disease

Until the arrival of the discussed important radiological and possibly infectious findings, the administration of non-steroidal anti-inflammatory *therapies* is quite sensible and necessary for symptom relief. This therapy would hardly delay diagnostics. Giving systemic steroid therapy to a possibly infectious inflammatory joint effusion should be very carefully/conservatively considered. Antibiotic therapy would require a similarly thorough infectious workup of the case (joint puncture and pathogen detection **before** the start of antibiotic therapy) in order to justify a targeted antibiotic therapy after an initial empirical therapy.

7.6 Further Course

In the 4-year-old girl, based on the clinical findings and the clear sonographic finding, which showed an echo-poor joint effusion, the diagnosis of a **Coxitis fugax** was defined; initially, a non-steroidal anti-inflammatory therapy (Ibuprofen 30 mg/kg body weight/day orally for 5 days) was given, which led to complete relief of symptoms within a few days. The child was clinically and sonographically checked again after a week, showing complete relief of symptoms and no further indications of abnormalities in the hip joint. The initially existing effusion was no longer detectable. Therefore, further diagnostics were waived and another check-up was only recommended in case of recurring symptoms.

7.7 Summary

7.7.1 Etiology

The acute transient arthritis of the hip joint (**Coxitis fugax**) is a transient arthritis of the hip joint of unclear etiology. It is the most common cause of hip pain in children aged 2 to 10 years. Synonyms are transient arthritis and hip cold. Possible causes for coxitis fugax are **viral infections** that occurred 1–2 weeks ago, a hypersensitivity reaction, or minimal trauma (Girschick and Huppertz 2022). The disease is self-limiting and can occasionally last longer than 6 weeks. The clinical symptoms are characterized by acute pain, limping, limited mobility, especially abduction and rotation in one hip joint. The pain is often projected distally, i.e., into the leg or knee joint, so that the hip joint must always be examined in case of knee pain. Children usually fall ill in pre-school or primary school age, are afebrile and otherwise healthy.

7.7.2 Diagnosis

Laboratory tests (determination of inflammation parameters, which are usually inconspicuous) are also part of the diagnosis. If a joint puncture is performed, a serous, slightly inflammatory finding is found (cell count usually < 20,000 cells/µl). The diagnosis is supported by the sonographic detection of free joint fluid. An X-ray of the hip in coxitis reveals an inconspicuous finding. It should only be performed in case of doubtful diagnosis or if the complaints persist. Also, a **Morbus Perthes** can be associated with joint effusion, this can be diagnosed early (also sonographically) and safely in the MRI examination and should therefore be carried out in any case if the disease persists for more than 2 weeks (Plesca et al. 2013). The most important differential diagnosis of coxitis fugax is septic arthritis: In the presence of fever, very severe rest pain despite relief, or significantly increased signs of inflammation, septic arthritis must be ruled out by joint puncture. Increasingly, septic arthritis and osteomyelitis, caused by **Kingella kingae**, complicate this traditional teaching, as these are associated with minor signs of systemic inflammation, often no temperature increase. Conventional cultivation methods are difficult, therefore without selective PCR-based detection the puncture remains "sterile". A microbiological long-term incubation of 10 days is absolutely necessary and should be standard today in diagnostic joint puncture (Girschick et al. 1998).

7.7.3 Therapy

The therapy for coxitis fugax is conservative, usually rest for a few days is sufficient, mobilization is carried out after the complaints have subsided, if children are not symptom-free after a few days, the diagnosis should be reconsidered. The use of non-steroidal anti-rheumatic drugs is helpful and is now standard. Splints and extensions are not indicated, they impair the child more than the disease. Therefore, long-term immobilizations should be avoided.

Conclusion

Parents often show great concern due to the severe pain in coxitis fugax. Therefore, a quick comprehensive diagnosis (laboratory and sonography) is very useful for rapid de-escalation. Consistent rest and symptomatic therapy then quickly lead to complete improvement.

References

Girschick H, Huppertz HI (2022) Reaktive Arthritis/Coxitis fugax und infektionsassoziierte Arthritiden bei Kindern und Jugendlichen. In: Wagner N, Dannecker G, Kallinich T (Eds). Pädiatrische Rheumatologie, Springer, Berlin/Heidelberg, pp 459–474

Girschick HJ, Harmsen D, Kreth HW (1998) Septische Arthritis durch Kingella kingae. Monatsschr Kinderheilkd 146:938–941

Plesca DA, Luminos M, Spatariu L, Balgradean M (2013) Postinfectious arthritis in pediatric practice. Maedica 8(Buchar):164–169

Tonsillitis—What Comes Next?

Christian Huemer

8.1 Medical History

The 8-year-old girl was referred by the pediatrician, the girl had swelling and pain in the area of the left knee joint for 4 weeks. According to the pediatrician, the child had suffered from a high-fever purulent tonsillitis 2 months ago, which was treated orally with a penicillin therapy for a week after a confirmed streptococcal detection (throat swab and rapid test) until the complete improvement of the condition. After a symptom-free interval, a sudden onset of gonarthritis on the left has been present for 4 weeks, no other symptoms. The referral was made to rule out a rheumatic disease. General medical history is otherwise unremarkable. Family medical history is unremarkable.

8.2 Examination Findings

8-year-old girl in good general and nutritional condition. Musculoskeletal status shows significant **gonarthritis** on the left with warming and slight redness of the knee joint, especially suprapatellar (◘ Fig. 8.1). Slight pain at the end range of flexion. Joint status and axial skeleton otherwise

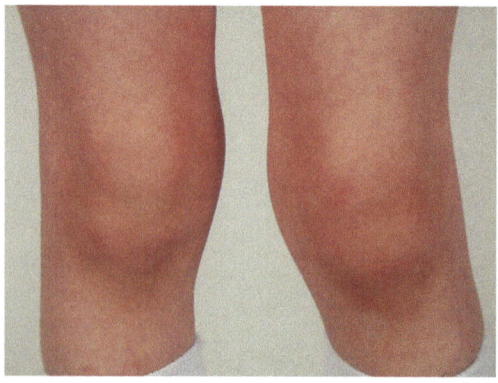

◘ **Fig. 8.1** Monarthritis in the left knee 3 weeks after a scarlet fever with detection of A-streptococci in the throat swab

unremarkable. Internal status completely unremarkable without focal signs of inflammation. Throat mucous membranes bland, tonsils hypertrophic, not coated, eardrums on both sides bland.

8.3 Laboratory Values

Blood count, CRP, ESR unremarkable. Liver function parameters, kidney function parameters, electrolytes unremarkable. Borrelia serology unremarkable. Urine findings unremarkable.

8.4 Educational Questions

1. What differential diagnoses would you consider in this constellation of a girl without fever with persistent gonarthritis?
2. What further diagnostic procedures can now provide additional information in the differential diagnosis?
3. What treatment concepts result from this?

8.5 Differential Diagnostic Considerations and Educational Answers

The *differential diagnoses* of arthritis, which occurs a few weeks after an acute infection in childhood, are broad. Generally, in this context, we speak of **reactive arthritides**, which manifest themselves from inflammatory joint diseases following infections in the genital area, urinary tract, gastrointestinal tract, but also other organs and tissues.

The pathogenetic boundaries to septic infections or autoimmune-caused arthritides are blurred. For the *further diagnostic approach*, it is therefore important to identify possible pathogens based on a detailed medical history and precise description of the preceding infection. This is usually not achieved as a direct pathogen detection, but in the sense of a post-infectious reaction e.g. through infection serological findings. The *treatment concept* for the treatment of a reactive arthritis therefore always results in the sense of an anti-inflammatory therapy. If a pathogenetically infectious agent is still to be assumed, there is a positive direct pathogen detection or a persistent clinical picture in the sense of an infection, especially fever and additional specific organ symptoms, then an anti-infective therapy should be used. The classic example for this would be joint borreliosis/Lyme arthritis.

8.6 Further Course

In the girl, further diagnostic tests were carried out due to the clear anamnestic indications for acute tonsillitis, including a serological test for streptococcal antibodies (**Antistreptolysin titer, Antistrepto-DNase-B titer**) and another direct pathogen detection using a throat swab. (Here, no positive finding for streptococcal colonization was found, but there was a significant increase in the antistreptolysin titer > 2000 and significantly increased antistrepto-DNase-B titer > 600).

Further infection serological findings (respiratory panel for EBV, adenovirus, coronavirus, influenza virus) were inconspicuous. Based on the clinical and existing infection serological findings, the **diagnosis of aPost-Streptococcal Arthritis(PSRA)** was made. An anti-inflammatory therapy with non-steroidal anti-inflammatory therapy was then recommended. Under ibuprofen therapy (daily dose 30 mg/kg body weight/day p.o.) for 4 weeks, the inflammation in the area of the left knee joint could be treated sustainably, further immunomodulatory therapy or even local anti-inflammatory therapy was discussed, but no longer had to be indicated. After 4 weeks of ther-

apy, the girl had a completely inconspicuous clinical finding and a normalization of the joint status functionally.

8.7 Summary

Reactive arthritis can occur after infections with a variety of both bacterial and viral infectious agents. Even if a cultivable infectious agent cannot usually be detected in the inflamed synovia or joint effusion, the pathogens still seem to play a direct role, as non-cultivable pathogen particles or their DNA or RNA have been detected. Especially in small children and school children, diarrheal diseases with Salmonella, Shigella, Yersinia and Campylobacter play a larger role than genital infections with Chlamydia (Huppertz and Scheurlen 1991; Buxton et al. 2002). In 80% of the affected children and adolescents, gastroenteritis is usually identified as the triggering infection, here the role of HLA-B27 for reactive arthritis was recognized pathogenetically very early, but the precise molecular immunological processes are still unclear. Only 20% (up to 60%) of those affected are HLA-B27 positive, this shows that reactive arthritis can also occur in the absence of HLA-B27. Reactive arthritis typically occurs especially in adolescents and young adults, the age of the clinical symptoms also depends on the type of infectious agent, Chlamydia and genital infections play a role especially in older adolescents and adults (Chen et al. 2003). In 70% of children with the symptom triad of arthritis, uveitis and urethritis, preceding diarrheal diseases were described (shigellosis, salmonellosis, yersiniosis or also Campylobacter infections).

Streptococcal infections as primary triggering infections for a reactive arthritis have already been described in a number of cohort studies. Mackie and Keat (2004) have already described this entity in a cohort of 180 patients with PSRA (Mackie and

8

Keat 2004). 83% of these patients had suffered from a disease with group A streptococci, about 2 weeks after infection a non-migrating arthritis of large and small joints occurred, which could also affect the axial skeleton. The response to non-steroidal anti-inflammatory drugs was described as slow, a chronic course as possible (Girschick and Huppertz 2022). The differentiation from acute rheumatic fever is difficult in individual cases (Tutar et al. 2002), HLA studies, however, showed that an association with HLA-B27 hardly exists here, so that the PSRA is pathogenetically rather located in the vicinity of acute rheumatic fever and not in the area of HLA-B27 reactive arthritis (Ahmed et al. 1998).

The therapy of PSRA is usually anti-inflammatory, an antibiotic therapy is initially recommended in individual cases with suspicion of further existing direct pathogen detection (Moorthy et al. 2009), then the conceptual transition to septic arthritis would exist. A cardiac involvement is described as rare.

The therapy of reactive arthritis is primarily based on an anti-inflammatory therapy, a rheumatism basic therapy should only be discussed for a short time and in a limited form. The study situation regarding the use of a rheumatism basic therapy in reactive arthritis is limited (Girschick and Huppertz 2022). As a rule, such a therapy is only considered if the reactive arthritis is assessed as enthesitis-associated arthritis or spondyloarthropathy due to a persistent chronic course. The use of sulfasalazine should be considered, especially if the patients are HLA-B27 positive (sulfasalazine in a dose between 20 and 50 mg/kg body weight/day p.o. for max. 3-6 months).

Conclusion

Any form of childhood arthritis with anamnestic indications for preceding infections requires a detailed differential diagnosis. If an arthritis initially assessed as reactive takes a chronic course, then an immunomodulatory therapy should be considered within the framework of a then rheumatological conception.

References

Ahmed S, Ayoub EM, Scornik JC, Wang CY, She JX (1998) Poststreptococcal reactive arthritis: clinical characteristics and association with HLA-DR allels. Arthritis Rheum 41:1096–1102

Buxton JA, Fyfe M, Berger S, Cox MB, Northcott KA (2002) Reactive arthritis and other sequelae following sporadic Salmonella typhimurium infection in British Columbia, Canada: a case control study. J Rheumatol 29:2154–2158

Chen T, Rimpilainen M, Luukainen R, Mottonen T et al (2003) Bacterial components in the synovial tissue of patients with advanced rheumatoid arthritis or osteoarthritis: analysis with gas chromatography-mass spectrometry and panbacterial polymerase chain reaction. Arthritis Rheum 49:328–334

Girschick HJ, Huppertz HI (2022) Reaktive und parainfektiöse Arthritiden. In: Wagner N, Dannecker G, Kallinich T (Eds) Pädiatrische Rheumatologie. Springer, Berlin/Heidelberg, pp 459–474

Huppertz HI, Scheurlen W (1991) Salmonella septic arthritis presenting as reactive arthritis. J Rheumatol 18:1112–1113

Mackie SL, Keat A (2004) Poststreptococcal reactive arthritis: what is it and how do we know? Rheumatology (Oxford) 43:949–954

Moorthy LN, Gaur S, Peterson MG, Landa YL, Tandon M, Lehman TJ (2009) Poststreptococcal reactive arthritis in children. Clin Pediatr 48:174–182

Tutar E, Atalay S, Yilmaz E, Ucar T, Kocak G, Imamoglu A (2002) Poststreptococcal reactive arthritis in children: is it really a different entity from rheumatic fever? Rheumatol Int 22:80–83

Worm-Like Movement, and the Tonsil was Inflamed

Ae-Rie Im-Schipolowski and Hermann Girschick

Contents

9.1 Medical History

Due to the broad spectrum of streptococcal sequelae, including **acute rheumatic fever** (ARF) in children and adolescents, the following presents two patients with their history:

▪▪ Monika

A 13-year-old girl presented to the emergency department with involuntary short twitches of the right hand that had been present for about 1 week. These occurred occasionally, mainly in rest or stress situations, and led to a perceived clumsiness of the girl. The travel and family history was unremarkable, no other pre-existing conditions known. Recent infections were initially denied. Over the course of 6 days, there was a progressive worsening of symptoms with now sudden, lightning-like movements of the right upper extremity, leading to forced left-handedness, an unsteady gait, and orofacially emphasized twitches.

▪▪ Anna

3 weeks after a clinical scarlet fever with evidence of A-streptococci and fever for the duration of 2 days, a clinically successful cephalosporin therapy (suspected penicillin allergy) was carried out. About 2 weeks later, a partially itchy rash appeared on the entire integument without fever. Symptomatic therapy with H2 antagonists was carried out. Another week later, changing joint complaints occurred in terms of location and duration. The girl is presented with severe neck pain and swelling of the left hand and knee joint. The child was otherwise always healthy. No rheumatic diseases/autoimmune diseases can be described in the family history.

9.2 Examination Findings

▪▪ Monika

The neurological examination showed a right-sided, subtle muscular hypotonia as well as hyperkinetic, choreatic movements of the upper extremity. The pediatric-internal whole body status was otherwise unremarkable except for subfebrile temperatures up to 37.9 °C. The child's mother now reported about a purulent tonsillitis about 6 weeks ago, which had "healed" without antimicrobial therapy. In recent weeks, the girl had complained of recurrent, but always only short-term joint pain. However, there were no clinical indications of arthritis. Therefore, the initial suspicion was a **Chorea minor** as part of a "rheumatic fever" after streptococcal infection.

▪▪ Anna

The 5-year-old girl presented in a reduced general condition. The skin showed a garland-shaped exanthema on the thorax, in the left axilla, also in the area of the face/nose, an Erythema marginatum was diagnosed (❑ Fig. 9.1). In part, this appeared as a factitious urticaria. Currently, there was no fever. Significant restriction of neck mobility with myalgic complaints, the thumb base joint was swollen and restricted in movement on the right, left knee and left wrist also painfully restricted with swelling and overheating, in the knee also effusion formation (❑ Fig. 9.2). Moderate conjunctivitis on both sides. The tonsils appeared somewhat hyperplastic, however without coatings and without current signs of inflammation.

9.3 Laboratory Values and Imaging

▪▪ Monika

Inflammatory parameters were elevated with a CRP of 73 mg/dl and an ESR of 40 mm/h, the A-streptococci rapid test was inconspicuous. No **β-hemolytic A-streptococci** could be detected in the throat swab either. However, the ASL titer was elevated at > 2100 IE/l above the highest measured value, other streptococcal-associated antibodies such as ADB (Anti-Deoxyribonucleotidase B) were not determined. Furthermore, a moderate

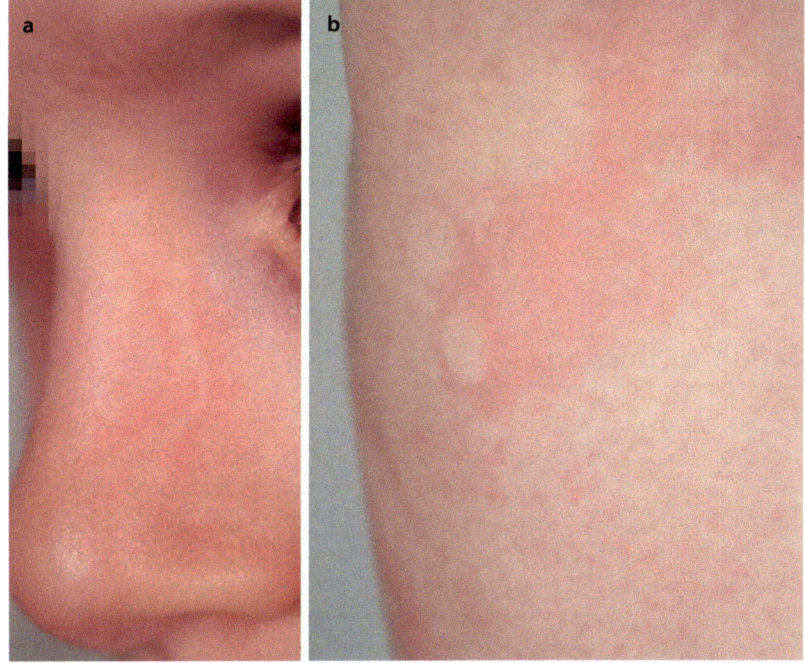

☑ **Fig. 9.1** **a,b** Anna, 5 years old, with skin rash of the entire integument: Erythema marginatum, partly urticarial. The images show the erythematous skin rash, which occurred parallel to a polyarthritis with a migratory character

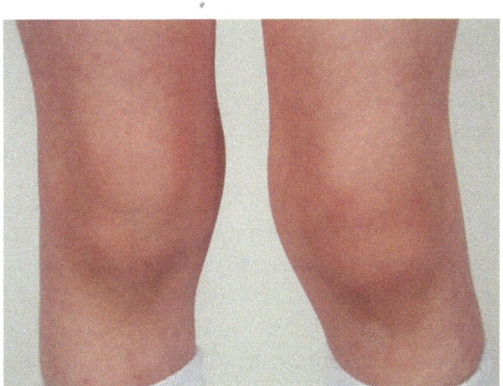

☑ **Fig. 9.2** Oligoarthritis and polyarthralgia involving the left knee. The image shows the arthritis in the left knee and the erythematous skin rash 3 weeks after a scarlet fever with evidence of A-streptococci in the throat swab

leukocytosis and a microcytic, hypochromic anemia were seen in the blood count. No bacterial growth could be led in the blood culture. A lumbar puncture was not performed. In the autoimmune diagnostics, ANA, ENA, ANCA, dsDNA were negative. Wilson's disease was unlikely with normal ceruloplasmin and total copper in the serum.

The echocardiography and sonography of the abdomen showed no abnormalities, a cranial magnetic resonance imaging and that of the extremities were inconspicuous. ECG and EEG also showed no abnormal findings.

■ ■ **Anna**

There were no significantly noticeable inflammatory parameters (CRP 1.3 mg/dl, ESR 25 mm/h, ferritin 62 µg/l), likewise the blood count and overview values for "liver, kidney, muscle, bone" were normal. Autoimmune diagnostics (ANA) were not indicative. The infection serologies for Parvovirus B19, EBV virus, Cytomegalovirus were each inconspicuous. No increase in the antistreptolysin titer or the anti-streptococcal DNAase.

Sonographically, a moderate knee joint effusion was shown on the left, slightly also on the right. No signs of measurable arthritis at the hip or wrist joints. An abdominal sonographic diagnosis was regular, as was an echocardiography. An ECG and an EEG examination were normal.

9.4 Educational Questions

1. What differential diagnosis do you consider for choreiform movement disorders?
2. What differential diagnosis do you consider for arthritis and exanthema?
3. How do you design the diagnostics, from laboratory to imaging, in case of suspicion of streptococcal sequelae?
4. What conceptual considerations are there for reactive streptococcal diseases from an immunological point of view?

9.5 Diagnostic Considerations for Rheumatic Fever

According to the revised **Jones diagnostic criteria** (Dajani et al. 1992; Gewitz et al. 2015), the diagnosis of rheumatic fever is confirmed in the presence of a positive streptococcal swab or rapid test and/or antibody detection **plus** 2 major criteria or 1 major and 2 minor criteria (see ◘ Tab. 9.1).

The prerequisite is a clinical reference to a possible infection with A-streptococci, their detection in the smear or the indirect indication by an increase of a streptococcal-associated antibody (Dajani et al. 1992). ARF is very rarely diagnosed in its full picture in Central Europe, incidences are below 1/100,000 school children. Recent reports from Southeast European countries, Asia, Africa, and South America show significantly higher incidences and thus the global significance and their disease burden (Carapetis et al. 2005; Keitzer 2005; Jackson et al. 2011).

◘ **Tab. 9.1** Revised Jones diagnostic criteria

Major criteria	Minor criteria
Migratory polyarthritis	Fever
Carditis	Arthralgia
Chorea minor	Increased ESR, CRP
Erythema marginatum/anulare	Extended QT or PR time in ECG

▪▪ Monika

Since the patient, apart from the chorea minor and the increased inflammation parameters, did not show any further major and no reliably detectable minor criteria, the diagnosis of rheumatic fever could not be conclusively made. However, the chorea minor could certainly be seen as an immunological consequence after an untreated streptococcal infection with a very high ASL titer.

▪▪ Anna

Anna showed a variably pronounced, indeed "migratory" arthritis of knees, wrist and finger joints, furthermore, an erythema was present, which could be described as erythema marginatum (◘ Fig. 9.1), so that she had "fulfilled" 2 major criteria. In addition, she showed moderately increased inflammation signs and arthralgia, so that also 2 minor criteria were considered fulfilled. Thus, Anna's disease was also formally classifiable/diagnosable as a streptococcal sequelae in the sense of a rheumatic "fever" according to Jones.

9.6 Further Progress

■■ Monika

Under oral therapy with Penicillin V (100,000 IU/kg body weight/day) and glucocorticoids (Prednisolone 2 mg/kg body weight/day), the symptoms quickly subsided and the inflammation parameters decreased. Intravenous immunoglobulin therapy was considered, but was not carried out due to the good response to the measures taken. After 10 days, the antimicrobial treatment could be stopped, and the glucocorticoid therapy could be reduced or phased out after 7 days. The girl was discharged home after a close pediatric and immunological control was established. A follow-up a few months later revealed an unremarkable course.

■■ Anna

The patient's migrating joint pain and oligoarthritis were well controlled with the use of NSAIDs, and the patient was symptom-free after a few days. The rash, which was partly mechanically induced, improved with the local application of antihistamines. There were no indications of an allergic diathesis at the beginning of care. However, the patient developed signs of a penicillin allergy over time, and she also had urticarial reactions to cephalosporins. Specific IgE antibodies against penicillins and cephalosporins could not be detected. The total IgE remained low normal and did not increase over a period of 2 years. It was agreed with the pediatrician that in the event of a possible recurrence of streptococcal disease, early diagnosis and antibiotic therapy would be carried out, which was the case about 1 to 2 times a year in the following years. Since the diagnosis of rheumatic fever without cardiac involvement was discussed, a limited infection prophylaxis was "agreed" with the parents. Certainly, if there was cardiac involvement, antibiotic infection prophylaxis would be pursued much more consistently with 10 years of continuous therapy.

9.7 Educative Answers

- **1. What differential diagnosis do you consider for choreiform movement disorders?**

Other differential diagnoses for choreiform movements include major chorea (Huntington), benign familial chorea, familial benign choreoacanthocytosis, and possibly drug-induced chorea. Wilson's disease should also be considered and differentially diagnosed. In the broadest sense, neuroinflammatory, possibly also oncological diseases should be considered. If chorea occurs with joint involvement, arthritic diseases such as reactive, septic or juvenile idiopathic arthritis and indeed rheumatic fever should be considered. In case of cardiac involvement, endocarditis of other origins should be considered.

- **2. What differential diagnosis do you consider for arthritis and exanthema?**

Historically, the Jones criteria referred to a migratory polyarthritis, with arthralgias being considered a minor criterion from 1992 onwards. After the revision of the Jones criteria in 2015, aseptic monoarthritis in populations at increased risk for ARF is also considered a criterion. Such high-risk populations include, for example, the indigenous population in Australia or New Zealand. Generally, an incidence in low-risk populations of < 2/100,000 school children and a "rheumatic" heart disease occurring in all age groups with a prevalence of less than 1/1000 persons is referred to. For high-risk populations, incidences of 500/100,000 children are sometimes reported. Both the diagnostic and therapeutic algorithms have not changed significantly in the last 20 years. Since echocardiography has become standard, the Jones criteria were modernized in 2015 with regard to imaging echocardiography, and a risk stratification according to the incidence of rheumatic heart disease was introduced. In this context, **monoarthritis and polyarthralgia** in high-risk groups were re-evaluated as **major** criteria. However, these new major criteria would not apply to Central Europe, where the incidence is reported to be less than 1/100,000. However, regional outbreaks, as reported in the USA or Slovenia, can reach relevant numbers. The differential diagnosis of arthritis, fever, and rash ultimately refers to the classic septic arthritis, which can also be associated with bacterial septic spread, e.g., in the area of the mitral valve. In the context of genuine viral infections, especially Parvovirus B19 infection, arthritis can occur. The classic reactive "hip cold" should also be considered in this context, with fever, rash, and arthritis. Classic peri-infectious arthritides such as Lyme borreliosis are also important. Post-infectious reactive arthritides in the context of, for example, diarrheal diseases, which are mostly HLA-B27-associated, should be considered. In the context of crystal arthropathy or inflammasome-associated autoinflammatory diseases, arthritis may be considered differential to ARF. Kawasaki disease should also be mentioned in this context. Various basic rheumatological diseases such as juvenile idiopathic arthritis (JIA) or systemic lupus erythematosus (SLE) should be considered. The JIA subgroup of the systemic form (sJIA), formerly also called Still's disease, is particularly important here. However, the ARF fever characteristic is quite different from Still's disease: In sJIA, the fever rises in the afternoon/evening to high peaks and is accompanied by a fine-spotted rash. The systemic fever episode is followed by a polyar-

thritic component, which can take a difficult course without therapy. In contrast, polyarthritis in the context of acute rheumatic fever often self-limits after weeks, it responds excellently to NSAIDs.

- **3. How do you conduct the diagnostics, from laboratory to imaging, in case of suspected streptococcal sequelae?**

A previous streptococcal infection can be assumed due to a recently occurred pharyngitis. Confirmation can be obtained through a culture, a positive throat swab, increased or preferably rising **antistreptolysin-O titers**, or a positive GAS antigen test in the presence of clinical symptoms. It should be noted that throat swabs and streptococcal rapid tests can often be inconspicuous during ARF manifestation, whereas the antistreptolysin test and anti-DNase B typically reach their maximum after 3–6 weeks. Approximately 80% of children with ARF have a significantly increased antistreptolysin-O titer (> 300 IU) (Keitzer 2005; Steer et al. 2015).

Increases in ESR and serum CRP are sensitive but not specific. Often, an increase in serum CRP > 30–70 mg/l is seen. Leukocytosis and "infection-" anemia are also common occurrences.

An ECG should be performed during the initial examination and the serum should be tested for heart markers. Normal troponin-I levels rule out severe myocardial damage. ECG anomalies such as PR prolongation are not proof of carditis.

Echocardiography is recommended for all patients with suspected or confirmed ARF to detect subclinical **carditis** even in the absence of heart murmur. Valve affections mainly affect the mitral- (80%) and less frequently the aortic valve (approx. 20%). However, not all echocardiographic anomalies indicate rheumatic carditis. To increase specificity, Doppler flow criteria and echocardiographic morphological criteria were developed (Gewitz et al. 2015).

A chest X-ray is not routinely performed, but it can possibly detect cardiomegaly. If skin manifestations are present, a biopsy may lead to an earlier diagnosis. Joint sonography is standard. If joint involvement is present, a puncture with microscopy and culture may be necessary to rule out infectious septic causes of arthritis. In case of CNS involvement, a cerebrospinal fluid analysis and a cranial MRI should be performed, extended by determination of serum copper and ceruloplasmin as well as antinuclear antibodies in the case of choreiform movement patterns.

- **4. What conceptual considerations are there for reactive streptococcal diseases from an immunological perspective?**

According to currently available evidence, ARF is caused exclusively by Group A Streptococci (GAS), *Streptococcus pyogenes*. Among these, types 1, 3, 5, 6, 14, 18, 19, and 24 are primarily associated with the disease (Keitzer 2005; Bessen et al. 1989). It is also estimated that about 3–6% of the population are genetically particularly susceptible to acute rheumatic fever. This is based on the observation of familial clusters and a concordance in identical twins (44% in monozygotic versus 12% in dizygotic twins). Some class II alleles of the human leukocyte antigen (HLA-DR7 and -DQ), specific B-cell alloantigens (D8/17), and gene polymorphisms for transforming growth factor (TNF-α, interleukins) are associated with increased susceptibility. In contrast, other class II alleles (HLA-DR) appear to have a protective function (Guilherme and Kalil 2010; Bryant et al. 2009; Guilherme et al. 2011).

The pathogenesis of ARF is not yet fully understood. The concept of **molecular mimicry** is the most widespread theory: After infection of the pharyngeal epithelium, both B and T cells are activated, leading to antibody production (IgM and IgG) and activation of primarily CD4 cells. However, the immune response, which is actually directed against antigens on the M-protein and the N-acetylglucosamine of the streptococcal carbohydrate, also attacks human tissue (especially endothelial cells of the heart, brain, joints, and skin) due to cross-reactivity. The lysis of the endothelial cells releases peptides such as laminin, keratin, and tropomyosin, which in turn activate further cross-reacting T cells. These migrate into the affected tissue and cause greater damage and thus the spread of the epitope (Carapetis et al. 2016). In the case of **rheumatic carditis**, the cross-reaction of IgG antibodies directed against valve endothelial cells leads to an increased activation and production of vascular cell adhesion protein 1 (VCAM1). This recruits activated lymphocytes. As the process continues, the normal endothelial cells die off and are converted into collagen (Chopra and Narula 1991). CD4$^+$- and CD8$^+$-T cells infiltrate the heart valves and produce inflammatory cytokines. The resulting lesions show **Aschoff nodules**. These are granulomas that contain high concentrations of T cells and macrophages and are indicative of a pronounced inflammation process (Aschoff 1906). During healing, the affected areas scar and sclerose (Keitzer 2005). In Sydenham's chorea, neurons of the basal ganglia are attacked by the cross-reactive antibodies. After activation of the calcium-calmodulin-dependent protein kinase II, there is an increase in tyrosine hydroxylase and thus ultimately an increased production of L-Dopa, the precursor of dopamine. This can lead to an altered cellular signal cascade as well as abnormal movements and behavior patterns (Carapetis et al. 2016). In the case of the erythema marginatum typical for rheumatic fever, antibodies react against keratin in the epidermis. The subcutaneous nodules are possibly caused by a delayed hypersensitivity to group A streptococcal antigens and histologically show granulomas, similar to

Aschoff's nodules (Carapetis et al. 2016). Another hypothesis postulates that during the invasion of the epithelial cells by the streptococci, the M-protein binds to type IV collagen, making the latter immunogenic (Dinkla et al. 2003a, b; Tandon et al. 2013).

9.8 Summary

9.8.1 Etiology

The etiology of Monika's and Anna's immunological diseases are most likely infections with A-streptococci.

9.8.2 Pathogenesis/Clinic

The immunological pathogenesis after the infection is, strictly speaking, still unclear. The following concepts are considered immunologically: In the immune response actually directed against the streptococcal antigens, the body's own endothelial cells, especially of the heart, CNS, joints, and skin, are also attacked and destroyed (**molecular mimicry**).

Possibly, during the invasion of the epithelial cells by the bacteria, the streptococcal M-protein could bind to type IV collagen, which thus becomes immunogenic and is subsequently "destroyed" by the antibodies.

9.8.3 Diagnosis

The precise descriptive clinical examination is flanked by the attempt to detect the streptococcal infection in a swab and serologically (ASL, ADB for example). Sonographic diagnostics of joints and heart are standard, as well as an ECG and possibly an EEG. In case of central nervous involvement, a cerebrospinal fluid analysis and a cranial MRI examination may be important.

9.8.4 Therapy

The therapy aims to suppress the clinical manifestation of the infection through antibiotic therapy and the subsequent inflammation, whether by the use of NSAID for arthritis/arthralgia or glucocorticoids for carditis. The therapy is supported by physiotherapeutic exercise treatment.

9.8.5 Diagnosis

The diagnosis is primarily based on the clinical picture of the disease, the detection of a streptococcal infection recently or currently, and the imaging detection methods sonography and MRI.

9.8.6 Prophylaxis

A reinfection prophylaxis to prevent the disease is extremely important. Penicillins, cephalosporins, and erythromycin are available for allergic diathesis. The duration depends on the primary manifestation. The WHO recommends a 10-year prophylaxis or until the age of 25 in the case of clear carditis. If there has been valve destruction or the need for cardiac surgery, lifelong antibiotic prophylaxis is recommended. For patients without carditis, a 5-year prophylaxis or alternatively one until the age of 18/21 is recommended.

> **Conclusion**
> ARF is very rarely diagnosed in its full form in Central Europe. However, current reports from Southeast European countries, Asia, Africa, Australia/New Zealand, and South America show its global significance and the associated disease burden. In particular, the late cardiac consequences with valve insufficiency, arrhythmias, and global heart failure

should be considered. In the course of international migration, ARF must also be recognized as a disease in pediatric consultations and wards in this country.

References

Aschoff L (1906) Myocarditisfrage. Verh Dtsch Path Ges 8:46–53

Bessen D, Jones KF, Fischetti VA (1989) Evidence of two distinct classes of streptococcal M protein and their relationship to rheumatic fever. J Exp Med 169:269–283

Bryant PA, Robins-Browne R, Carapetis JR, Curtis N (2009) Some of the people, some of the time. Susceptibility to acute rheumatic fever. Circulation 119:742–753

Carapetis JR, Steer AC, Mulholland EK, Weber M (2005) The global burden of group A streptococcal diseases. Lancet Infect Dis 5:685–694

Carapetis JR, Beaton A, Cunningham MW, Guilherme L, Karthikeyan G et al (2016) Acute rheumatic fever and rheumatic heart disease. Nat Rev Dis Primers 2:15084

Chopra P, Narula JP (1991) Scanning electron microscope features of rheumatic vegetations in acute rheumatic carditis. Int J Cardiol 30:109–112

Dajani AS, Ayoub E, Bierman FZ et al (1992) Guidelines for the diagnosis of rheumatic fever. JAMA 268:2069–2073

Dinkla K, Rohde M, Jansen WT, Carapetis JR, Chhatwal GS, Talay SR (2003a) Streptococcus pyogenes recruits collagen via surface-bound fibronectin: a novel colonization and immune evasion mechanism. Mol Microbiol 47:861–869

Dinkla K, Rohde M, Jansen WT, Kaplan EL, Chhatwal GS, Talay SR (2003b) Rheumatic fever—associated Streptococcus pyogenes isolates aggregate collagen. J Clin Invest 111:1905–1912

Gewitz MH, Baltimor RS, Tani LY, Sable CA, Shulman ST, Carapetis JR, Remenyi B et al (2015) Revision of the Jones criteria for the diagnosis of acute rheumatic fever in the era of doppler echocardiography. A scientific statement from the American Heart Association. Circulation 131:1806–1818

Guilherme L, Kalil J (2010) Rheumatic fever and rheumatic heart disease: cellular mechanisms leading autoimmune reactivity and disease. J Clin Immunol 30:17–23

Guilherme L, Köhler KF, Khalil J (2011) Rheumatic heart disease: mediation by complex immune events. Adv Clin Chem 53:31–50

Jackson SJ, Steer AC, Campbell H (2011) Systematic review: Estimation of global burden of non-suppurative sequelae of upper respiratory infection: rheumatic fever and post-streptococcal glomerulonephritis. Tropical Med Int Health 16:2–11

Keitzer R (2005) Acute rheumatic fever (ARF) and poststreptococcal reactive arthritis (PSRA)—an update. Z Rheumatol 64:295–307

Steer AC, Smeesters PR, Curtis N (2015) Streptococcal serology, secrets for the specialist. Pediatr Infect Dis J 24:1250–1252

Tandon R, Sharma M, Chandrashekhar Y, Kotb M, Yacoub MH, Narula J (2013) Revisiting the pathogenesis of rheumatic fever and carditis. Nat Rev Cardiol 10:171–177

Rheumatism and the Tick—How are they Connected? A 10-Year-Old Girl with Pronounced Knee Swelling

Christian Huemer

Contents

C. Huemer and H. Girschick (eds.), *Clinical Examples in Pediatric Rheumatology*,
https://doi.org/10.1007/978-3-662-68732-1_10

10.1 Medical History

The 10-year-old girl is presented in the pediatric outpatient clinic with a joint swelling in the left knee that has been present for a few days. The child was referred by the pediatrician with suspicion of left gonarthritis. In the medical history, there is no indication of preceding trauma or febrile infections. Pain is not reported. However, the child's mother has the impression that the knee joint is significantly warmer. No other joint complaints. No further symptoms, especially no fever.

General medical history of the child is unremarkable, no pre-existing diseases, once questionable tick exposure.

10.2 Examination Findings

10-year-old girl in excellent general and nutritional condition, afebrile. Musculoskeletal status shows a massive **gonarthritis** on the left (◘ Fig. 10.1) with significant swelling not only on the actual knee, but also descending dorsally into the lower leg, without tenderness on pressure. Pain on movement only at the end range of flexion. Slight warming, no redness. Further joint status unremarkable. Internal status summarizing completely unremarkable without focal signs of inflammation.

10.3 Laboratory Values and Imaging

10.3.1 Laboratory Values

Blood count and CRP unremarkable, ESR 3, interleukin-6 and procalcitonin unremarkable, rheumatoid factor negative, **antinuclear antibodies 1:320 positive.**

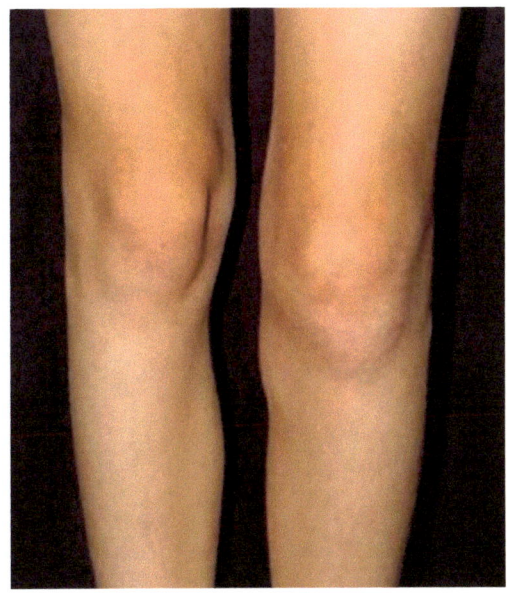

◘ **Fig. 10.1** Image of the lower extremities with pronounced swelling of the left knee joint and also the left distal lower extremity, here due to a ruptured Baker's cyst

10.3.2 Imaging

Plain radiography of the left knee joint shows soft tissue swelling, otherwise unremarkable findings.

Sonography shows a clear, echo-free fluid collection, there is synovial proliferation.

Magnetic resonance imaging of the left knee joint (◘ Fig. 10.2): Shows a voluminous knee joint effusion. Thickened and increased contrast-enhancing synovia. Additionally, elongated **Baker's cyst**, which is partially ruptured. Diffuse edematous changes in the periarticular soft tissues.

10.4 Educational Questions

1. What differential diagnoses should be discussed given the current clinical and laboratory findings?

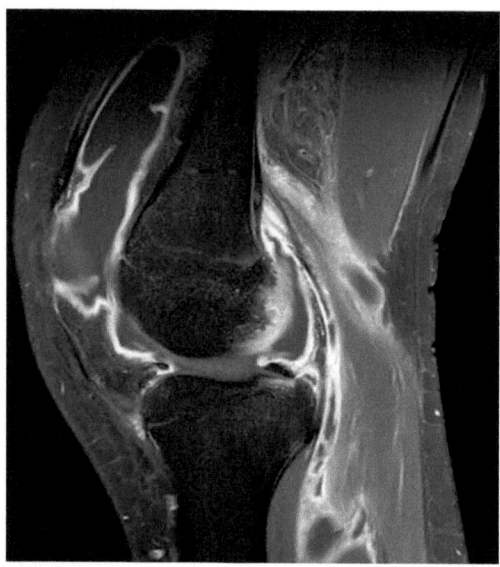

◘ Fig. 10.2 Magnetic resonance imaging of the left knee joint. Voluminous knee joint effusion. Thickened and increased contrast-enhancing synovia. Additionally, elongated Baker's cyst, partially ruptured. Diffuse edematous changes in the periarticular soft tissues. (With kind permission from Dr. A. Schuster, Radiological Department LKH Bregenz)

10

2. Are there any missing historical clues to further specify the diagnosis?
3. What further laboratory diagnostics would be useful and what therapy steps would result from it?

10.5 Differential Diagnostic Considerations

The clinical finding of joint swelling, in this case of the knee joint in a child, is a very common problem in medical practice. Crucial in an acutely occurring monoarthritis is the initial assessment regarding an infectious process: fever, especially touch sensitivity, immediate movement pain, high inflammatory parameters and sonographic evidence of significant echogenicity of the described effusion can be indications to perform a diagnostic joint puncture to rule out a purulent-**septic arthritis**. In a history of a few days, a native radiological finding is only of "relative" importance, but an osseous trauma, a non-inflammatory (e.g., neoplasia, bone dysplasia, malformations) diagnosis can certainly already impress in simple native radiography. Ultimately, it is crucial to quickly plan to rule out an infectious process using joint puncture: A clear, serous joint puncture without increased cell count (the cut-off for the diagnosis of purulent arthritis is given as > 20,000 cells/μl) makes the probability of a purulent arthritis very low. In our case, there was no fever, no inflammatory activity in the laboratory and also sonographically no echogenicity of the described effusion. Therefore, a diagnostic joint puncture was decided against. The only anamnestic clue in the child was a possible tick exposure last summer, which naturally led to considering the differential diagnosis of a **Lyme arthritis**. It should be noted that often even with confirmed Lyme arthritis, the history regarding tick exposure is negative. This diagnosis should therefore always be considered for epidemiological reasons in tick-prevalent regions: The laboratory diagnostic of choice is the performance of an ELISA for Borrelia-specific antibodies, followed by a confirmation using Immunoblot examination (two-step diagnostics) in case of positivity. Further infection serological examinations should be oriented towards the prehistory. If in doubt, a magnetic resonance imaging of the knee joint should certainly be discussed—even before the definition of a suspected diagnosis of juvenile idiopathic arthritis. Also, rarer diagnoses with monoarthritis of a knee joint, such as villonodular synovitis, intra-articular tumors, malformations would thus be ruled out. In chronic monoarthritis, a second imaging beyond sonography is always to be considered.

10.6 Further Course

In the further course, an extended laboratory diagnosis, supplemented by infection serological findings, was planned for the 10-year-old girl: The antistreptolysin titer, as well as Borrelia antibodies (IgM and IgG), were determined. Borrelia IgG showed 240 AU/ml: highly positive, Borrelia IgM: negative; Borrelia Immunoblot IgG and IgM: both highly positive for Borrelia-specific antigens. Based on the clinical picture and these infection serological findings, the diagnosis of **Lyme arthritis** was confirmed in this girl. Subsequently, in addition to the NSAID therapy, an oral antibiotic therapy (**Doxycycline** 4 mg/kg body weight/day: 1 time 200 mg/day p. o.) was started for 4 weeks. In a clinical follow-up after the end of the antibiotic therapy, there was a significant improvement in the findings, but not yet complete normalization of the joint findings. The NSAID therapy (Ibuprofen) was therefore continued for a few more weeks.

10.7 Educative Answers

- **1. What differential diagnoses should be discussed based on the present clinical and laboratory findings?**

See differential diagnostic considerations (▶ Sect. 10.5).

- **2. Are there any missing anamnestic clues for a more precise diagnosis?**

It is important to capture a possible time of tick exposure and the question of a rash occurring after tick exposure. However, this history would only provide additional information and would not be conclusive for Lyme arthritis.

- **3. What extended laboratory diagnostics would be useful and what therapy steps would result from this?**

Crucial for the diagnosis of Lyme arthritis is the performance of an ELISA and in case of positivity a confirming immunoblot for **Borrelia species (*B. burgdorferi*, *B. garinii*, *B. afzelii* and *B. spielmanii*)** in a manifest oligoarthritis. With sufficient preclinical probability for Lyme arthritis, this laboratory diagnostics may be purposeful. For example, in a pronounced polyarthritis involving the fingers, a positive serology may not even make a significant pathogenetic "contribution" because the clinical disease picture would not be typical. Nevertheless, in individual cases, antibiotic therapy may seem sensible, but the main diagnosis of "rheumatic polyarthritis" would be in the foreground.

10.8 Summary

10.8.1 Definition and Frequency

Lyme disease is an inflammatory disease caused by Borrelia species (*B. burgdorferi*, *B. garinii*, *B. afzelii* and *B. spielmanii*). Lyme arthritis was first described in 1977, the incidence of Lyme disease has varied over the years from 26 to 41 per 100,000 inhabitants in Germany, in some regions 200 per 100,000 inhabitants, e.g. in the Bavarian Forest region. (Enkelmann et al. 2018)

10.8.2 Classification

For the classification of Lyme disease, case definitions (Huppertz et al. 1998, 2012) are provided:

1. Lyme disease is present when an **Erythema migrans** is observed, this skin lesion slowly spreads centrifugally over a period of days to weeks and shows central pallor in the course. A serological proof is not necessary, the clinical picture is decisive.
2. For the later manifestations, the serological or possibly even microbiological proof of infection is additionally required. Lyme disease can be divided into different clinical stages, which can overlap. The *first two stages* within a few weeks or months after infection represent the early phase of the infection, they are often not correctly temporally separable in childhood. The *"third" or late phase* occurs after several months to years. In the stage of *early manifestations*, there are essentially a summer flu similar to influenza, an Erythema migrans, a lymphocytoma or a lymphocytic meningitis with or without cranial nerve paralysis in childhood. In the *late stage*, an Acrodermatitis atrophicans, an episodic or chronic Oligoarthritis (**Lyme disease**—described after the region of the first discovery), a Uveitis and Keratitis and rarely a Meningoradiculoneuritis, an Encephalomyelitis and a cardiomyopathy have been described in children.

10.8.3 Clinic

After Erythema migrans, Lyme arthritis is the most common manifestation in childhood. Arthralgia or myalgia can occur within a few days to weeks after an infection, possibly as part of a "summer flu". However, the actual arthritis typically occurs months to a few years after the infection (Huppertz et al. 1995). Large joints such as the knee are affected in about two-thirds of cases. The diagnosis of Lyme arthritis requires additional criteria to the clinical

symptoms, these are essentially based on the performance of serological laboratory tests.

10.8.4 Diagnosis

In addition to detailed history taking, tick exposure can be reported months or years ago, possibly together with a simultaneously occurring Erythema migrans. However, in large cohorts, these criteria do not apply to a large number of patients. As a rule, serological evidence is provided for the diagnosis, usually the serological detection of IgM and IgG class antibodies in the serum, in most patients depending on serological tests of the duration of the disease and the clinical manifestation in early stages up to 50% a detection of IgM antibodies, in late stages the seropositivity of 70 to 90% indicates, a seroconversion from IgM to IgG can then be detected. As a rule, an ELISA test for IgG and IgM is first carried out, if this shows a positive result, a confirmatory Western blot is attached. In most cases, Lyme arthritis is associated with a highly positive IgG serology in all tests, if it is negative, then this usually excludes late Lyme disease. A seronegative Lyme arthritis is an absolute rarity and should be discussed with specialist centers. This currently represents the international recommendation for the performance of the diagnosis of Lyme arthritis (Steere 2001; Huppertz et al. 2012).

10.8.5 Therapy

Lyme arthritis should generally be treated symptomatically with nonsteroidal anti-inflammatory drugs, and in Europe, the antibiotic therapy usually recommended for children up to 8 years old is intravenous antibiotic therapy with either ceftriaxone, cefotaxime, or penicillin G for **2** to a maximum of 4 weeks (Huppertz et al. 1995). If the child is older than 8 years, an alternative oral antibiotic therapy with amoxicillin or doxycycline can be carried out for a duration of 28–30 days. If there is no or insufficient response to a first cycle of antibiotic therapy, a repetition of the antibiotic therapy is recommended. If the arthritis continues to persist, an intra-articular steroid application or therapy with methotrexate can then be considered (Dressler et al. 2005; Girschick et al. 2009).

10.8.6 Prognosis

As a rule, Lyme arthritis is treated with antibiotic therapy. Anecdotally, however, there are also indications for a different approach: If Lyme arthritis is not treated with antibiotics, it may still have a "hopeful" prognosis: of 46 children with Lyme arthritis who did not receive antibiotic therapy within the first 4 years after a tick bite, 10 were still suffering from up to 2 episodes of arthritis after these 4 years, 10 years later no child had arthritis anymore (Dressler et al. 2005). In rare cases, however, a persistent and also therapeutically stubborn arthritis can persist. The therapy then follows rheumatic algorithms. Pathogenetically, it is assumed that immune stimulations maintained by pathogen components locally in the joint (Morbach et al. submitted 2022).

Conclusion

Lyme arthritis in children is an important differential diagnosis especially for monoarthritis e.g. of the knee joint. The history of tick exposure is of little relevance for the diagnosis, what is important is the clinical finding and a two-stage diagnosis of the serological findings.

References

Dressler F, Hobusch D, Girschick HJ, Huppertz HI (2005) Lyme-Arthritis. Urban&Fischer, München
Enkelmann J, Böhmer M, Fingerle V, Siffczyk C, Werber D, Littmann M, Merbecks SS, Helmeke C et al (2018) Incidence of notified Lyme borreliosis in Germany 2013–2017. Sci Rep 8(1):14976
Girschick HJ, Morbach H, Tappe D (2009) Treatment of Lyme borreliosis. Arthritis Res Ther 11:e258
Huppertz HI, Karch H, Suschke HJ (1995) Lyme arthritis in European children and adolescents. The Pediatric Rheumatolgy Collaborative Group. Arthritis Rheum 38:361–368
Huppertz HI, Bentas W, Haubitz I et al (1998) Diagnosis of pediatric Lyme arthritis using a clinical score. Eur J Pediatr 157:304–308
Huppertz HI, Bartmann P, Heininger U, Fingerle V, Kinet M, Klein R, Korenke GC, Nentwich HJ (2012) Rational diagnostic strategies for Lyme borreliosis in children and adolescents: recommendations by the Committee for Infectious Diseases and Vaccinations of the German Academy for Pediatrics and Adolescent Health. Eur J Pediatr 171(11):1619–1624
Steere AC (2001) Lyme disease. N Engl J Med 345:115–125

First Weeks of Joint Pain, Then a Severe Rash

Annette Holl-Wieden

Contents

11.1 Medical History

▪▪ Sophie

The 16-year-old girl presented herself because she had been experiencing recurring **pain in the elbow joints** for 4 weeks. There were no other complaints. Previous illnesses reported included hypothyroidism and medication with L-thyroxine.

▪▪ Leni

12-year-old Leni had been experiencing recurring **pain and swelling of various joints** for 2 months. The affected areas were the ankle joints, knee joints, left wrist, right middle finger, right thumb. At her first presentation, she reported that she had had a "rash" on her feet for a few days. She currently had pain and especially swelling in the area of both ankle joints and feet. Walking was hardly possible.

11.2 Examination Findings

▪▪ Sophie

Sophie had **arthritis** of the right elbow joint with swelling and severely painful restricted flexion. The rest of the examination findings were unremarkable.

▪▪ Leni

The clinical examination showed **arthritis** of the right thumb base joint with swelling and tenderness to pressure, and also arthritis of the right knee joint with slight swelling. Leni had a few **petechiae** and many palpable **purpura efflorescences** in the area of the feet and legs. Notable were severe swellings in the area of the dorsum of the foot and distal lower legs (◻ Fig. 11.1a, b). The rest of the examination findings were unremarkable.

11.3 Laboratory Values and Apparative Diagnostics

11.3.1 Laboratory Values

▪▪ Sophie

The inflammation parameters were slightly elevated (**ESR 31 mm/h, CRP 0.64 mg/l** [normal value < 0.5]). The blood count was normal. The Borrelia serology was negative.

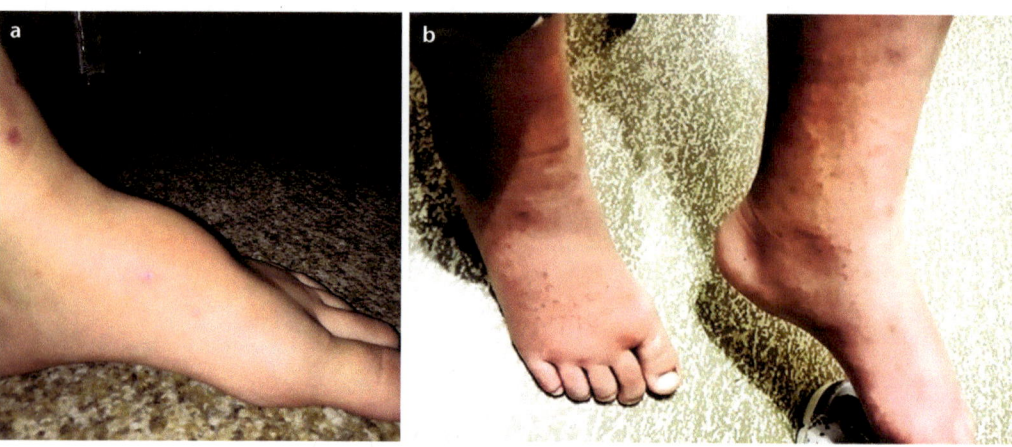

◻ **Fig. 11.1**   **a, b** Leni, 12 years old: Clinical findings of the skin. Swelling of the dorsum of the foot and the distal lower legs as well as some petechiae and purpura efflorescences

Complement C3 was slightly elevated (143 mg/dl [normal value 80–120]), C4 within the normal range. Immunoglobulin G (IgG) was elevated (**IgG 2390 mg/dl** [normal value 690–1600]), IgA and IgM within the normal range. The thyroid values TSH, T3, T4 were within the reference range. Thyroid peroxidase antibodies (TPO antibodies) were negative, **thyroglobulin antibodies** elevated (**249 U/ml** [normal value up to 100]). The findings suggested Hashimoto's thyroiditis. The antinuclear antibodies (ANA) and antibodies against double-stranded DNA (Anti-dsDNA-AB) were elevated (**ANA speckled > 1:10240** [normal value <1:80], **Anti-dsDNA-AB in immunofluorescence 1:320** [normal value <1:10], **Anti-dsDNA-AB in ELISA 325 IU/ml** [normal value <30], **Anti-dsDNA-AB in RIA 138 IU/ml** [normal value <7]). The **rheumatoid factor** was elevated (30 U/ml [normal value 0–14]).

▪▪ Leni

The erythrocyte sedimentation rate was elevated (**ESR 28 mm/h**), the CRP was negative. The blood count showed leukopenia and lymphopenia (**leukocytes 3870/μl** [normal value 4500–14,500], **lymphocytes 1110/μl** [normal value 1200–6500]) as well as a slight normochromic, normocytic anemia (**Hb 11.1 g/dl** [normal value 11.5–15.5]). The **direct Coombs test was positive**. Reticulocytes, haptoglobin, indirect bilirubin, and LDH were within the normal range, thus there was no indication of hemolysis. There was a **complement**reduction (**C3 24 mg/dl** [normal value 80–120], **C4 < 2 mg/dl** [normal value 10–34]). The overview values of coagulation were normal (PTT, Quick, fibrinogen). When determining the **antiphospholipid antibodies** a slight increase of anti-β2-glycoprotein-1-antibody-IgG (35.8 U/ml [normal value < 20]) was found, anti-β2-glycoprotein-1-antibody-IgM, lupus anticoagulant and anti-cardiolipin antibodies were not elevated. The urine examination showed an unremarkable particle count

and a normal total protein/creatinine ratio. The thyroid values and thyroid antibodies were within the normal range. The ANAs and Anti-dsDNA-AB were highly elevated (**ANA homogenous/speckled > 1:10240** [normal value <1:80], **Anti-dsDNA-AB in immunofluorescence ≥ 1:2560** [normal value <1:10], **Anti-dsDNA-AB in ELISA 911 IU/ml** [normal value <30], **Anti-dsDNA-AB in RIA 296 IU/ml** [normal value <7]). ENA and ANCA were not detectable.

11.3.2 Apparative Diagnostics

▪▪ Sophie

The sonography of the right elbow joint showed an effusion. The sonography of the thyroid was normal. ECG - Electrocardiogram, echocardiography, a sonography of the abdomen, a lung function test, and an ophthalmological examination showed no abnormalities.

▪▪ Leni

Due to the swelling of the feet, a sonography of the leg veins was performed, there was no indication of a thrombosis. Sonographically, a small effusion was seen in the right knee joint, no effusion in the left knee joint and in the ankle joints.

ECG and echocardiography, a sonography of the abdomen and the thyroid were normal. Also, a lung function test, chest X-ray, and ophthalmological examination showed no pathological findings.

11.4 Educational Questions

1. What differential diagnoses are considered for Sophie based on the anamnesis, examination, and laboratory findings?
2. What differential diagnoses should be considered for Leni based on the petechiae and purpura as well as arthralgia/arthritis?

3. What diagnosis is to be made for Leni based on the examination findings, laboratory values, and instrumental diagnostics?
4. What therapy and further procedure is necessary for Leni?

11.5 Differential Diagnostic Considerations

■ ■ **Sophie**

In the case of arthritis, a differential diagnosis must consider a variety of diseases such as septic arthritis, malignant diseases, reactive arthritis, juvenile idiopathic arthritis/rheumatoid arthritis, but also collagenoses such as systemic lupus erythematosus. For Sophie, the presence of rheumatoid arthritis was also considered. However, the high ANA titer and the detection of anti-dsDNA-AB suggested systemic lupus erythematosus (SLE). The ACR/EULAR classification criteria for SLE were not met. Although the ANA titer was positive as an entry criterion, as required, no clinical criterion was present. For the clinical criterion "joint involvement", the presence of arthritis in at least 2 joints is necessary. The patient only had 6 of the required 10 points (6 points for detection of anti-dsDNA-AB) (Aringer et al. 2019). Often, patients with SLE develop further organ manifestations over time, so that then a classification of the patient's disease based on classification systems may possibly succeed more precisely in terms of the diagnosis, ultimately the diagnosis can be made more clearly.

■ ■ **Leni**

In the case of petechiae and purpura as well as arthralgia/arthritis, various differential diagnoses must be considered. Petechiae and Purpura can be caused by thrombocytopenia, but also by a **vasculitis** in the broadest sense. The blood count showed no thrombocytopenia, so a vasculitis of the small vessels was to be assumed, especially because the purpura was palpable. There are a variety of vasculitides in childhood. According to the EULAR/PReS classification criteria for vasculitides in childhood, vasculitides are primarily distinguished into large vessel vasculitides, medium vessel vasculitides, small vessel vasculitides, and other vasculitides (Ozen et al. 2006). The last group includes secondary vasculitides caused by infections, malignant diseases, medications, and vasculitides in the context of collagenoses. Various vasculitides also cause arthralgia and arthritis. In the case of suspected vasculitis, a comprehensive investigation must be carried out.

This requires extensive organ diagnostics, but also immunological diagnostics with determination of antinuclear antibodies (ANA), antibodies against extractable nuclear antigens (ENA), antibodies against double-strand DNA (anti-dsDNA-AB) and antineutrophil cytoplasmic antibodies (ANCA). In unclear cases, a skin biopsy is also indicated. In Leni, there was no indication of an infectious disease or malignant disease. She also had not taken any medications. In the case of a palpable vasculitis, one should primarily think of a purpura according to Schönlein-Henoch. However, in the girl, not only the skin efflorescences (petechiae/palpable purpura) and the arthritis, but also the leukopenia, lymphopenia, the complement reduction and above all the high ANA titer along with detection of anti-dsDNA-AB already suggested SLE at the first presentation. The ACR/EULAR classification criteria for SLE were met (ANA positive as entry, presence of 2 clinical criteria, presence of 19 of the required 10 points). The diagnosis of SLE could thus be made with good rationale. The activity determination resulted in a SLEDAI-2K index value of 17.

11.6 Further Course

▪▪ Sophie

Initially, the joint pain was only intermittently present, and the family did not want therapy. After 3 months, there was a deterioration, the patient had persistent arthritis of the right elbow joint and recurrent arthralgia of the left elbow joint. We decided on a therapy with **MTX,** bridged with **Naproxen** and a low-dose **glucocorticoid therapy**. In the course of time, Sophie was symptom-free. 6 months after the start of therapy, the patient developed **leukopenia** and severe **lymphopenia** (leukocytes 3670/µl [normal value 4500–13,000], lymphocytes **280/µl** [normal value 1200–6500]) as well as **diffuse alopecia**. During a summer vacation, the patient showed pronounced redness on the trunk after a short stay in the **sun,** despite applying high sun protection factor cream, a large-scale infiltrated erythema with fine whitish scaling and some post-inflammatory hyperpigmentation on the chest and abdomen (◘ Fig. 11.2). The findings were consistent with an **acute cutaneous SLE.** Now the ACR/EULAR classification

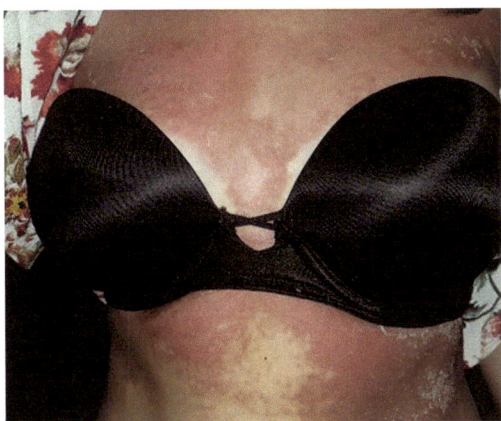

◘ **Fig. 11.2** Sophie, 16 years old, with skin rash after sunbathing: After sun exposure, large-scale infiltrated erythema and whitish scaling and some post-inflammatory hyperpigmentation

criteria for SLE were met (ANA positive as entry, presence of 3 clinical criteria from 2 domains (leukopenia, alopecia, acute cutaneous SLE), presence of 15 of the required 10 points). The SLEDAI-2K index was 7. A short-term low-dose glucocorticoid therapy and a therapy extension with **hydroxychloroquine** and **Vitamin D** were initiated. It was again pointed out that sun exposure can lead to a recurrence of SLE and should therefore be avoided.

The skin manifestations completely regressed, the hair loss improved. The blood count still showed a slight leukopenia and lymphopenia. One year after diagnosis, Sophie is largely symptom-free, the SLEDAI-2K index is currently at 3.

▪▪ Leni

After Leni was diagnosed with SLE, a therapy with **hydroxychloroquine, low-dose glucocorticoids** and **Vitamin D** was started. Due to the assessment of a moderate severity of the disease, it was decided to also start a csDMARD therapy ("conventional synthetic disease modifying antirheumatic drugs"). The goal was to save the use of glucocorticoids. Due to the arthralgia/arthritis and vasculitis, a therapy with **MTX** was chosen. In the course of time, there was a rapid improvement of the joint complaints, petechiae and purpura did not occur anymore. The oral prednisolone therapy was ended after 8 weeks. Notably and quite expectedly, there was still a complement reduction in the sense of a subclinical activity of the SLE. Therefore, close follow-up checks were carried out. 8 months after diagnosis, a slight **erythrocyturia** and **proteinuria** were noticed for the first time (spontaneous urine: erythrocytes 63/µl [normal value < 25], total protein/creatinine ratio 462 mg/g creatinine [normal value < 100]). Within a few weeks, there was an increase in proteinuria and albuminuria (24-hour collected urine: total protein/day 862 mg/day [normal value < 150], albumin/day 566 mg/dl [normal value < 30]). Under the suspicion of nephritis, the indication for kidney biopsy was made. Just before the planned kidney biopsy, there was a clinical and laboratory deterioration. Leni developed purpura on her legs again. The proteinuria and erythrocyturia increased (spontaneous urine: total protein/creatinine ratio 1154 mg/g creatinine [normal value up to 100], erythrocytes 1800/μl [normal value up to 25], acanthocytes 35% [normal value 0]), the kidney retention parameters increased (**creatinine 0.94 mg/dl** [norm 0–0.68], urea 54 mg/dl [normal value 10–50]). Sonographically, the kidneys appeared slightly enlarged on both sides with increased echogenicity. The therapy with MTX was ended. The histological examination of the kidney biopsy showed a **membranoproliferative glomerulonephritis** of the SLE-associated **immune complex type** with small focal, partly scarred, partly florid extracapillary component (**lupus nephritis IV-A**) (Fig. 11.3). Even during the stationary

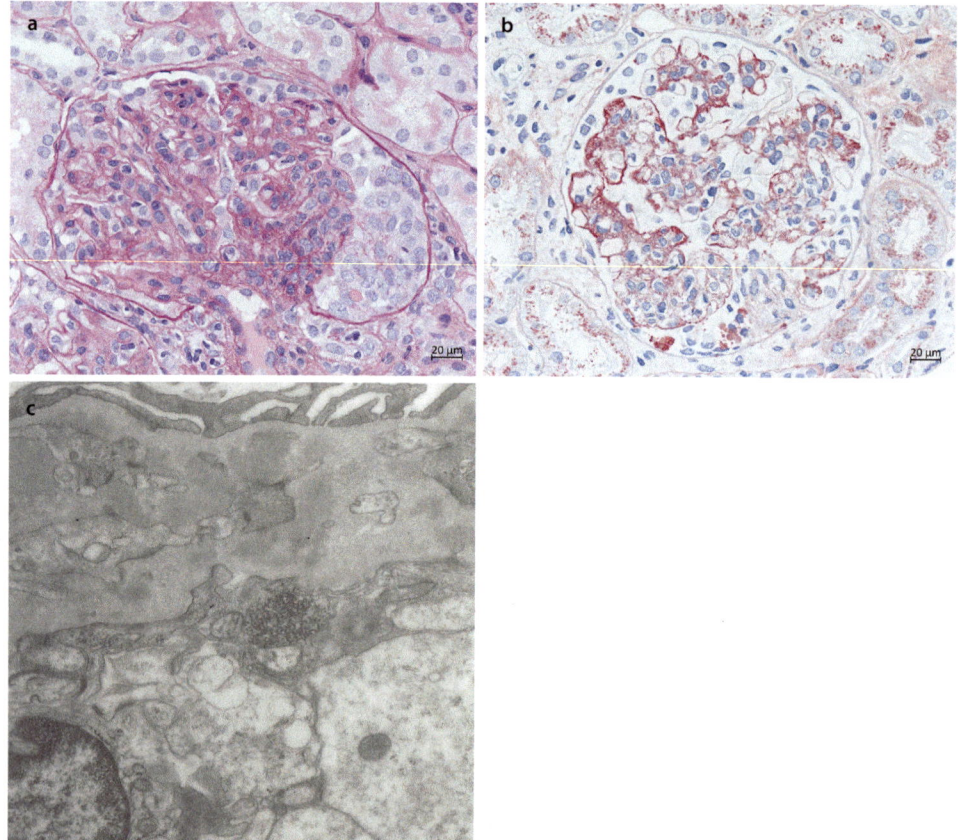

□ **Fig. 11.3   a–c** Leni, 12 years: Diffuse proliferative lupus glomerulonephritis (IV). **a** Light microscopy: Glomerulus with segmental cellular capsule proliferation (crescent), cell-increased mesangium, capillaries with partly double-contoured capillary walls with interposed cells and with increased mononuclear cells and few granulocytes. **b** Immunohistology: Pronounced granular deposits of IgG in the mesangium and on the peripheral glomerular capillary walls. **c** Electron microscopy: Electron-dense material (immune deposits) in the mesangium and subendothelial. (With kind permission of Prof. Dr. med. Thorsten Wiech, ► Institute for Pathology, University Medical Center Hamburg-Eppendorf)

stay for kidney biopsy, the patient developed the full picture of a **nephrotic syndrome** as well as temporary renal insufficiency (Proteinuria 5093 g/day, Albuminuria 3722 g/day, Serum albumin 2.4 g/dl [normal value 3.5–5.5], GFR according to Schwartz of 40 ml/min/1.73 m^2 [normal value > 80ml/min/1.73 m^2], Creatinine 1.58 g/dl [normal value 0–0.68], Cystatin C 2.7 mg/l [normal 0.61–0.95]). The SLEDAI-2K index was 21. A **methylprednisolone pulse therapy** (20 mg/kg body weight/day) was carried out over 4 days, followed by an **oral therapy with prednisolone** (1 mg/kg body weight/day). After the methylprednisolone pulse therapy, a therapy with **cyclophosphamide i.v.** (750 mg/m^2 BSA) was carried out with a total of 3 doses at intervals of 4 weeks each. During the therapy with cyclophosphamide, ovarian protection was carried out with a GnRH analog (Enantone s.c.), a *Pneumocystis jirovecii* prophylaxis with cotrimoxazole, and thrombosis prophylaxis with low molecular weight heparin (Clexane s.c.). The blood pressure values were always within the age-appropriate normal range. In addition, a nephroprotective treatment with the ACE inhibitor Ramipril was carried out. Over time, the protein ratios in the urine and serum normalized, the renal retention parameters decreased, and the complement factors C4 and C3 increased to the lower normal range. 4 weeks after the third cyclophosphamide pulse, a remission maintenance with **mycophenolate mofetil (MMF)** (1100 mg/m^2 BSA/day) was initiated. The therapy with prednisolone was reduced over the next months. 12 months after the diagnosis of SLE nephritis IV-A, Leni is symptom-free under a therapy with MMF, hydroxychloroquine, Ramipril, and low-dose prednisolone therapy (5 mg/day). The urine examination, blood count, laboratory values, ESR are inconspicuous. There is no longer any complement reduction. The ANA titer has dropped (ANA homogen/speckled 1:5120), anti-dsDNA antibodies are no longer detectable. The SLEDAI-2K index is at 0. A discontinuation of the prednisolone therapy is planned.

11.7 Educational Answers

- **1. What differential diagnoses should be considered for Sophie based on her medical history, examination, and laboratory findings?**

The most important differential diagnoses for Sophie are rheumatoid arthritis and systemic lupus erythematosus. The high ANA titer and the detection of anti-dsDNA-AB most likely suggest SLE.

- **2. What differential diagnoses should be considered for Leni based on the petechiae and purpura as well as arthralgia/arthritis?**

In the case of petechiae/purpura and arthralgia/arthritis, primary vasculitides, but also secondary vasculitides in the context of infections, malignancies, and collagen diseases should be considered.

- **3. What diagnosis should be made for Leni based on the examination findings, laboratory values, and instrumental diagnostics?**

For Leni, the diagnosis of SLE was made based on the clinical picture with petechiae/purpura and arthritis as well as the laboratory findings (leukopenia, lymphopenia, complement reduction, detection of ANA and anti-dsDNA-AB).

- **4. What therapy and further action is necessary for Leni?**

Therapy with hydroxychloroquine and glucocorticoids should be started. Due to the assessment of a moderate severity of the disease, the use of a csDMARD such as MTX or mycophenolate mofetil is also advisable. Regular follow-up checks are important to detect further organ involvement, especially kidney involvement, in a timely manner.

11.8 Summary

11.8.1 Definition

SLE is a chronically inflammatory systemic autoimmune disease that occurs in flares. The phenotype, course, and prognosis are **very variable** and differ between patients, genders, ethnicities, and age groups (Aringer et al. 2019).

11.8.2 Pathogenesis

The pathogenesis of SLE is not yet fully understood. In addition to a genetic predisposition, environmental influences, hormonal and epigenetic factors contribute to the development of the disease. It is assumed that a disturbed clearance of cell components, especially nuclear components and/or "Neutrophil extracellular traps" (NETs, essentially these are DNA-containing nets) are crucially involved in the development of SLE. The release of cell components ultimately leads to a pathological activation of autoreactive B cells, differentiation into plasma cells, production of pathogenic autoantibodies, formation of immune complexes, which in turn activate dendritic cells to produce **Interferon-α**. Interferon-α is particularly elevated in patients with SLE, especially during flares, and contributes significantly to the dysregulation of the immune system. Disturbances in T-cell functions lead to a loss of tolerance to autoantigens. Especially in early childhood, mutations in Type-I-Interferon(T1IFN)-associated genes play a role in a monogenetically inherited variant of SLE. Particularly in phagocytically active cells, the demon-

stration of an activated interferon signature is successful—it describes the activation of these signaling pathways involving several involved genes (Alexander and Hedrich 2022; Trindade et al. 2021).

11.8.3 Clinic

Most children with SLE have **general symptoms** such as loss of appetite, weight loss, fatigue, fever at the onset of the disease. In addition, there are general signs of immune system activation such as lymphadenopathy and hepatosplenomegaly. SLE can start in one organ, but ultimately manifests as a multisystem disease. The most commonly affected in children in the first year after diagnosis are the skin (60–80%), musculoskeletal system (arthritis 60-88%) and kidney (nephritis 20-80%) (Klein-Gitelmann and Lane 2016).

▪▪ Skin and Mucosal Manifestations
There are different skin manifestations. These include the classic butterfly erythema, photosensitive rashes, discoid lupus, lupus tumidus, bullous lupus, Raynaud's phenomenon, Perniones, subungual erythema with abnormalities in the nail fold microscopy, Livedo reticularis, thrombocytopenic or **vasculitic petechiae and purpura**, urticaria, alopecia (Klein-Gitelmann and Lane 2016).

▪▪ Musculoskeletal Symptoms
Children with SLE often have **arthralgia** and **myalgia.** Often there are **arthritides** of the finger joints, but also of other peripheral joints. Myositis is also observed less frequently (Klein-Gitelmann and Lane 2016).

▪▪ Nephritis
Kidney involvement plays a crucial role in morbidity and mortality. Findings in **lupus nephritis** can be: isolated asymptomatic hematuria and/or proteinuria, an acute

nephritic syndrome with hematuria usually also arterial hypertension and proteinuria or a nephrotic syndrome with proteinuria, hypoalbuminemia, hyperlipidemia and edema. If there is evidence of lupus nephritis, a kidney biopsy is usually necessary, exceptions would be e.g.: only one kidney is present or there is a renal vein thrombosis or a coagulation pathology exists as a contraindication. Histologically, lupus nephritis is divided into 6 types according to the WHO. The classification is based on light microscopic, electron microscopic and immunofluorescence findings. Particularly WHO class IV nephritis, as in our patient, can be associated with increased morbidity and mortality (Klein-Gitelmann and Lane 2016).

11.8.4 Diagnosis

The diagnosis is made based on clinical and immunological criteria. In the majority of children and adolescents with SLE, increased antinuclear antibodies (ANA) and antibodies against double-stranded DNA (anti-dsDNA-AB) are found. Anti-dsDNA-AB are also suitable for monitoring the disease. There are 3 classification criteria for SLE that are used in clinical practice, research and clinical studies: The **ACR classification criteria,** which were modified in **1997** (1997-ACR), the **SLICC classification criteria of 2012** (2012-SLICC) and the **ACR/EULAR classification criteria of 2019** (2019-EULAR/ACR) (Hochberg 1997; Petri et al. 2012; Aringer et al. 2019).

The criteria have also been evaluated for childhood in various studies. The criteria all have good sensitivity and specificity. One study showed the same sensitivity for the 2019-EULAR/ACR criteria as for the 2012-SLICC criteria (97.4%) and a higher sensitivity compared to the 1997-ACR criteria (87.2%) as well as a similar specificity for the 2019-EULAR/ACR criteria and

the 2012-SLICC criteria (99.7% and 98.4%) (Ma et al. 2020). It is recommended to regularly determine the disease activity in a standardized way with the **Lupus erythematosus Disease Activity Index 2000 (SLEDAI 2K)** or the pediatric **BILAG**-Index 2004 (pBILAG-2004) (Groot et al. 2017a). Also, subsequent damage should be recorded in a standardized way with the **Systemic Lupus International Collaborating Clinics/American College of Rheumatology Damage Index (SDI) for children** (Gutierrez-Suarez et al. 2006).

11.8.5 Therapy

For the diagnosis and treatment of children with SLE, there are European evidence-based recommendations (SHARE initiative) (Groot et al. 2017a). Based on the good evidence in adults, all children with SLE are recommended to be treated with **Hydroxychloroquine**. In adults with SLE, higher remission rates, fewer relapses, and less organ damage were demonstrated under therapy with Hydroxychloroquine. **Glucocorticoids** are often necessary to achieve rapid disease control, but their use should be limited in time and dose. If a dose reduction of glucocorticoids is not possible under therapy with Hydroxychloroquine and glucocorticoids, the therapy should be extended by a DMARD. DMARDs that are often used are **Azathioprine, MMF and MTX**, in severe cases **Cyclophosphamide** (Groot et al. 2017a). In practice, a DMARD is initially used in more severe diseases when it seems unlikely that therapy with Hydroxychloroquine and glucocorticoids will be sufficient. This is also recommended in the 2019 revised EULAR recommendations for adult SLE (Fanouriakis et al. 2019).

For the individual organ involvements, there are special recommendations (Groot et al. 2017a; Fanouriakis et al. 2019). In patients with refractory disease, **Belimumab** or

Rituximab is used. Belimumab is the only biologic approved for the treatment of juvenile SLE in Germany. It is a monoclonal antibody against the B-lymphocyte stimulator (BLyS). Belimumab is approved for children from 5 years of age with active SLE (without severe kidney involvement) who have a high disease burden despite standard therapy. For the diagnosis and treatment of children with lupus nephritis, there are also European evidence-based recommendations (SHARE initiative). For lupus nephritis WHO class III and IV, a therapy with **Cyclophosphamide or MMF and intravenously applied glucocorticoids** as induction therapy and **MMF or Azathioprine** as remission-maintaining therapy for 3 years is recommended (Groot et al. 2017b). Studies are underway on further therapeutic approaches such as further anti-B-cell therapies and anti-interferon therapies (Trindade et al. 2021).

It is also important to lead a healthy lifestyle, avoid **sunlight**exposure that triggers disease flares, apply high sun protection factor and carry out all recommended **vaccinations**, as the risk for infections is generally increased. Usually, as an immunomodulatory and especially osteoprotective therapy, a **Vitamin-D-substitution** is carried out (Fanouriakis et al. 2019).

11.8.6 Prognosis

The 5-year survival rate has significantly improved through treatment. Children and adolescents with SLE have a higher disease activity than adults with SLE and it is assumed that they have more disease damage than adults (Alexander and Hedrich 2022).

> **Conclusion**
>
> SLE is very variable. Even with petechiae/purpura or arthritis, which are relatively common in childhood for various reasons, SLE must be considered in the differential diagnosis.

References

Alexander T, Hedrich CM (2022) Systemic lupus erythematosus – are children small adults? Z Rheumatol 81(1):28–35. ▶ https://doi.org/10.1007/s00393-021-01116-x

Aringer M, Costenbader K, Daikh D, Brinks R, Mosca M, Ramsey-Goldman R, Smolen JS, Wofsy D, Boumpas DT, Kamen DL, Jayne D, Cervera R, Costedoat-Chalumeau N, Diamond B, Gladman DD, Hahn B, Hiepe F, Jacobsen S, Khanna D, Lerstrom K, Massarotti E, McCune J, Ruiz-Irastorza G, Sanchez-Guerrero J, Schneider M, Urowitz M, Bertsias G, Hoyer BF, Leuchten N, Tani C, Tedeschi SK, Touma Z, Schmajuk G, Anic B, Assan F, Chan TM, Clarke AE, Crow MK, Czirjak L, Doria A, Graninger W, Halda-Kiss B, Hasni S, Izmirly PM, Jung M, Kumanovics G, Mariette X, Padjen I, Pego-Reigosa JM, Romero-Diaz J, Rua-Figueroa Fernandez I, Seror R, Stummvoll GH, Tanaka Y, Tektonidou MG, Vasconcelos C, Vital EM, Wallace DJ, Yavuz S, Meroni PL, Fritzler MJ, Naden R, Dorner T, Johnson SR (2019) 2019 European League Against Rheumatism/American College of Rheumatology classification criteria for systemic lupus erythematosus. Ann Rheum Dis 78(9):1151–1159. ▶ https://doi.org/10.1136/annrheumdis-2018-214819

Fanouriakis A, Kostopoulou M, Alunno A, Aringer M, Bajema I, Boletis JN, Cervera R, Doria A, Gordon C, Govoni M, Houssiau F, Jayne D, Kouloumas M, Kuhn A, Larsen JL, Lerstrom K, Moroni G, Mosca M, Schneider M, Smolen JS, Svenungsson E, Tesar V, Tincani A, Troldborg A, van Vollenhoven R, Wenzel J, Bertsias G, Boumpas DT (2019) 2019 update of the EULAR recommendations for the management of systemic lupus erythematosus. Ann Rheum Dis 78(6):736–745. ▶ https://doi.org/10.1136/annrheumdis-2019-215089

Groot N, de Graeff N, Avcin T, Bader-Meunier B, Brogan P, Dolezalova P, Feldman B, Kone-Paut I, Lahdenne P, Marks SD, McCann L, Ozen S, Pilkington C, Ravelli A, Royen-Kerkhof AV, Uziel Y, Vastert B, Wulffraat N, Kamphuis S, Beresford MW (2017a) European evidence-based recommendations for diagnosis and treatment of childhood-onset systemic lupus erythematosus: the SHARE initiative. Ann Rheum Dis 76(11):1788–1796. ▶ https://doi.org/10.1136/annrheumdis-2016-210960

Groot N, de Graeff N, Marks SD, Brogan P, Avcin T, Bader-Meunier B, Dolezalova P, Feldman BM, Kone-Paut I, Lahdenne P, McCann L, Ozen S, Pilkington CA, Ravelli A, Royen-Kerkhof AV, Uziel Y, Vastert BJ, Wulffraat NM, Beresford MW,

Kamphuis S (2017b) European evidence-based recommendations for the diagnosis and treatment of childhood-onset lupus nephritis: the SHARE initiative. Ann Rheum Dis 76(12):1965–1973. ▶ https://doi.org/10.1136/annrheumdis-2017-211898

Gutierrez-Suarez R, Ruperto N, Gastaldi R, Pistorio A, Felici E, Burgos-Vargas R, Martini A, Ravelli A (2006) A proposal for a pediatric version of the Systemic Lupus International Collaborating Clinics/American College of Rheumatology Damage Index based on the analysis of 1015 patients with juvenile-onset systemic lupus erythematosus. Arthritis Rheum 54(9):2989–2996. ▶ https://doi.org/10.1002/art.22048

Hochberg MC (1997) Updating the American College of Rheumatology revised criteria for the classification of systemic lupus erythematosus. Arthritis Rheum 40(9):1725. ▶ https://doi.org/10.1002/art.1780400928

Klein-Gitelmann M, Lane JC (2016) Systemic lupus erythematosus. In: Petty RE (Ed) Textbook of pediatric rheumatology, 7. edn. Elsevier, Philadelphia, pp 285–317

Ma M, Hui-Yuen JS, Cerise JE, Iqbal S, Eberhard BA (2020) Validation of the 2019 European League Against Rheumatism/American College of Rheumatology Criteria compared to the 1997 American College of Rheumatology Criteria and the 2012 Systemic Lupus International Collaborating Clinics Criteria in pediatric systemic lupus erythematosus.

Arthritis Care Res (Hoboken) 72(11):1597–1601. ▶ https://doi.org/10.1002/acr.24057

Ozen S, Ruperto N, Dillon MJ, Bagga A, Barron K, Davin JC, Kawasaki T, Lindsley C, Petty RE, Prieur AM, Ravelli A, Woo P (2006) EULAR/PReS endorsed consensus criteria for the classification of childhood vasculitides. Ann Rheum Dis 65(7):936–941. ▶ https://doi.org/10.1136/ard.2005.046300

Petri M, Orbai AM, Alarcon GS, Gordon C, Merrill JT, Fortin PR, Bruce IN, Isenberg D, Wallace DJ, Nived O, Sturfelt G, Ramsey-Goldman R, Bae SC, Hanly JG, Sanchez-Guerrero J, Clarke A, Aranow C, Manzi S, Urowitz M, Gladman D, Kalunian K, Costner M, Werth VP, Zoma A, Bernatsky S, Ruiz-Irastorza G, Khamashta MA, Jacobsen S, Buyon JP, Maddison P, Dooley MA, van Vollenhoven RF, Ginzler E, Stoll T, Peschken C, Jorizzo JL, Callen JP, Lim SS, Fessler BJ, Inanc M, Kamen DL, Rahman A, Steinsson K, Franks AG Jr, Sigler L, Hameed S, Fang H, Pham N, Brey R, Weisman MH, McGwin G Jr, Magder LS (2012) Derivation and validation of the Systemic Lupus International Collaborating Clinics classification criteria for systemic lupus erythematosus. Arthritis Rheum 64(8):2677–2686. ▶ https://doi.org/10.1002/art.34473

Trindade VC, Carneiro-Sampaio M, Bonfa E, Silva CA (2021) An update on the management of childhood-onset systemic lupus erythematosus. Paediatr Drugs 23(4):331–347. ▶ https://doi.org/10.1007/s40272-021-00457-z

When the Skin Just Won't Heal

Hermann Girschick

Contents

12.1 Medical History

The 5 $^1/_2$-year-old Luzie developed an **Oligoarthritis** of the left knee, left wrist, and left ankle after an inconspicuous infancy and toddler period, which improved to symptom-free within a few weeks under anti-inflammatory medication with Ibuprofen. At the same time, a variably pronounced MRSA-related **Impetigo** with partial blistering of the skin occurred. The histology of a bullous ulcerating lesion initially gave no direct indication of the presence of vasculitis. Rheumatological diagnostics at this time revealed a positive low antinuclear antibody titer of 1:200. Antibodies against native DNA were not detectable. Perinuclear antibodies against granulocytes (p-ANCA) were present in low concentrations, c-ANCA were absent.

At the age of 6 $^1/_2$ years, the arthritis flared up as a **polyarthritic** picture with symmetrical involvement of the metacarpophalangeal joints I to IV, furthermore the proximal interphalangeal joints III and IV on both sides as well as the left knee. A low-dose oral glucocorticoid use (Prednisolone 10 mg in the morning) in combination with continuous Ibuprofen administration improved the findings again to remission. The impetigo lesions remained a clinical problem. Domestic hygiene deficiencies were evident, eradication measures were not successful.

In her Seventh year of life, the patient developed a severe **Acute Respiratory Distress Syndrome** (ARDS) in the context of pneumonia. In addition, there was a hemorrhagic pulmonary edema, a pericardial effusion, and a transfusion-dependent Anemia (◘ Fig. 12.1).

12.2 Examination Findings

The girl had a high fever of 40 °C, showed significant respiratory distress and bronchial obstruction. The circulatory conditions were centralized, there was respiratory insufficiency.

Simultaneously with the severe **ARDS/Pneumonia**, the **Polyarthritis** on the left knee and left wrist was reactivated, also the PIP joints of the middle fingers on both sides and the base joint of the index finger on the right were affected. The patient

12

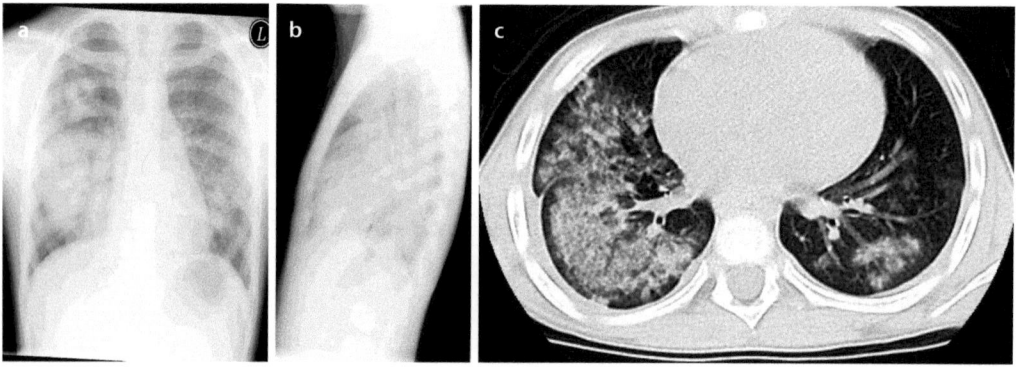

◘ **Fig. 12.1** **a–c** Conventional chest X-ray p.a. (**a**) and lateral (**b**), furthermore computed tomography of the thorax (**c**) in the context of severe pneumonia/ARDS in the Seventh year of life. **a,b** Initial X-rays in severe intensive care pneumonia with hemorrhagic pulmonary edema, respiratory insufficiency, pericarditis, and transfusion-dependent anemia. **c** In the computed tomogram, the coarse infiltrates are impressive. (With kind permission from Prof. Dr. J. Wagner, Institute for Radiology and Interventional Therapy, Vivantes Klinikum im Friedrichshain, Berlin)

had to be mechanically ventilated for several weeks. The clinical examination still focused on the **Impetigo**. In the armpit area, an erythema consistent with an **Erythema exsudativum multiforme** was visible, in the finger area there were papular changes without ulcers (◘ Fig. 12.2). Medially on the thigh, a deep **skin ulcer** of unclear origin could be documented. A histological confirmation from this ulcer (◘ Fig. 12.2a) revealed a **vasculitis of the small arterial vessels and arterioles**.

12.3 Labor Values and Imaging

12.3.1 Laboratory Values

The blood count showed a normal leukocyte count and differentiation, further-more a microcytic-hypochromic (MCV 72 fl, MCH 23 pg) anemia (Hb 9.6 g/dl). There was a thrombocytosis of 641,000/µl. The CRP was initially moderately elevated (13.4 mg/l), but it rose to a maximum value of 102 mg/l. The erythrocyte sedimentation rate was massively accelerated. Extensive microbial diagnostic procedures such as blood culture, wound swabs, bronchoalveolar lavage, urine culture, gastric juice analysis, provocation sputum did not detect any pathogens, including a multiplex PCR for bacterial pathogens in the bronchoalveolar lavage. Serological examinations regarding Legionella or *Coxiella-burnetii* infections (Q fever) were inconspicuous. An intracutaneous tuberculin skin test was inconspicuous. The girl had previously had an EBV virus infection. A multimodal antibiotic therapy with vancomycin, imipenem, clarithromycin, subsequently ciprofloxacin,

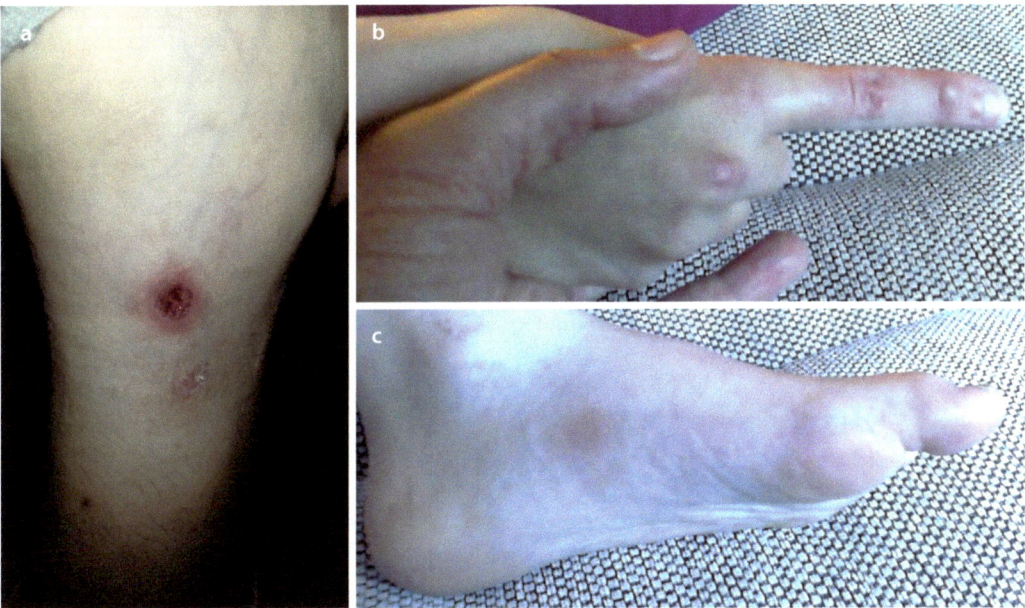

◘ **Fig. 12.2 a–c** Skin findings at 7.5 years: Vasculitis, acral papules, ulcers, and acrocyanosis. **a, b** show a persistent, non-healing ulcer, in which MRSA pathogens were repeatedly detected, but which histologically showed signs of vasculitis. At the same time, Luzie also developed peripheral firm papules on the fingers and hands, which were identified as "Gottron's papules". **c** On the feet and lower legs, there was acrocyanosis from autumn to spring, individual blisters on the toes occurred and healed ulcerating with scar formation cotrimoxazole, caspofungin was carried out calculatedly.

Peripheral IgG, IgA, IgM were each within the normal range. A moderate reduction of the Quick value to 59% with a slight increase in D-dimers and inconspicuous overview values was interpreted as moderate coagulation activation. Autoimmunologically, the **antinuclear antibody titer had risen to 1:640** and for the first time **antibodies against free double-stranded DNA** could be detected at a low concentration of 43 U/ml (< 20). However, DNA-AB were not detectable in the Crithidia assay. An ENA screening was inconspicuous. Again, a positive p-ANCA-AB (c-ANCA-negative) was found, antiphospholipid-AB (cardiolipin, lupus anticoagulant, β2-glycoprotein-1-AB) were not detectable. A moderate complement reduction C3 with inconspicuous C4 was detected. Rheumatoid factors-IgM were not detectable.

12.3.2 Imaging

12

Conventional radiology showed a **severe pneumonia** with coarse infiltrates and the development of a "white lung", consistent with ARDS (◘ Fig. 12.1). The computed tomography of the thorax showed infiltrative changes mainly in the area of the entire right lung with emphasis on the caudal subfields (◘ Fig. 12.1c). A **hemorrhagic pulmonary edema** component could also be clinically suspected with bloody bronchial secretions. Echocardiographically, a moderate pericardial effusion was shown, myocardial hypertrophy was described.

12.4 Educational Questions

1. What suspected diagnosis can be considered with recurring ulcerative skin lesions, a changing polyarthritis, positive ANA-AB?
2 Can a prioritization of possible differential diagnoses be carried out at this point in the course of ARDS?
3. Should the diagnosis of a macrophage activation syndrome be considered in the context of the intensive medical deterioration?
4. What acute therapeutic steps could be considered in addition to the previously used NSAID, low-dose glucocorticoids?

12.5 Differential Diagnostic Considerations

The patient had already undergone 2 years of a "rheumatological" medical history. Various arthritides, ulcerative skin changes, impetigo, and now a febrile event with pneumonia, ARDS, perimyocarditis, and anemia were described. The involvement of the skin is unusual for a classic childhood joint rheumatic disease from the area of juvenile idiopathic arthritis (JIA). Since the initial arthritides were not accompanied by fever attacks and general skin rashes, systemic JIA, Morbus Still, was not to be considered in the differential diagnosis. Rather, the positive antinuclear antibody titer and then the detection of antibodies against DNA seemed to be diagnostically significant. At the same time, there was a reduction in complement (C3) and repeated detection of antibodies against granulocytes (p-ANCA). This shifts the pathophysiological assessment in the direction of a general **autoimmune disease** from the area of lupus erythematosus with concurrent **vasculitis**. At the time of disease manifestation, the concepts of autoinflammatory diseases and especially in the area of interferonopathies were just emerging. No familial background for SLE was described in the family. Difficult social conditions and staphylococcal-associated **impetigo** had to be considered as additional pathogenesis factors. A "classic" fever syndrome-autoinflammatory disease seemed unlikely (TNF-α-, interleukin-1- or interleukin-6-associated).

Within the classification criteria of the American Rheumatism Association ARA (Perez-Gutthann et al. 1991), the following criteria could be described: arthritis, serositis, hematological symptoms, autoantibodies against native DNA, antinuclear antibodies, and ultimately also a cutaneous SLE. Oral mucosal lesions and aphthae were added later in the course.

Thus, 6 out of 11 criteria in the ARA classification of the patient's symptomatology were given as systemic lupus erythematosus (Perez-Gutthann et al. 1991).

Ultimately, in the case of an unclear autoimmune disease with recurrent cutaneous infections, an immune defect diagnosis, a **primary immune defect** (PID), is possible. This was ruled out in the patient by extensive immunocytological and chemical analysis of the peripheral blood including granulocyte function tests ("respiratory burst"). However, a C3 complement deficiency in the patient, which is most likely to be interpreted as secondary, still had to be considered in terms of a genetic predisposition. HIV serology was unremarkable in the differential diagnosis PID.

12.6 **Further Course Including Therapy**

After the suspected diagnosis of SLE with arthritic and pulmonary involvement, a systemic steroid therapy (prednisolone 10 mg/ kg body weight i.v. daily) was initiated. This led to a rapid improvement with fever reduction, reduction of ventilation and circulatory support. A basic therapy with mycophenolate mofetil (500 mg daily, corresponding to 25 mg/kg body weight/day) was started. An antibiotic prophylaxis with cotrimoxazole and aminopenicillin for pulmonary protection was initiated.

In the Ninth year of life, the acral papules (Gottron's papules) increased, also recurrent nail bed inflammations, a winter-associated **acrocyanosis and telangiectasias** in the finger area were added. At this time, the patient received NSAID, a low-dose glucocorticoid therapy with 5 mg prednisolone on 3 days per week and the continuation of the mycophenolate therapy. In the 9th year of life, 2 moderately occurring pneumonias were described, a concomitant bronchodilator-inhalation therapy was carried out. Intermittently, the patient's arthritis flared up as dactylitis of the middle finger.

For the first time at the age of 10 $^1/_2$, **skin lesions** were found on the anterior left elbow, then also on the olecranon, which were erosive and **ulcerative**. No infectious agents could be detected in the skin swab. At this time, the ANA-AB titer was 1:2560, p-ANCA-AB were still detectable, a complement deficiency no longer existed. Antiphospholipid-AB were negative. Hematological abnormalities no longer existed. At this time, it could not be ruled out that the patient was also inflicting self-injuries mechanically (◙ Fig. 12.3a–h). The skin lesions sometimes appeared as if artificially inflicted or caused by chronic rubbing. To assess this more accurately, a hospital admission was also made and an attempt at skin transplantation into the chronically non-healing wound on the anterior elbow (◙ Fig. 12.3c). Unfortunately, it could not be ruled out that the patient had mechanically removed the skin graft herself (◙ Fig. 12.3a, right picture).

Under the assumption that glucocorticoids delay wound healing, the immunosuppressive therapy was gradually reduced, which, however, led to a worsening of the skin lesions. Consequently, the mycophenolate therapy was increased to 2 times 500 mg/day in the Twelfth year of life, while continuing a daily low-dose prednisolone therapy (5 mg/day).

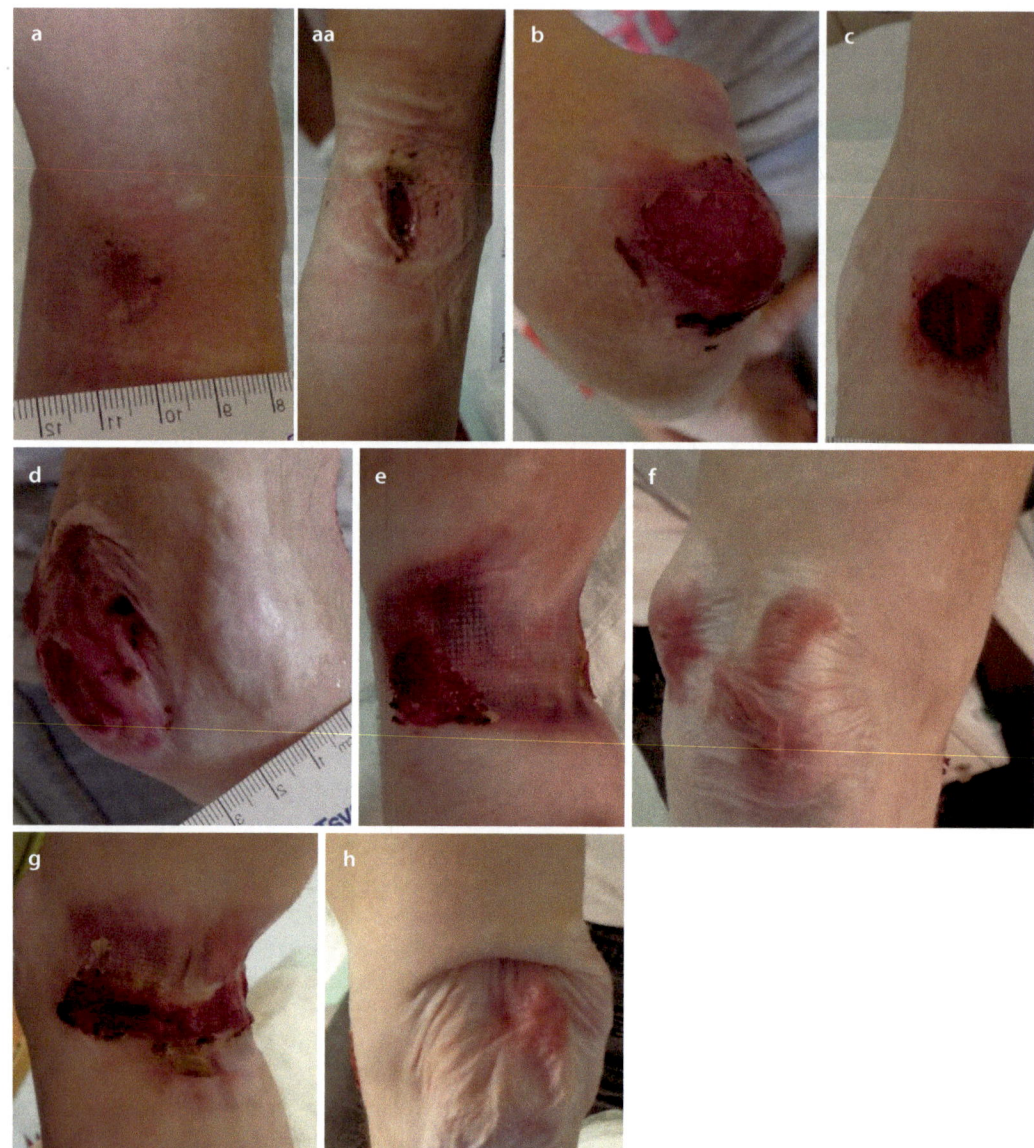

◘ **Fig. 12.3 a–d** Skin findings at 13 years on both elbows (right: **a–b**; left: **c–d**): chronic deep ulcers. **e–h** Findings at 16.5 years after 1.5 years of belimumab therapy (right: **e–f**; left: **g–h**). The images show the development of anterior and dorsal elbow ulcers. Although there was a tendency towards epithelialization, it repeatedly broke open ulceratively. A reduction of the immunosuppressive basic therapy with mycophenolate mofetil worsened the findings. In addition, mechanical-artificial alteration could not be ruled out (**a** right picture; at 13.5 years). Ultimately, the additional therapy with belimumab enabled healing (**e–h**)

Infection events, especially in the pulmonary area, also seemed to significantly worsen the skin findings clinically. At this time, an increase in antibodies against native DNA was measured immunologically (dsDNA-ELISA 180 international units/ml (< 100 normal);

Crithidia assay positive). Antibodies against ribonuclear proteins U1 were also detectable for the first time.

Despite the involvement of a multiple weekly nursing service, wound care was difficult because the bandage changes carried out always "tore" the wounds again. Accompaniment with a professional wound manager was continuously implemented. The intensification of immunosuppressive therapy ultimately seemed urgently necessary, even though the pulmonary pathology, the polyarthritis, the impetigo, the skin lesions outside the elbows no longer had any clinical relevance, respectively were inconspicuous. The start of cytotoxic medication with e.g. chemotherapy/cyclophosphamide did not seem opportune in the overall assessment.

Instead, the start of a costimulation blockade with **belimumab** was more appropriate. This was started at the age of 15 and, with continuous 4-weekly application, could contribute to increasing wound closure and partial healing of the lesions after another year (◘ Fig. 12.3). Clinically, no further manifestations of systemic lupus erythematosus have occurred. The patient's tendency to skin infections no longer existed. The arthritis was in remission. A lung function/body plethysmography has been able to document no respiratory restriction except for a seasonal obstruction as part of a sensitization to grasses and early bloomers.

12.7 Educational Answers

- **1. What suspected diagnosis can be considered for recurrent ulcerative skin lesions, a changing polyarthritis, positive ANA-AB?**

In the differential diagnosis of an ANA-positive polyarthritis in early childhood, juvenile idiopathic arthritis should be considered. Cutaneous skin ulcers and pro-

longed fever suggest a "more complex" autoimmune disease, systemic lupus erythematosus. However, the first manifestation in the 5th year of life is to be seen as very early and suggests the presence of a **genetic predisposition**.

- **2. Can a prioritization of possible differential diagnoses be carried out at this point in the context of ARDS?**

Due to the significant symptom expression, systemic lupus erythematosus with co-manifestation of cutaneous vasculitis and pulmonary vasculopathy was already prioritized in the context of severe ARDS/pneumonia, and consequently, a basic immunosuppressive therapy was started. A pulmonary infection event was to be considered, but was not diagnostically tangible.

- **3. Should the diagnosis of a macrophage activation syndrome be considered in the context of intensive medical deterioration?**

Since the girl had already serologically undergone an EBV virus infection, macrophage activation was to be considered in the context of systemic lupus, anemia, leukopenia, and fever. However, the ferritin level of 500 ng/ml, which was also determined as a marker for this disease, argued against the presence of a significantly severe macrophage activation syndrome (MAS).

- **4. What acute therapeutic steps could be considered in addition to the previously used NSAID, low-dose glucocorticoids?**

In the situation of a febrile pneumonia with ARDS and perimyocarditis, a moderate glucocorticoid pulse therapy was decided upon (10 mg/kg body weight/day), as well as the start of a basic immunosuppressive therapy with mycophenolate mofetil. The use of a cytotoxic therapy with cyclophosphamide did not seem justified. A selective cytokine blockade against interleukin-1 or TNF-α appeared contraindicated in the context of the prioritized basic diagnosis of SLE. The targeted influence of interferon signaling pathways was considered experimental at this point and not accessible for children and adolescents.

12.8 Summary

12.8.1 Etiology

For the classic systemic lupus erythematosus in childhood and adolescence, manifestation at 5 years of age is considered early. Therefore, a genetic predisposition had to be assumed for this patient. Just as tissue/structure disorders of the skin (◘ Fig. 12.3) increasingly manifested, the diagnostics were expanded again. An examination of peripheral monocytes with regard to interferon-stimulated genes (◘ Fig. 12.4) was interpreted as a moderately pronounced **interferon signature**.

A genetic fine typing on the one hand towards type-1 interferonopathies (Aicardi-Goutières syndrome I–VII; *TMEM173* gene), revealed no informative genetic change. A **whole-genome sequencing approach** with extended panel diagnostics towards interferonopathy and SLE could not confirm a genetically inherited complement deficiency. On the other hand, a molecular association with a mutation in the area of integrins, the **complement receptor 3b** (CD11 integrin beta; *ITGAM*-locus) could be demonstrated (Fagerholm et al. 2013; Järvinen et al. 2010) (Mutation detection *ITGAM* c.1141T>C; p.Tyr381His, heterozygosity). CD11 binds to iC3b, ICAM-1 and other ligands. This binding contributes to the phagocytosis of complement-opsonized particles, such as pathogens, immune complexes or apoptotic material. A disturbance of this process is associated with increased inflammation. Since this specific mutation of the patient in the complement receptor 3/*ITGAM*-locus/CD11 b had not been described before, its clinical

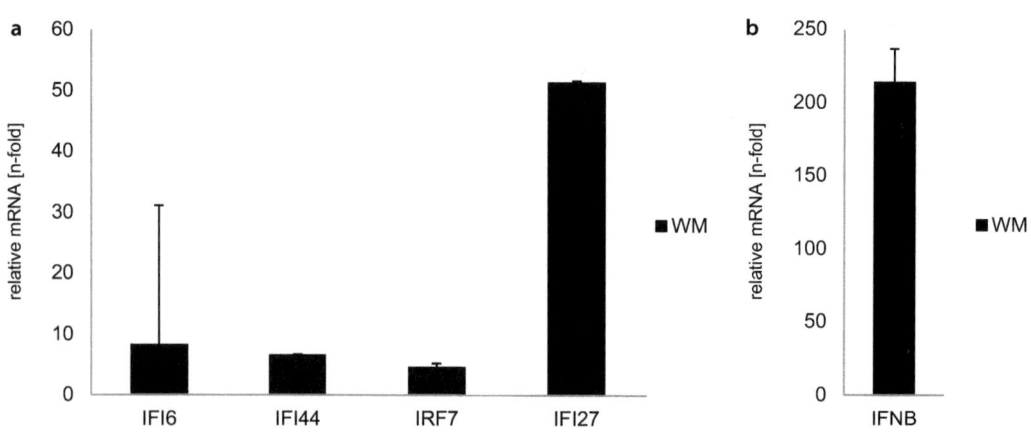

◘ **Fig. 12.4** **a, b Relative expression of interferon-stimulated genes and IFNB concentration in monocytes. a** Expression of interferon-stimulated genes *IFI6*, *IFI44*, *IRF7* and *IFI27* analyzed in peripheral blood monocytes and **b** of *IFNB*. The mRNA expression was normalized to the *GAPDH*-expression in the cells. Shown is the relative gene expression compared to the average of two wild-type controls *(WM)*. The gene expression was determined by quantitative RT-PCR, shown is the average of a triple experiment. Interpretation: **strong IFN signature.** (With kind permission from Prof. Dr. Min Ae Lee-Kirsch, Clinic for Pediatrics and Adolescent Medicine, Medical Faculty Carl Gustav Carus, Technical University Dresden)

significance in the findings could only be suspected, but seems very likely.

12.8.2 Pathogenesis/Clinic

Meanwhile, a genetically altered *ITGAM* gene locus has been described with a particular tendency towards a discoid cutaneous lupus (Järvinen et al. 2010). Mutations in the *ITGAM* gene have been described with disturbed **phagocytosis** and increased Toll-like receptor-dependent inflammation (Faridi et al. 2017; Roberts et al. 2014).

12.8.3 Diagnosis

We were ultimately unable to define evidence of an immune defect/PID in the classical sense as the basis of this severe autoimmune disease in our patient, however, the defect in complement receptor 3 (CD11 b) can certainly be described as a moderate immune defect. Indicative for the diagnosis of lupus erythematosus were the classic parameters ANA titer, detection of antibodies against free DNA, positive detection of antibodies against ribonuclear proteins U1 (SM antigen). Luzie did not have hypergammaglobulinemia. At the age of 15, part of the interferon type I signature was determined with the determination of **SIGLEC1** (Sialic acid-binding immunoglobuline-like lectin 1) on monocytes. This antigen is considered a regulator for both innate and adaptive immune cell function, especially in monocytes and macrophages. In Luzie, the expression on monocytes could not be determined as elevated (Stuckrad et al. 2020; Greenan-Barrett et al. 2021). Additional autoimmune phenomena, e.g. on kidney, thyroid, CNS, heart or lung, we did not see in the patient during the course. The particularly pronounced **skin fragility and mucosal instability with recurrent tendency to**

aphthae were in the foreground. Thus, the diagnosis of SLE was possible throughout the course, with cutaneous and mucosal lesions dominating in the end.

12.8.4 Therapy

The systemic component of lupus erythematosus could be stabilized therapeutically with conventional immunosuppressive therapy (glucocorticoids, mycophenolate mofetil). Additional immunosuppression was necessary to address the skin manifestation. Belimumab has recently proven effective in the long-term use of mucocutaneous SLE disease (Akbar et al. 2020), as well as in Luzie.

The use of **Janus kinase inhibitors** can currently only be speculated in childhood. Based on pathophysiological considerations, it can be assumed that targeted interferon-blocking therapy could also have a positive effect on Luzie.

12.8.5 Diagnosis

Systemic lupus erythematosus based on genetic background with mutation in complement receptor 3b (CD11 b).

12.8.6 Prophylaxis

Careful skin hygiene and avoidance of cutaneous infections seem important to reduce the chronicity of skin lesions. This also includes warming measures in winter and pressure-avoiding footwear for **acrocyanosis** (◘ Fig. 12.2c). Wound healing disorders should be addressed early. Regular monitoring, especially of the organs kidney, lung, heart and thyroid within the framework of rheumatological-autoimmunological care is essential.

Conclusion

Next generation sequencing and targeted panel diagnostics for autoimmune diseases and specifically SLE allowed the diagnosis of **monogenetically predisposed SLE**. This explained at least in large parts the lupus symptomatology of Luzie, which occurred particularly early in childhood.

References

Akbar L, Alsagheir R, Al-Mayouf SM (2020) Efficacy of a sequential treatment by belimumab in monogenic systemic lupus erythematosus. Eur J Rheumatol 7:184–189. ► https://doi.org/10.5152/eurjrheum.2020.20087

Fagerholm SC, MacPherson M, James MJ, Sevier-Guy C, Lau CS (2013) The CD11b-integrin (ITGAM) and systemic lupus erythematosus. Lupus 22:657–663. ► https://doi.org/10.1177/0961203313491851

Faridi MH, Khan SQ, Zhao W, Lee HW, Altintas MM, Zhang K, Kumar V, Armstrong AR, Carmona-Rivera C, Dorschner JM, Schnaith AM, Li X, Ghodke-Puranik Y, Moore E, Purmalek M, Irizarry-Caro J, Zhang T, Day R, Stoub D, Hoffmann V, Khaliqdina SJ, Bhargava P, Santander AM, Torroella-Kouri M, Issac B, Cimbaluk DJ, Zloza A, Prabhakar R, Deep S, Jolly M, Koh KH, Reichner JS, Bradshaw EM, Chen J, Moita LF, Yuen PS, Li Tsai W, Singh B, Reiser J, Nath SK, Niewold TB, Vazquez-Padron RI, Kaplan MJ, Gupta V (2017) CD11b activation suppresses TLR-dependent inflammation and autoimmunity in systemic lupus erythematosus. J Clin Invest 127:1271–1283. ► https://doi.org/10.1172/jci88442

Greenan-Barrett J, Doolan G, Shah D, Virdee S, Robinson GA, Choida V, Gak N, de Gruijter N, Rosser E, Al-Obaidi M, Leandro M, Zandi MS, Pepper RJ, Salama A, Jury EC, Ciurtin C (2021) Biomarkers associated with organ-specific involvement in juvenile systemic lupus erythematosus. Int J Mol Sci 22. ► https://doi.org/10.3390/ijms22147619

Järvinen TM, Hellquist A, Koskenmies S, Einarsdottir E, Panelius J, Hasan T, Julkunen H, Padyukov L, Kvarnström M, Wahren-Herlenius M, Nyberg F, D'Amato M, Kere J, Saarialho-Kere U (2010) Polymorphisms of the ITGAM gene confer higher risk of discoid cutaneous than of systemic lupus erythematosus. PloS One 5:e14212. ► https://doi.org/10.1371/journal.pone.0014212

Perez-Gutthann S, Petri M, Hochberg MC (1991) Comparison of different methods of classifying patients with systemic lupus erythematosus. J Rheumatol 18:1176–1179

Roberts AL, Thomas ER, Bhosle S, Game L, Obraztsova O, Aitman TJ, Vyse TJ, Rhodes B (2014) Resequencing the susceptibility gene, ITGAM, identifies two functionally deleterious rare variants in systemic lupus erythematosus cases. Arthritis Res Ther 16:R114. ► https://doi.org/10.1186/ar4566

Stuckrad SLV, Klotsche J, Biesen R, Lieber M, Thumfart J, Meisel C, Unterwalder N, Kallinich T (2020) SIGLEC1 (CD169) is a sensitive biomarker for the deterioration of the clinical course in childhood systemic lupus erythematosus. Lupus 29:1914–1925. ► https://doi.org/10.1177/0961203320965699

12

A 2-Year-Old Toddler with Painful Bluish-Livid Discolorations of the Hands and Feet

Christian Huemer

Contents

13.1 Medical History

The 2 $\frac{1}{2}$-year-old boy is presented in the rheumatology outpatient clinic of the children's hospital, the patient has been experiencing significant changes in the area of the forefeet on both sides since infancy, induced by cold. This symptomatology has significantly intensified in the past 12 months. The main complaints are the child's pronounced cold hands and feet, associated with significant **redness**, but also **swelling** in the area of the toes and **blistering**, especially with **cold exposure**. Individual episodes with blue-purple discoloration and then significant pain symptoms on the forefeet were reported (**Acrocyanosis**). Due to very similar symptoms in the child's mother, there was a suspicion of a hereditary disease from the beginning. General medical history is otherwise unremarkable. Growth and development are normal. Extended family history is also unremarkable, except for very similar symptoms in the child's mother: The child's mother (38 years old) has had similar symptoms of the hands for years, with livid-blue color changes and particular cold sensitivity. She also has noticeable redness of the cheeks; she has not been thoroughly examined so far, but feels completely healthy.

13.2 Examination Findings

2 $\frac{1}{2}$-year-old boy, extremely cooperative, in excellent general and nutritional condition. The **skin findings** show significant redness, partly livid discoloration in the area of the forefeet on both sides as well as the entire toe region on both sides. In individual sections, especially in the area of the acra of the First and Second toe on both sides, small areas of necrosis and also desquamative skin changes (● Fig. 13.1). Peripheral pulses are symmetrical and palpa-

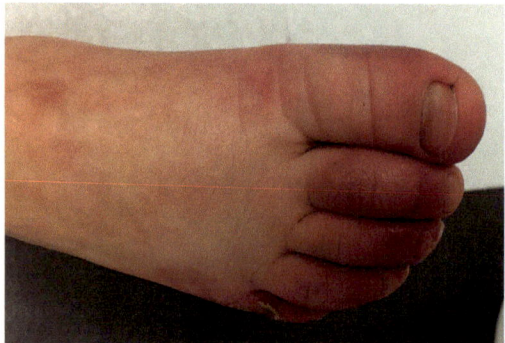

● **Fig. 13.1   Skin findings of the patient with Chilblain Lupus at the time of diagnosis.** Significant livid blue changes in both forefeet, partly also desquamative lesions. (Fifth toe)

ble. Musculoskeletal status is unremarkable with no evidence of synovitis or enthesopathy. Internal status: Heart, lungs auscultation unremarkable. Abdomen unremarkable. ENT findings without focal signs of inflammation.

13.3 Laboratory Values

Inflammatory parameters (ESR, CRP, ferritin) as well as the blood count and serum chemical findings (liver, kidney, muscle and bone parameters) were normal. Autoimmunological diagnostics (ANA, ENA, dsDNA antibodies, C3, C4, Cardiolipin antibodies, cryoglobulins) were all unremarkable. Urine findings unremarkable.

13.4 Educational Questions

1. What further diagnostic steps would you suggest?
2. What differential diagnoses should be discussed?
3. In case of a positive family history, what genetic investigations would you suggest?

13.5 Differential Diagnostic Considerations and Educational Answers

With this very specific medical history and clinical picture of a toddler with bluish-livid changes on the extremities and a **positive family history**, it is obvious to primarily consider a genetically predisposed cutaneous or vascular disease. The already longer medical history of > 12 months makes infectious causes no longer likely. Therefore, diseases with chronic inflammatory or autoinflammatory presentations (**collagenoses, vasculitides, cryoglobulinemia and autoinflammatory interferonopathys**) should be discussed. The clear indications of a positive family history with very similar symptoms in the child's mother make further molecular genetic investigation seem sensible.

13.6 Further Course

In the detailed examination of the child, there was no indication of further organ-specific symptoms, there was only cutaneous symptomatology. The diagnosis of a collagenosis and also of a systemic vasculitis therefore seemed clinically and also—with completely unremarkable autoimmune laboratory findings—very unlikely. The diagnosis of cryoglobulinemia could already be ruled out in the laboratory findings.

The child was then presented to the pediatric dermatologists: The joint clinical suspicion for the child (also for the child's mother) was **familial Chilblain Lupus**.

In a subsequent laboratory examination, the child's "interferon signature" was examined: This revealed a strong type-1 interferon activation in our patient (the expression of the interferon-stimulated genes

IFI127, IFI44m, UFI44L, IFIT1, ISG15, RSAD2 and SIGLEC1 was examined, Laboratory for Molecular Pediatrics, Prof. Dr. Min Ae Lee-Kirsch, University Hospital Dresden). The mother of the child also had this finding. A subsequent mutation analysis (chain termination reactions according to Sanger) in the selected genes TREX1, SAMHD1 or TMEM173 showed no abnormalities. An additional whole-exome sequence analysis was now planned to confirm the clear clinical picture. Together with Pediatric Dermatology, a hydroxychloroquine therapy was initially indicated, which led to a significant stabilization of the cutaneous findings in a follow-up period of 6 months. A therapy with a Janus kinase (JAK) inhibitor (Baricitinib) was discussed with the parents of the child, this active substance would be another option.

13.7 Summary

Type-1 interferonopathies comprise a group of heterogeneous disease patterns that are due to a malfunction of the innate immune system (Crow and Stetson 2022), the **familial Chilblain Lupus** is part of this spectrum of diagnoses.

13.7.1 Clinical Symptoms

Familial Chilblain Lupus represents a monogenically inherited form of cutaneous lupus erythematosus that begins in early childhood (Lee-Kirsch 2006, 2017; d'Angelo et al. 2021). It is characterized by cold-induced bluish-red plaques and papules in acral areas such as fingers, toes, nose, cheeks, and ears. The lesions are painful and can ulcerate. Histologically, perivascular inflammatory infiltrates with deposition of immunoglobulins or complement along the basement membrane are found. An "interferon signature" of activated genes is constitutively increased detectable.

13.7.2 Frequency and Genetics

The prevalence is estimated at < 1:1000,000. Familial Chilblain Lupus is caused by autosomal dominant inherited mutations in the genes TREX1, SAMHD1 or TMEM173 (Bienias et al. 2018).

13.7.3 Therapy/Prognosis

Symptomatic therapy includes the local and systemic administration of anti-inflammatory steroids or Hydroxychloroquine as well as a circulation-promoting therapy with e.g. Nifedipin. Cold protection measures serve for prophylaxis. Case reports have shown a clinical improvement under the therapy with the JAK inhibitors Tofacitinib and Baricitinib (Bienias et al. 2018). However, long-term observations from randomized studies are not available. Patients with familial Chilblain Lupus tend to show an improvement of symptoms with increasing age.

Conclusion

The symptomatology of bluish-livid discoloration of hands and feet in childhood is indeed a common problem and in pediatric rheumatology a differential diagnostic challenge: In addition to the very benign acrocyanoses and the important differential diagnosis Raynaud's phenomenon, the possible diagnosis of an interferonopathy—especially with a positive family history—is relevant, because it can be treated specifically therapeutically.

References

Bienias M, Brück N, Griep C et al (2018) Therapeutic approaches to type I interferonopathies. Curr RheumatolRep 20:32

Crow YJ, Stetson DB (2022) The type I interferonopathies: 10 years on. Nat Rev Immunol 22(8):471–483. ► https://doi.org/10.1038/s41577-021-00633-9. Epub 2021 Oct 20. PMID: 34671122; PMCID: PMC8527296

d'Angelo DM, Di Filippo P, Breda L, Chiarelli F (2021) Type I interferonopathies in children: an overview. Front Pediatr 31(9):631329. ► https://doi.org/10.3389/fped.2021.631329

Lee-Kirsch MA (2006) Familial chilblain lupus, a monogenic form of cutaneous lupus erythematosus, maps to chromosome 3p. Am J Hum Genet 79:731–737

Lee-Kirsch MA (2017) The type I interferonopathies. Annu Ref Med 68:297–315

13

When Every Movement and Even Laughter Becomes Agony

Hermann Girschick

Contents

14.1 Medical History

Starting at the age of 16, Ida first felt a weakness in her legs, then also in her arms. This finding was gradually increasing, so that at the age of 17 she could no longer sit up from a lying position. In addition, she experienced pain in her knee and wrist joints. She noticed that her fingers were repeatedly turning white, and she was losing hair. Difficulties swallowing solid food eventually led to a **weight loss** of 12 kg in the last year, and in the last 6 weeks before presentation, the situation had further intensified and Ida lost an additional 5 kg. At the age of 17 10/12, she presented at our institution. In her past medical history, there were no abnormalities, not even in the skin, mucous membranes, or joints. In her family, Hashimoto's thyroiditis and multiple sclerosis in her mother were reported.

14.2 Examination Findings

Ida could hardly stand alone, she needed support for this. There was a general overall **muscle weakness** of practically all muscles, emphasized in the upper extremities and also in the thoracic back muscles. The gross strength in the arms and legs was reduced to a power grade of 2/5. The Childhood Myositis Assessment Scale (**CMAS**) only yielded 22 out of a possible 51 points. Her voice was quiet and also somewhat **hoarse**. Ida could only swallow food with great difficulty. The active and passive movement of both wrists was painful, she showed flexion contractures in the metacarpophalangeal and also proximal interphalangeal joints. However, no particular swelling was visible here (◘ Fig. 14.1b, c).

Occasionally, **capillary telangiectasias** were visible in the nail bed area (◘ Fig. 14.1b). Skin microscopy confirmed this finding. Finger tip ulcers were initially not present, but these appeared on the middle finger over time. The face showed a significant rarefaction of the **facial expressions**, the skin appeared pale, generally tense in the face, a mild heliotrope was described (◘ Fig. 14.1a). The eyebrows—as well as the eyelids—were inconspicuous, but overall there was a reduced density of the hair. The facial expressions, especially in the mouth area, appeared somewhat restricted. The skin in other body regions appeared normal, no signs of vasculitis. The joints of the lower extremities and also the larger joints of the upper extremities, as well as the spine, appeared normal.

14.3 Laboratory Values and Imaging

14.3.1 Laboratory Values Part 1

The blood sedimentation rate was 35 mm/h, the ferritin was slightly elevated at 182 μg/l, the CRP was unremarkable at 3.2 mg/l. Blood count and differential blood count were technically unremarkable except for a moderate monocytosis of 11%. A coagulation analysis showed a slight aPTT prolongation of 48.4 s, with a normal factor-sensitive PTT of 32 s (normal value 25–33 s). The thrombin time and fibrinogen were normal. There was a slight increase in D-dimers of 2.4 mg/l (< 0.5). The **creatine kinase** (CK) was **3132 U/l (< 167 U/l)**, with a CK-MB fraction of 19% (586 U/l) (normal < 24 U/l). In addition, there was a significant increase in **proBNP** to **1286 ng/l (< 97 ng/l)**. The **troponin** was also significantly elevated at **1723 ng/l (< 50 ng/l)**. The transaminase-AST was elevated at 140 U/l (< 35 U/l) and ALT at 76 U/l (< 31 U/l), the GGT and alkaline phosphatase were unremarkable, the LDH was elevated at 952 U/l.

When Every Movement and Even Laughter Becomes Agony

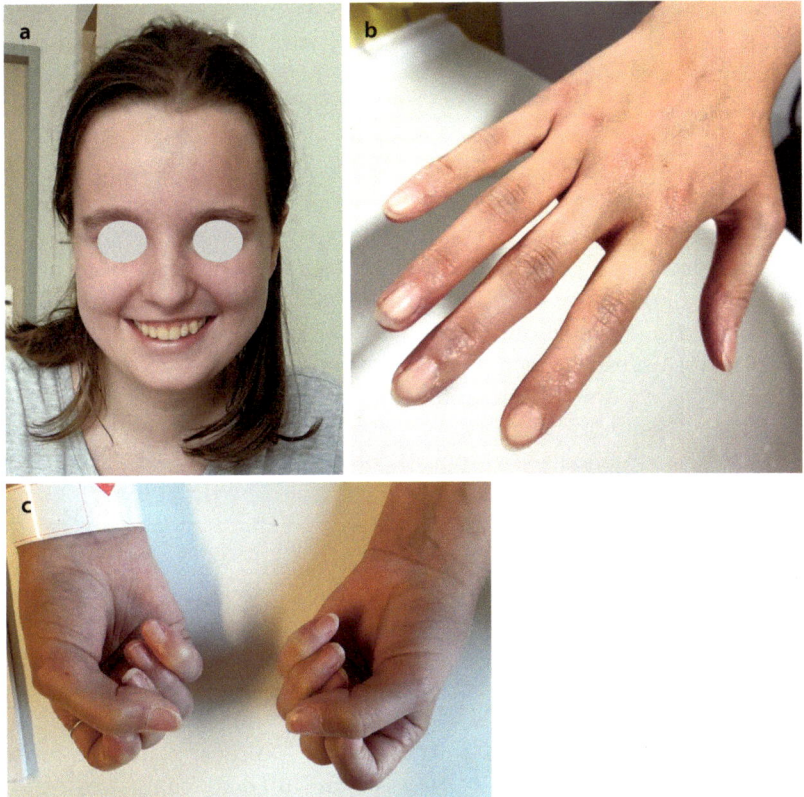

◘ Fig. 14.1 a–c Ida's clinic at 17.5 years: Hypomimia, Gottron's sclerodactyly, acrocyanosis, polyarthritis, **a** shows the hypomimia and the suggested heliotrope of the patient (consent of the patient is available for showing the whole face and covering the eyes). **b** At the same time, Ida also showed peripheral firm thickening/sclerodactyly, not yet papules on the fingers and hands, which were rated as beginning "Gottron's papules", there was a periungual skin lesion on the middle finger, consistent with ulcerated vascular lesion/telangiectasia. Acrocyanosis was present in all seasons. **c** The maximum finger extension and also flexion was not possible due to pain, consistent with polyarthritis

14.3.2 **Educational Questions**

1. What differential diagnosis would you consider for severe diffuse muscle weakness, difficulty swallowing, acrocyanosis, fingertip ulcers, facial abnormalities, and a significant restriction of movement in the finger joints, most likely fitting with polyarthritis?

2. Is it possible to prioritize the differential diagnosis based on the clinical picture alone?

3. How would you design the laboratory diagnostics with the aim of analyzing a complex autoimmune disease in the tension field between dermatomyositis and systemic lupus?

4. What strategic therapeutic considerations should be taken into account, especially including classification considerations?

14.3.3 Laboratory Values Part 2

Since the main symptoms of severe diffuse muscle weakness, difficulty swallowing, acrocyanosis, fingertip rarefaction, hypomimia, and polyarthritis, especially a myositis with scleroderma component, were in the foreground due to the multi-year history, we have particularly positioned the autoimmune diagnostics here. From the perspective of dermatomyositis/polymyositis, an antibody profile with 15 antigens was tested. **Dermatomyositis-/Myositis-specific antibodies (MSA)** from the area of **amino-RNA synthetases** (PL-7, PL-12, EJ, OJ, Jo-1), SRP, TIF-1γ, NXP-2, MI2a/b, MDA5, SAE1 were however not detectable. **Myositis-associated antibodies (MAA)**, which are especially important for the diagnosis of **scleroderma**, were on the other hand highly positive (PM100-antibodies, PM75-antibodies, Ro-52-MB-antibodies). **Antinuclear antibodies** (ANA) were also highly positive with a titer of 1:2560. They could be divided "positive" with an anti-dsDNA-ELISA. However, the Crithidia-immunofluorescence antibody test for dsDNA antibodies was negative. ENA-related nuclear antibodies were not detectable.

A **Rheumatoid factor-IgM** was solidly elevated (62 U/ml [< 20]), as were rheumatoid factors IgA (56 U/ml [< 20 U/ml]). Accordingly, antibodies against citrullinated proteins (**ACPA**) were also found, they were significantly elevated with 27 U/ml (< 20 U/ml). **Antiphospholipid-AB** (Cardiolipin, Beta-2-Glycoprotein-1-AB, Lupus anticoagulant) were not detectable. The B-cell compartment showed no general immune stimulation, IgG, IgA, IgM were normal in serum. The complement analysis C3,

C4 was inconspicuous. There were no indications of celiac disease (transglutaminase-IgA and -IgG antibodies).

Infection serologically, hepatitis B, hepatitis C, HIV 1/2 and cytomegalovirus could be excluded. An older serology was present for EBV virus without detection of IgM. Ida was vaccinated against chickenpox. There were no indications of Lyme disease in the ELISA and immunoblot. The kidney and thyroid function were inconspicuous.

14.3.4 Imaging and Functional Examinations

The initial whole-body MRI in strong edema/T2-weighted TIRM sequence with fat saturation impressively showed a diffuse **myositis** with emphasis on the shoulder girdle, the M. erector spinae, and in the region of the M. quadratus femoris (◘ Fig. 14.2). The nail fold capillaroscopy revealed occasional tuft-like capillaries with branches, also noticeable dilations with caliber jumps and occasional megacapillaries, consistent with a **microangiopathy** in the context of the underlying disease. A fluorescence angiography/rheuma scan (Xiralite®) revealed a symmetrical **polyarthritis** of all PIP and interphalangeal joints. In addition, there were indications of **acrocyanosis/Raynaud's phenomenon** (Apitz and Girschick 2021). The lung function analysis with body plethysmography revealed a severe **restriction** (vital capacity 1.5 l [47%], FEV 1 1.4 l [49%], total lung capacity 3.2 l (70%), see ◘ Fig. 14.3a, c). The carbon monoxide diffusion measurement revealed a restriction to 5.0 mmol/min/kPa (63%), indicating a slightly restricted CO diffusion capacity (◘ Fig. 14.3b, d). Consistent with the significantly reduced CMAS myositis score, the biodynamic jump test showed a significantly reduced jump force of 16 W/kg body weight (◘ Fig. 14.4). An ECG revealed a

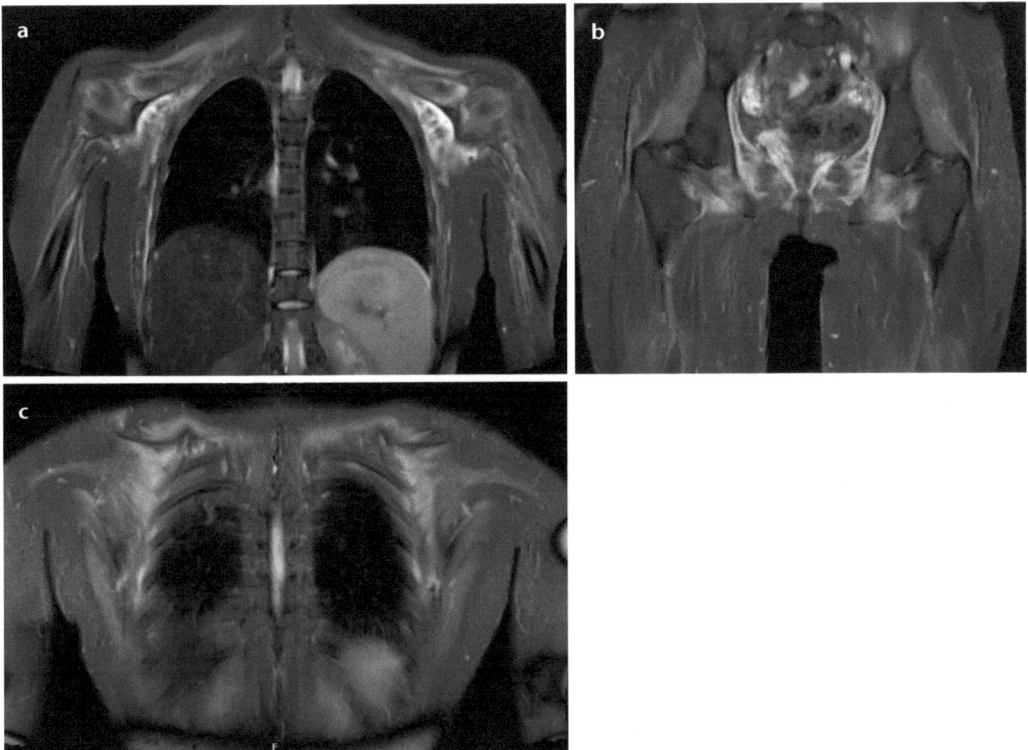

□ **Fig. 14.2** **a–c** Initial whole-body MRI in strong edema/T2-weighted TIRM sequence with fat saturation. The diffuse myositis of the shoulder girdle, the M. erector spinae, and in the region of the M. quadratus femoris is impressive. (With kind permission from Prof. Dr. J. Wagner, Institute for Radiology and Interventional Therapy, Vivantes Klinikum im Friedrichshain, Berlin)

sinus bradycardia of 45/min without signs of repolarization disorders, in the long-term recording a heart rate of 72/min was shown. A transthoracic echocardiography revealed no significant cardiac restriction in the left ventricular function and also not in the diastolic filling phase. In the case of a moderately increased pulmonary arterial hypertension, a moderate tricuspid and mitral insufficiency, a cardiac MRI (CK-MB increased) was performed. This showed a slightly **impaired systolic left ventricular function** without regional wall motion abnormalities, no evidence of intramural edema, myocardial scar, or fibrosis. Contrast agent administration revealed a normal muscular enhancement without late accumulation.

Contrary to the clinical assessment, with a significant restriction of the swallowing act, the radiologically measured esophageal passage time was unremarkable at 3 s.

The sonographic representation of the finger and wrist, knee and ankle joints revealed a synovitis in the area of all PIP/IP joints and both wrists. The sonography of the musculature showed an increase in echogenicity, fan-like and flat, in the area of the proximal musculature. An abdominal sonographic screening was unremarkable.

An ophthalmological examination revealed no evidence of uveitis or retinal vasculopathy/bleeding signs.

A chest X-ray examination was rated as unremarkable. There were no indications of

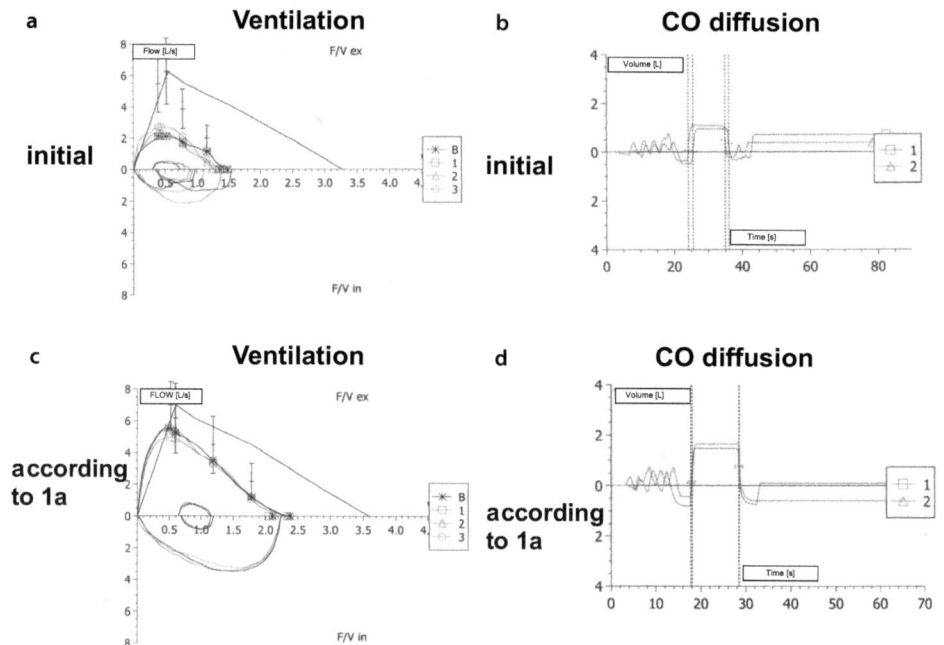

◘ Fig. 14.3 **a–d** Ida's positive development of ventilation and diffusion restriction initially (**a, c**) and after one year of therapy (**b, d**). The maximum vital capacity improved from 1.7l to 2.33l (52%, resp. 66% of the target). The CO diffusion improved from carbon monoxide transfer factor (TLCO) 4.2 mmol/min/kPa (52% of the target) to TLCO 6.0 mmol/min/kPa (65% of the target). (With kind permission from Dr. Jakob Borchardt, Clinic for Pneumology, Vivantes Klinikum im Friedrichshain, Berlin)

14

tuberculosis in either the intracutaneous tuberculin skin tests or an interferon-γ release assay.

14.4 Differential Diagnostic Considerations

For the patient, the primary concerns were severe **diffuse muscle weakness, difficulty swallowing** with weight loss, and **hypomimia**. In terms of differential diagnosis, dermatomyositis is primarily considered. The clinical signs of systemic scleroderma are second in priority. Since the patient also has polyarthritis in the hands and thus a significant systemic component in addition to skin, muscles, and joints, the clinical suspicion is an **overlap syndrome** between these

complex autoimmune diseases. For systemic lupus erythematosus (SLE), the classification criteria of antinuclear antibodies, dsDNA antibodies, and joint pain/polyarthritis have been identified. Thus, 3 out of 11 of the ACR classification criteria would be present (Perez-Gutthann et al. 1991; Rider et al. 2013; Hochberg 1990). However, due to the severe myositis and skin changes, dermatomyositis and systemic scleroderma, including cardiac involvement, were in the foreground.

Based on this then classic MRI finding for dermatomyositis, we refrained from a muscle biopsy. We could infer a pulmonary involvement with presumed interstitial changes from the lung function analysis. Even though the echocardiographic examinations and the cardio-MRI showed mod-

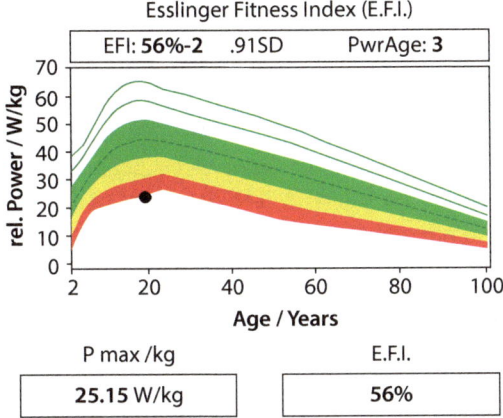

Esslinger Fitness Index (E.F.I.)

P max /kg	E.F.I.
25.15 W/kg	56%

■ **Fig. 14.4** Muscular strength/performance testing initially and one year after therapy. The figure shows the positive development of performance in the "Esslinger Fitness Index" with a significant increase in total performance/kg body weight from 16.9 to 25.15 W/kg. The maximum jump force increased from 2.17 kN to 2.7 kN, and the maximum jump speed from 1.2 to 1.6 m/s. (Leonardo-Mechanography, Novotec Medical, Esslingen)

erate signs of carditis in line with the significantly elevated cardiac muscle enzymes, it was still surprising that these imaging examinations of the heart were moderate and that Ida, apart from bradycardic episodes without hemodynamic impairment, showed no signs of cardiac dysfunction/insufficiency.

The targeted autoimmune diagnostics towards juvenile myositis/dermatomyositis did not yield any MSA (Rider et al. 2013; Shah et al. 2013; Leclair and Lundberg 2018). Rather, **MAA** were shown (Mende et al. 2019), which mainly suggested the presence of an overlap syndrome.

14.5 Further Course

Therapeutically, the patient immediately received intravenous **methylprednisolone pulse therapy** (15 mg/kg body weight/day) for 3

days, followed by oral prednisolone 1 mg/kg body weight/day and the immediate start of basic immunological therapy with methotrexate 20 mg subcutaneously/week. To reduce arthralgia and myalgia, naproxen was used at a daily dose of 750 mg. This was supplemented by an antacid therapy with pantoprazole, folic acid support with 5 mg on 3 days after methotrexate administration, and a **vitamin D administration** of 500 IU/day. Intensive daily physiotherapy complemented the medicinal concept. Steroid pulses were applied 6 times at intervals of 4 weeks. Due to the differential diagnostic proximity to lupus erythematosus, **hydroxychloroquine** was also started at a daily dose of 200 mg. Under this, physical activity and muscle strength gradually improved significantly. The cardiac functional abnormalities and also enzymatic abnormalities were significantly reduced after 2 steroid pulses (creatine kinase 640 U/l, CK-MB 109 U/l, troponin 281 ng/l, NT-proBNP normalized, AST 50 U/l, ALT 34 U/l). After 4 methylprednisolone pulses, the creatine kinase was 241 U/l, CK-MB 35 U/l, troponin was still moderately elevated at 88 ng/l, the transaminases, and further NT-proBNP were normalized. After 6 glucocorticoid pulse therapies, the CK was normalized at 16 U/l, only the troponin was still moderately elevated at 51 ng/l. The oral glucocorticoid therapy could be ended after 12 months.

Within a year, the patient had gained 12 kg in weight. This was due to the now normalized food intake with no longer restricted swallowing. At the end of a long school day, the patient complained of general **muscular exhaustion**, but the general muscle strength was no longer restricted, the voice phonation was unremarkable, and there was still a moderate **rarefaction of the fingertips**. The nail fold was normal. There were subtle signs of previous glucocorticoid therapy.

14.6 Educative Responses

- **1. What differential diagnosis do you consider for severe diffuse muscle weakness, difficulty swallowing, acrocyanosis, fingertip ulcers, facial abnormalities, and polyarthritis?**

If we go back to the classification criteria for polymyositis and dermatomyositis first established in 1975 (Bohan and Peter 1975), then the First criterion of symmetrical muscle weakness including the pelvic girdle, the 3rd criterion of significantly increased skeletal muscle enzymes, and the Fifth criterion of skin abnormalities with signs of Raynaud's phenomenon would be positive (muscle biopsy and electromyography not performed). The diagnosis of dermatomyositis would be possible. However, the skin findings were ultimately suggestive of dermatomyositis, with minimal heliotrope, "beginning" Gottron's signs, and existing dry scaling of the back of the hand. However, the rarefaction of the fingertips, the capillary ectasias, and the Raynaud's issues were more indicative of systemic scleroderma.

Since the introduction of this classification, there has been an increasing attempt, especially at the beginning of this millennium, to include the **myositis-specific autoantibody pattern (MSA)** in the diagnosis and classification. Over the past 20 years, the clinical description of disease patterns associated with particular autoantibody patterns has become much more concrete (Pinto et al. 2019; Leclair and Lundberg 2018; Rider et al. 2013), so that currently the subgroups of the **antisynthetase syndromes** are most likely associated with severe course and especially interstitial lung disease. Patients with **anti-SRP antibodies** primarily show peripheral muscle weakness, a tendency to fall, and Raynaud's phenomenon. Here, immobility is indeed a threat. The creatine kinase values are considered particularly high. Similarly, in the case of **anti-MI-2 antibodies**, myositis, possibly necrotizing, is in the foreground. Heliotrope, Gottron's papules, and the reddish skin rash in the area of the cheeks/butterfly erythema have been described. In contrast, patients with **TIF-1γ antibodies** show mild muscle weakness and low morbidity. Patients with **anti-MDA5 antibodies** show the classic picture of dermatomyositis also in the area of the fingers, an interstitial lung disease, and overall somewhat less myositis, but with clearly present arthritis and arthralgia (Yamasaki et al. 2021).

Newer classification efforts at the European level (Lundberg et al. 2017) are now again focusing on clinical characteristics for the classification of juvenile idiopathic inflammatory myopathies. A summation score was developed: Our patient had a score (no muscle biopsy performed) of 12.8 points out of a total of 22.3 points and would be classifiable as dermatomyositis according to this classification. However, this classification does not do justice to the **overlap syndrome**, which was most likely present in our patient. The MAA autoantibody pattern clearly indicates overlap with systemic scleroderma. For these patients, the risk of developing Raynaud's phenomenon and interstitial lung disease is particularly seen.

These two clinical diseases were present in our patient, Dermatomyositis/Scleroderma/Overlap Syndrome (Aringer 2019; Chiang et al. 2021).

According to the now current new classification by Aringer for SLE (Aringer 2019), the classification of Ida with positive antinuclear antibody and polyarthritis, furthermore myocarditis and anti-dsDNA antibodies in ELISA would not have been clearly classifiable. Nevertheless, we decided for a co-medication with hydroxychloroquine in the sense of the overlap also to SLE.

14

- **2. Is it possible to prioritize the differential diagnosis based on the clinical picture?**

Thus, we prioritized an overlap syndrome with the clinical symptoms of dermatomyositis and systemic scleroderma, accompanied by polyarthritis, in the differential diagnosis.

- **3. How do you design the laboratory diagnostics with the aim of analyzing a complex autoimmune disease in the tension field between dermatomyositis and systemic lupus?**

The laboratory diagnostics had to ultimately include all these complex autoimmune diseases according to newer criteria due to the described differential diagnosis. In the course, however, already under basic drug therapy, diagnostics for a possible "interferon signature" (SIGLEC expression on monocytes) were not conspicuous (**CD 169**; **SIGLEC I**) (Stuckrad et al. 2020).

- **4. What strategic therapeutic considerations should be taken into account, especially with regard to classification considerations?**

Due to the predominant dermatitis and myositis component, as well as systemic scleroderma with cardiac and pulmonary involvement, intravenous glucocorticoid pulse therapy was an option, as well as the immediate use of basic therapy with methotrexate (Bellutti Enders et al. 2017). The patient benefited from this, so an expansion of the anti-inflammatory therapy, e.g., towards cyclophosphamide, was not necessary.

Following the recommendations, the glucocorticoids were eventually switched to oral after 6 months, further reduced and discontinued after one year. Methotrexate was continued unchanged. The patient had almost achieved remission when transitioning into adulthood. According to the current EULAR recommendations for the management of juvenile dermatomyositis, this therapy should be continued for another year before considering a reduction or discontinuation of methotrexate. The clinical facets of scleroderma (Raynaud's phenomenon, rarefaction of the fingertips) did not progress, so the therapeutic concept seemed adequate.

14.7 Summary

14.7.1 Etiology

The etiology of Ida's complex autoimmune disease is ultimately unknown. It is assumed to be a complex disorder, primarily of the humoral immune system, with the development of measurable autoantibodies. Recent findings suggest that signaling pathways in the area of **interferon-α/type-I-interferon** are also involved. A monogenetic cause, as is discussed in rare cases of SLE, is not considered for dermatomyositis and scleroderma.

14.7.2 Pathogenesis/Clinic

The complex inflammatory disorder of skin, muscles, vessels, and joints ultimately leads to severe organ disorders, including permanent muscle weakness, heart failure, interstitial lung disease with pulmonary insufficiency, polyarthritis, and restrictions, including dermal and myogenic calcifications. In the overlap with SLE, all organs can ultimately be involved in the pathogenesis (Saito et al. 2021).

14.7.3 Diagnosis

In addition to a detailed history and clinical examination, the determination of myositis-specific antibodies and myositis-associated autoantibody patterns are relevant. Antibodies against nuclear components, against phospholipids, and also, for example, thyroid structures, complete the diagnosis.

14.7.4 Therapy

According to current EULAR recommendations, glucocorticoids and immunosuppressive therapy with methotrexate are the mainstay for both mild juvenile dermatomyositis and the onset of a severe course. Depending on the assessment and manifestation, other basic therapeutics, such as cyclophosphamide, are considered for pulmonary and cardiac involvement, as well as severe ulcerative skin disease. If there is no improvement, further therapy supplements, such as B-cell blockade with **anti-CD20** antibodies, TNF blockade, and the addition of therapy with intravenous immunoglobulins (Hyper-IgG) should be considered (Bellutti Enders et al. 2017).

Newer therapeutic strategies, such as **Janus kinase (JAK)-** or **IL-6 inhibitors**, appear promising in patients with therapy-resistant course (Ll Wilkinson et al. 2021) (author's experience).

14.7.5 Diagnosis

The diagnosis is primarily based on the clinical picture of the disease, it is supported in the context of classification efforts and modern laboratory diagnostics including MSA, MAA, and SLE-associated autoantibodies. The determination of an interferon signature or laboratory markers, which indicate an activation of the interferon signaling pathway (SIGLEC I/CD 169), can be additionally helpful in differential diagnosis. In childhood and adolescence, the algorithm for tumor exclusion existing in adult medicine is not in the foreground.

14.7.6 Prophylaxis

There is no prophylaxis to prevent the disease. Attention should be paid to the tendency for bacterial infections in the context of the underlying diseases, to exacerbations of pulmonary and cardiac manifestations in the context of viral infections, but also to the development of, for example, oral fungal infections (as also in our patient). Close connection to a specialized interdisciplinary center for autoimmunity is highly desirable.

Conclusion

Patients with complex autoimmune disease often have a long journey behind them until a diagnosis is more clearly graspable, as was the case with Ida with a 2-year history. Modern MSA and MAA autoantibody determinations are available, which allow a classification of the clinical picture of dermatomyositis in addition to classification efforts. A multidisciplinary interactive care strategy is based, among other things, on the use of a multi-topical anti-inflammatory medication as the basis for therapy. This is flanked by intensive physiotherapy and respiratory therapy, promotion of musculoskeletal fitness, and local skin care.

References

Apitz C, Girschick H (2021) Systemic sclerosis-associated pulmonary arterial hypertension in children. Cardiovasc Diagn Ther 11:1137–1143. ▶ https://doi.org/10.21037/cdt-20-901

Aringer M (2019) EULAR/ACR classification criteria for SLE. Semin Arthritis Rheum 49:S14–s17. ▶ https://doi.org/10.1016/j.semarthrit.2019.09.009

Bellutti Enders F, Bader-Meunier B, Baildam E, Constantin T, Dolezalova P, Feldman BM, Lahdenne P, Magnusson B, Nistala K, Ozen S, Pilkington C, Ravelli A, Russo R, Uziel Y, van Brussel M, van der Net J, Vastert S, Wedderburn LR, Wulffraat N, McCann LJ, van Royen-Kerkhof A (2017)

14

Consensus-based recommendations for the management of juvenile dermatomyositis. Ann Rheum Dis 76:329–340. ▶ https://doi.org/10.1136/annrheumdis-2016-209247

Bohan A, Peter JB (1975) Polymyositis and dermatomyositis (first of two parts). N Engl J Med 292:344–347. ▶ https://doi.org/10.1056/nejm197502132920706

Chiang HL, Tung CH, Huang KY, Hsu BB, Wu CH, Hsu CW, Lu MC, Lai NS (2021) Association between clinical phenotypes of dermatomyositis and polymyositis with myositis-specific antibodies and overlap systemic autoimmune diseases. Medicine (Baltimore) 100:e27230. ▶ https://doi.org/10.1097/md.0000000000027230

Hochberg MC (1990) Systemic lupus erythematosus. Rheum Dis Clin North Am 16:617–639

Leclair V, Lundberg IE (2018) New myositis classification criteria – what ee have learned since Bohan and Peter. Curr Rheumatol Rep 20:18. ▶ https://doi.org/10.1007/s11926-018-0726-4

Ll Wilkinson MG, Deakin CT, Papadopoulou C, Eleftheriou D, Wedderburn LR (2021) JAK inhibitors: a potential treatment for JDM in the context of the role of interferon-driven pathology. Pediatr Rheumatol Online J 19:146. ▶ https://doi.org/10.1186/s12969-021-00637-8

Lundberg IE, Tjärnlund A, Bottai M, Werth VP, Pilkington C, Visser M, Alfredsson L, Amato AA, Barohn RJ, Liang MH, Singh JA, Aggarwal R, Arnardottir S, Chinoy H, Cooper RG, Dankó K, Dimachkie MM, Feldman BM, Torre IG, Gordon P, Hayashi T, Katz JD, Kohsaka H, Lachenbruch PA, Lang BA, Li Y, Oddis CV, Olesinska M, Reed AM, Rutkowska-Sak L, Sanner H, Selva-O'Callaghan A, Song YW, Vencovsky J, Ytterberg SR, Miller FW, Rider LG (2017) 2017 European League Against Rheumatism/American College of Rheumatology classification criteria for adult and juvenile idiopathic inflammatory myopathies and their major subgroups. Ann Rheum Dis 76:1955–1964. ▶ https://doi.org/10.1136/annrheumdis-2017-211468

Mende M, Borchardt-Lohölter V, Meyer W, Scheper T, Schlumberger W (2019) Autoantibodies in myositis. How to achieve a comprehensive strategy for serological testing. Mediterr J Rheumatol 30:155–161. ▶ https://doi.org/10.31138/mjr.30.3.155

Perez-Gutthann S, Petri M, Hochberg MC (1991) Comparison of different methods of classifying patients with systemic lupus erythematosus. J Rheumatol 18:1176–1179

Pinto B, Janardana R, Nadig R, Mahadevan A, Bhatt AS, Raj JM, Shobha V (2019) Comparison of the 2017 EULAR/ACR criteria with Bohan and Peter criteria for the classification of idiopathic inflammatory myopathies. Clin Rheumatol 38:1931–1934. ▶ https://doi.org/10.1007/s10067-019-04512-6

Rider LG, Shah M, Mamyrova G, Huber AM, Rice MM, Targoff IN, Miller FW (2013) The myositis autoantibody phenotypes of the juvenile idiopathic inflammatory myopathies. Medicine (Baltimore) 92:223–243. ▶ https://doi.org/10.1097/MD.0b013e31829d08f9

Saito S, Endo Y, Nishio M, Uchiyama A, Uehara A, Toki S, Yasuda M, Ishikawa O, Muro Y, Motegi SI (2021) Anti-polymyositis/Scl antibody-positive overlap syndrome of diffuse cutaneous systemic sclerosis, dermatomyositis, systemic lupus erythematosus, and antiphospholipid syndrome. J Dermatol. ▶ https://doi.org/10.1111/1346-8138.16219

Shah M, Mamyrova G, Targoff IN, Huber AM, Malley JD, Rice MM, Miller FW, Rider LG (2013) The clinical phenotypes of the juvenile idiopathic inflammatory myopathies. Medicine (Baltimore) 92:25–41. ▶ https://doi.org/10.1097/MD.0b013e31827f264d

Stuckrad SLV, Klotsche J, Biesen R, Lieber M, Thumfart J, Meisel C, Unterwalder N, Kallinich T (2020) SIGLEC1 (CD169) is a sensitive biomarker for the deterioration of the clinical course in childhood systemic lupus erythematosus. Lupus 29:1914–1925. ▶ https://doi.org/10.1177/0961203320965699

Yamasaki Y, Kobayashi N, Akioka S, Yamazaki K, Takezaki S, Nakaseko H, Ohara A, Nishimura K, Nishida Y, Sato S, Kishi T, Hashimoto M, Mori M, Okazaki Y, Kuwana M, Ohta A (2021) Clinical impact of myositis-specific autoantibodies on long-term prognosis of juvenile idiopathic inflammatory myopathies: multicentre study. Rheumatology (Oxford) 60:4821–4831. ▶ https://doi.org/10.1093/rheumatology/keab108

When the Skin Hardens and Calcifies

Hermann Girschick

Contents

15.1 Medical History

Due to the complexity of **scleroderma** in childhood and adolescence with localized and systemic course, the following presents two patients with their history:

▪▪ Pia

Pia is a 10-year-old girl who has shown noticeable tough skin changes on the trunk and lower legs for 1 year, these are purple in the peripheral area, the face is spared. The general practitioner had initiated a *Borrelia burgdorferi* serology, which was inconspicuous. Nevertheless, a penicillin therapy was decided for a duration of 3 weeks with 5000,000 units intravenously daily. However, there was no significant change in the clinical findings. The lesions gradually increased over the next year, and the patient was then presented to pediatric rheumatology 2 $^1/_2$ years after the onset of the problem.

▪▪ Klara

At the age of 5, the family first noticed a weakness in the area of both hands and knee movement. In general, the mobility of the fingers and hands was limited. The **facial features** were "not very lively". Due to the significantly increasing **joint mobility restriction**, especially of the middle and end joints of the fingers, both elbows, a restricted shoulder abduction, jaw joint mobility, spine mobility with a thoracic hump/weak posture, further circulatory disorders in the area of the fingers and also narrowed finger tips, the child was presented at the age of 9.

15.2 Examination Findings

▪▪ Pia

Pia showed a clear spread of depigmented, in their **toughness** intensified skin lesions, which showed a slight redness and also purple discoloration at the edge, centrally a silvery scaling. There was no acrocyanosis. Mucosal pathologies were not present. The trunk and lower legs were affected. Upper arms and face were spared (◖ Fig. 15.1a–d; e–f shows the long-term findings).

▪▪ Klara

There was a clear **hypomimia** with narrow vermilion, the multiple joint mobility restrictions were confirmed, e.g. clearly in both elbows with flexion and extension deficit of 45 degrees each. There were subcutaneous nodular calcifications on the extensor sides of the upper arms and lower legs/knees. These repeatedly opened to the outside, discharging whitish, crumbly, chalk-like material. A **Raynaud's syndrome** was present (◖ Fig. 15.2a–c).

15.3 Laboratory Values and Imaging

15.3.1 Laboratory Values

▪▪ Pia

Inflammatory parameters (erythrocyte sedimentation rate, ferritin, CRP) were normal, as were the blood count and overview values of liver, kidney, muscle, and bone. Autoimmune diagnostics: Antinuclear antibodies (ANA) were positive with a titer of 1:160. They could not be divided into anti-dsDNA and ENA-related nuclear antibodies.

▪▪ Klara

Inflammatory parameters (erythrocyte sedimentation rate, ferritin, CRP) were normal, as were the blood count and overview values of liver, kidney, muscle, and bone. The autoimmune diagnostics (ANA, ENA, dsDNA antibodies, C3, C4, cardiolipin antibodies) were all unremarkable, thus no evidence of antibodies relevant for the di-

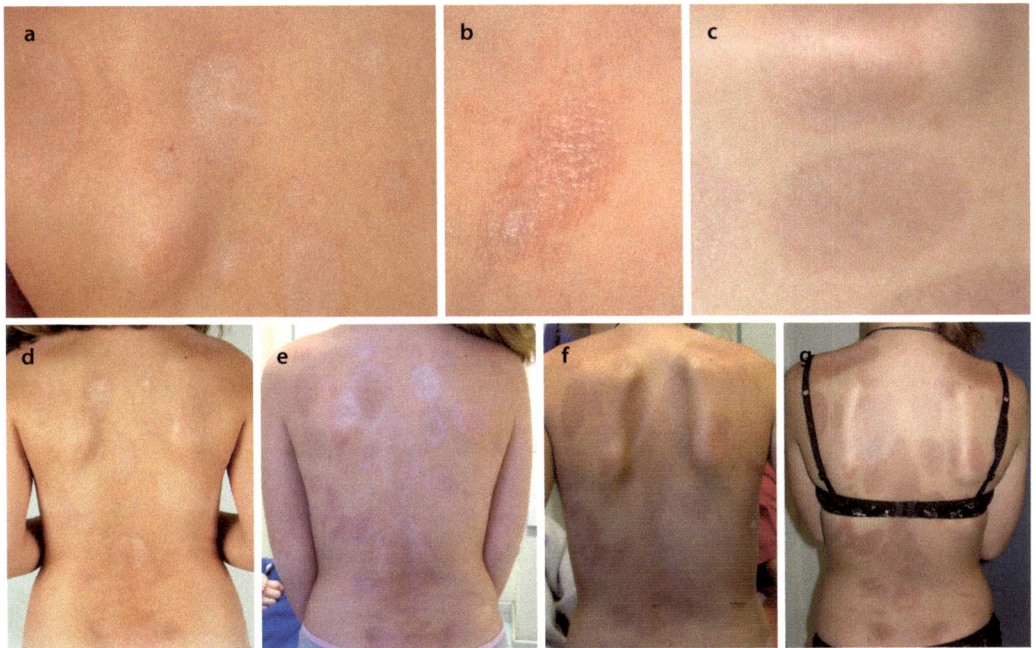

◘ Fig. 15.1   a–g Pia's clinic at 10 years: localized scleroderma in the form of generalized morphea. a, b, d show the circumscribed scleroderma/generalized morphea at initial presentation. At this time, the clinic had already existed for one year. There was no acrocyanosis. **e** After 1.5 years, **f** after 2 years and **c, g** after 3 years, the number and spread of the lesions did not increase anymore, the pigmentation of the lesion was increasing, but not their toughness

agnosis of scleroderma (scleroderma-associated antibodies [SAA], e.g., PM100 antibodies, PM75 antibodies, Ro-52-MB antibodies).

15.3.2 Imaging and Functional Examinations

▪▪ Pia

The sonography of the heart, abdomen, joints, conventional X-ray examinations (thorax, barium swallow analysis), the magnetic resonance imaging of the head, and a lung function test were unremarkable. An ophthalmological examination revealed no abnormalities on the retina. Evidence of the involvement of internal organs in the inflammatory process was not found.

▪▪ Klara

A barium swallow showed a significantly prolonged passage time, but the esophageal motility was essentially preserved. A gastroesophageal reflux was not documented (◘ Fig. 15.3a, b). Subcutaneous calcifications could be documented in the lower leg area (◘ Fig. 15.3c). The conventional X-ray image showing the hands and fingertips (◘ Fig. 15.3d, e) showed general osteoporosis and osteolysis of the distal phalanges (◘ Fig. 15.3d, e).

15.4 Educational Questions

1. What differential diagnosis do you consider for hypomimia, acrocyanosis, fingertip rarefaction, and a significant re-

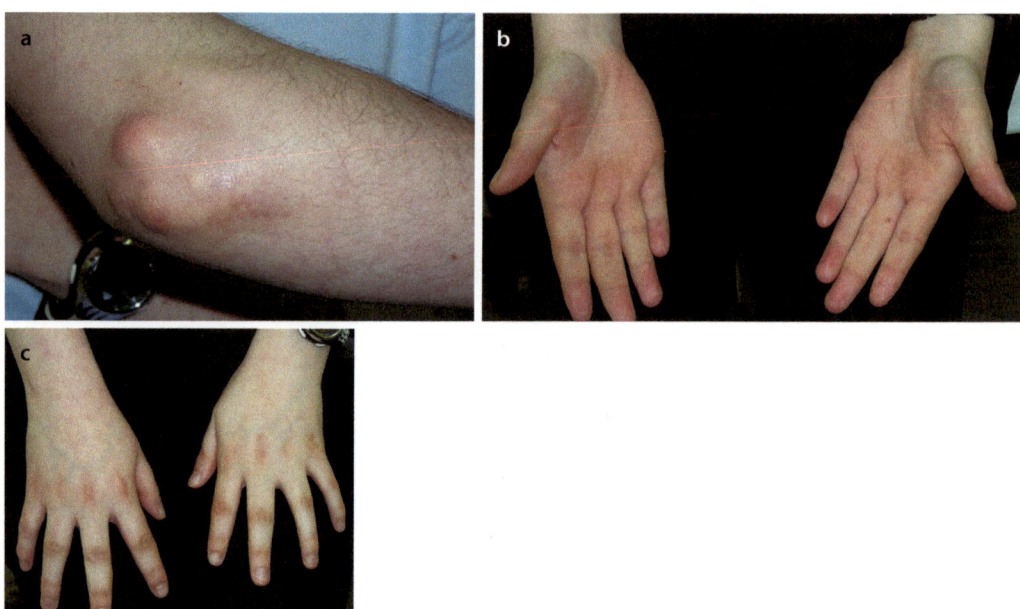

☐ Fig. 15.2   a–c Klara's clinic at 11 years: CREST syndrome, limited cutaneous systemic scleroderma with subcutaneous calcifications. a–c show the clinic after about 5 years of course at the age of 11. Subcutaneous calcifications had shown up especially on the extremities, e.g. on the elbow extensor side (**a**) reaching the joint capsule and also periosteum. The fingers show a rarefaction of the tips (**c**, see also radiology in ☐ Fig. 15.3d) and a reduced perfusion, which showed as Raynaud's phenomenon (**b**)

striction of movement in the finger joints?
2. Is the clinical description of the skin findings/clinical picture relevant for the classification of scleroderma?
3. How do you design the laboratory diagnostics with the aim of analyzing the various forms of scleroderma as a complex autoimmune disease?
4. What strategic therapeutic considerations should be taken into account, especially including target-defined therapy (treat-to-target) protocols?

15.5 Immunology and Classification

15.5.1 Immunology

Both localized and systemic scleroderma are considered complex autoimmune dis-

eases, both of which can impair the function of the skin, subcutis, and fascia with induration to the course of affection and fibrosis of internal organs. Often, the symptoms begin with general skin/finger swelling, a **Raynaud's phenomenon**, and nail fold capillary changes. There is an increased occurrence of autoimmune diseases in families. Ultimately, this inflammatory immunological pathology results in increased collagen formation and fibroblast proliferation. There are indications that the immune system in localized scleroderma is somewhat prematurely aged (Torok et al. 2019). In the pathogenesis of the systemic variant, microvascular endothelial damage, a proliferative vasculopathy is also discussed (Stevens et al. 2019). In addition to the activation of innate immunity, the formation of **autoantibodies against nuclear components** is also in the foreground. The pathogenesis of scleroderma itself is ultimately still unclear in its

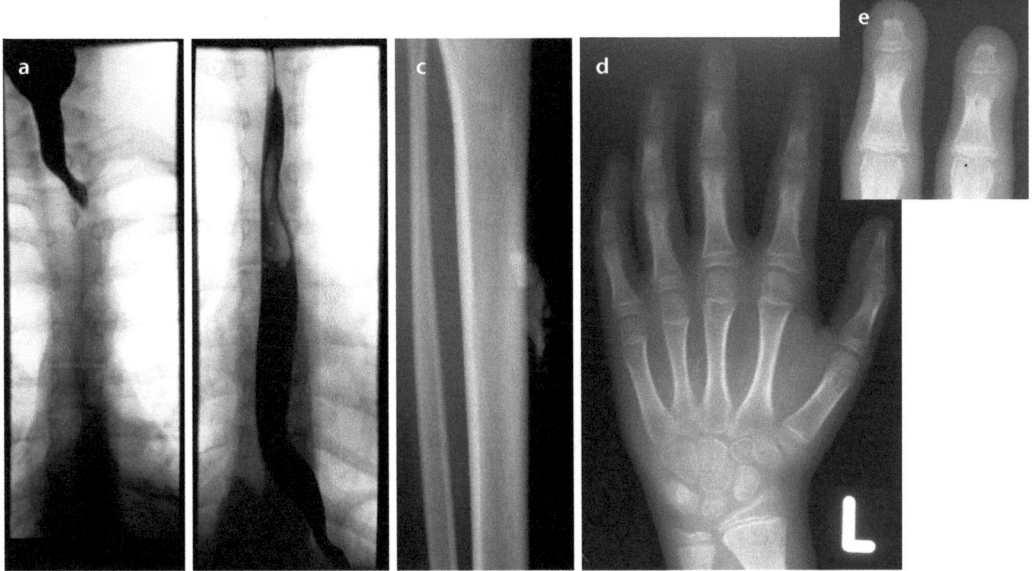

■ **Fig. 15.3　a–e Klara's conventional radiological diagnostics. a, b** Klara's barium swallow with extended transit time. **c** Deep subcutaneous calcifications pretibial. **d, e** Caused by the accompanying polyarthritis, a reduced bone density was evident, especially near the joint spaces and in the carpus (**d**). The distal phalanges showed distal osteolysis (**e**). (With kind permission from Prof. Dr. J. Wagner, Institute for Radiology and Interventional Therapy, Vivantes Klinikum im Friedrichshain, Berlin)

etiology. An immunopathogenesis is suspected: Certain HLA patterns - similar to rheumatoid arthritis - are present (Stevens et al. 2016), a characteristic autoantibody pattern is mainly described in the systemic form. Messenger substances, which are associated with increased T-cell activity and activation of the interferon-γ pathway, are measurable. Inflammatory lymphocytic/monocytic/macrophage infiltrates are found in the skin lesions. In childhood systemic scleroderma, the pathophysiological analyses are still very limited compared to adults. Early in the inflammation phase, TH1 and TH17 cells and their cytokines (IL-1, TNF-α, interferon-γ, IL-17) are attributed an important role. In the later phase, TH2 cells and their cytokine pattern (IL-4, IL-13, IL-33–35) play an important role in the profibrotic development. Interferon-γ-associated chemokines (MCP-1, IP-10) contribute, like the cytokines, to the fact that

fibroblasts and endothelial cells produce Transformimg growth factor β (**TGF-β)** and Connective tissue growth factor (**CTGF**), which contribute to the increased collagen production (Stevens et al. 2019).

The role of the innate immune system with monocytes, macrophages, dendritic cells, as well as endothelial cells and myofibroblasts is not yet properly understood, but is considered relevant. Overall, the findings on the immunopathogenesis of both localized and systemic scleroderma remain very "general", they describe the activation of "classical inflammation pathways", which lead to significant fibrosis of the skin and organs on a not yet clearly defined genetic basis (Di Battista et al. 2021). Within twin studies, the simultaneous occurrence of systemic scleroderma is described in about 5% of adults. In families with patients with systemic sclerosis, there was up to a 16-fold increased risk for another affected person, with siblings the risk increased up to about 27-fold (Stevens et al. 2019). Due to the rarity of the disease in childhood and adolescence with prevalence rates of only single children of 100,000 in the localized form and a few per 1 million in the systemic form, studies on etiology are generally limited, cohort analyses necessarily refer to small groups.

15.5.2 Classification

Based on these limited cohorts, attempts have been made through classification efforts of both linear and systemic scleroderma to provide assessment aids to attending physicians in order to be able to name scleroderma as such. Classification efforts are generally not suitable for actual diagnosis, they often arise in the context of expert consensus procedures, which naturally lead to a concentration and simplification of symptom enumerations. Based on this, algorithms are sought for classifying the symptoms of a patient as an entity. The reevaluation of these preliminary classification algorithms on larger case cohorts would be the next step. For example, in the latest classification of **childhood systemic sclerosis** (Zulian et al. 2007) from 48 clinical symptoms, 9 organ-related affection groups are formed, from which ultimately **3 main criteria (Raynaud's phenomenon, skin sclerosis proximal to the metacarpophalangeal/tarsophalangeal joint, and sclerodactyly)** were selected as relevant along with another 18 minor criteria. From this, the experts finally indicated *one major* criterion (skin sclerosis proximal to the MCP joint) and additionally *2 minor* criteria from the mentioned organ groups as, if present, sufficient for the diagnosis of systemic sclerosis.

In adulthood, the current classification of 2013 for systemic sclerosis indicates the same main criterion, but it also provides the possibility to consider 7 cumulative symptoms, e.g. skin thickening, rarefaction of the fingertips, telangiectasias, nailfold capillaries, interstitial lung disease, Raynaud's phenomenon, and scleroderma-associated autoantibodies (SAA), as sufficient for the diagnosis of systemic sclerosis (van den Hoogen et al. 2013).

For the diagnosis of **localized/circumscribed scleroderma**, various classification attempts have been developed, which from the author's point of view essentially capture the same entities (manifestation images), but group them slightly modified. The most recent, the **Padua classification** (Laxer and Zulian 2006), describes purely descriptively on the one hand the *linear form* of localized/circumscribed scleroderma related to the **extremities** or on the other hand to the special form on the head with the **"saber sheath stroke form ("en coup de sabre")"**. The greater involvement of the face with progressive unilateral facial atrophy is referred to as Parry-Romberg syndrome. The second group is the *limited form*, mainly described with various morphea variants (superficial and deep). The third form is referred to as the *generalized form* with involvement of at least 3 anatomical areas. The particularly pronounced sclerotic (pansclerotic) morphea can lead to atrophy of an entire extremity. If the fascia is particularly extensively affected, this is referred to as **eosinophilic fasciitis** (Kreuter et al. 2009).

15.6 Further Progress

▪▪ Pia

Due to the progressing **generalized morphea** the patient received an immunosuppressive basic therapy with methotrexate once weekly orally 20 mg, furthermore daily

Hydroxychloroquine at a dosage of 200 mg/day. Local skin care and lipid-replenishing measures were taken. Under this, there was a stagnation of the findings, the skin lesions decreased in their hardening, from the 2nd year no further lesions were added, however, they showed an increased pigmentation (◘ Fig. 15.1e–g). After about 6 years of stable course, the patient presented again at the age of 16, new lesions had recently appeared in the neck area, a local therapy with tacrolimus ointment 0.03% and in the course clobetasol propionate (Dermoxin®) ointment application was carried out. The patient was then transferred in the transition to adult dermatology. She continued to show an inconspicuous autoantibody pattern. Internal organs were not affected, her quality of life did not appear to be restricted

■■ **Klara**

After 7 years of clinical course control with continuous physiotherapy without systemic drug therapy (desired by the family), a decreasing hypomimia was observed in the face. Local skin care, lipid-replenishing measures were taken. The **calcinosis cutis** was regressive, but basically still existed. The finger mobility still showed a moderate restriction, as did the wrists. The flexion and extension deficit in the area of the elbows was 30 degrees. There were no indications of active arthritis at this time either. Involvement of the heart, lung, kidney could not be diagnosed in annual status surveys. Laboratory chemically, the autoantibody pattern remained inconspicuous in the course, ANA, dsDNA or ENA antibodies were not detectable, antiphospholipid antibodies were also not. A complement consumption did not occur. The patient had completed training as a medical assistant, she described her quality of

life in everyday life as not significantly restricted.

15.7 Educative Answers

■ **1. What differential diagnosis do you consider for hypomimia, acrocyanosis, fingertip rarefaction and a significant movement restriction in the area of the finger joints?**

Strictly speaking, Klara's differential diagnosis is limited. A **Raynaud's phenomenon/acrocyanosis,** which is associated with a **hypomimia** and **fingertip rarefaction** in the sense of digital atrophy/ulcer formation, can be assigned to other differential diagnoses only in the area of systemic lupus erythematosus, dermatomyositis or overlap syndromes. Since Klara also had sclerodactyly with transition into the metacarpus, the diagnosis of a **limited cutaneous form of systemic scleroderma** was possible according to the new classification (Zulian et al. 2007), according to the older descriptive assessment the diagnosis was made as **CREST syndrome**. Systemic manifestations on internal organs usually do not occur without cutaneous manifestations, which is also reflected in the classification of systemic scleroderma in childhood. These organ manifestations, particularly in the area of the lung and heart, which are decisive for the long-term prognosis, must be analyzed regularly every year with sonographic, conventional radiological examinations, and lung function tests. Attention must be paid to the development of pulmonary arterial hypertension (Apitz and Girschick 2021). It usually goes hand in hand with an interstitial inflammatory lung disease or left ventricular heart involvement. Interdisciplinary, multiprofessional diagnostic and therapeutic accompaniment is urgently required.

- **2. Is the clinical description of the skin findings/clinical picture relevant for the classification/clinical categorization of scleroderma?**

The classification of a sclerodermic skin lesion into a **localized** or also called circumscribed scleroderma as opposed to a **systemic** form is of crucial importance in terms of diagnosis, therapy, and prognosis. In individual cases, however, a clear separation between these groups cannot always be achieved, or internal organ involvement can be detected, e.g., in localized scleroderma. The major criterion (systemic sclerosis) of a sclerosis located proximal to the MCP/MTP joint is also only partially applicable, as it can also occur in a localized form. Internal, "systemic" manifestations (eye/retina, vascular structures of the regional head up to meningitis and vasculitis) have been described for the "en-coup-de-sabre form" in this demarcation (Holl-Wieden et al. 2006). **Thus, localized scleroderma also requires a "systemic" diagnostic approach.** A skin biopsy can help confirm the diagnosis in individual cases. The differential diagnosis of circumscribed scleroderma is quite diverse. It ranges from an infection with *Borrelia burgdorferi*, cutaneous mastocytosis, drug reactions to various granuloma or lichen forms, lipodystrophy, scarring, myxedema, further dermal manifestations of lupus erythematosus or dermatomyositis (Kreuter et al. 2009; Zulian et al. 2019).

- **3. How do you design the laboratory diagnostics with the aim of analyzing the various forms of scleroderma as a complex autoimmune disease?**

In addition to classic inflammation parameters differential blood count, CRP, ESR, ferritin, IgG, the determination of the autoantibody pattern in patients with sclerodermic skin changes is of great importance. Both in localized and systemic scleroderma, antinuclear antibodies are present in a high percentage (42–73%), but often an assignment to nuclear structures cannot be achieved except for anti-histone antibodies in the localized linear form (Torok et al. 2019). In adults, ssDNA antibodies are reported in up to 50% (overview in Torok et al. 2019). In addition to anti-histone antibodies, rheumatoid factor-IgM is also positive in childhood in the linear localized form of the extremities, but an association with arthritis is not given. The differential diagnosis towards systemic scleroderma requires additional screening for extractable nuclear antigens (ENA)/antibodies and in particular the determination of **Anti-Centromere** (in 2–16% of patients), **Anti-Scl 70** (Anti-Topoisomerase 1) (in 20–34% of patients), Anti-Fibrillarin, **Anti-Pm-Scl** (Polymyositis-Scleroderma-Antibodies) (2–16%), Anti-Histone-Antibodies and Anti-RNA-Polymerase-(1- or 3-)Antibodies. In terms of a possible **Overlap Syndrome**, the determination of Anti-U1-RNP-Antibodies (2–16%) is important (Torok 2012). In everyday life, such an autoantibody pattern as in our patient Klara may also be completely absent. In about 20–23% of ANA-positive children with systemic scleroderma form, the subdivision of the ANA is not successful (Torok 2012).

- **4. What strategic therapeutic considerations should be taken into account, especially including target-defined therapy (Treat-to-Target) protocols?**

For *localized scleroderma* in childhood, various consensus-based treatment plans are now available. Both American and European professional societies have published their recommendations (Li et al. 2012; Zulian et al. 2019). In addition to local anti-inflammatory applications (see below), systemic immunosuppressive basic therapy with **methotrexate** and glucocorticoids can also be considered for generalized *localized form*, linear or pansclerotic forms. Whether glucocorticoids are administered orally or intravenously as a pulse depends certainly

15

on the clinical severity of the manifestation and the stage of the disease. Early use with still significant local inflammatory signs appears systemically sensible. In case of intolerance, methotrexate can be switched to mycophenolate. Local therapy includes topically applied glucocorticoids, **calcipotriol** 0.005%, **phototherapy** with ultraviolet light A1, furthermore **topical calcineurin inhibitors** (Tacrolimus 0.1%) and the immunostimulator imiquimod. The previously quite frequently used D-penicillamine or oral calcitriol for the treatment of circumscribed scleroderma are no longer recommended. Likewise, hydroxychloroquine plays a role only in overlap syndromes at best. Intravenous immunoglobulins play no role in the therapy of circumscribed scleroderma (Torok 2012; Kreuter et al. 2009; Li et al. 2012; Rabinovich 2011; Zulian et al. 2019). Recording the disease activity within a **Scleroderma Skin Damage Index** can facilitate therapy monitoring (Arkachaisri et al. 2010). With regard to the various systemic manifestations in *systemic scleroderma*, the involved organ system is at the forefront of the therapy strategy. For Raynaud's phenomenon and digital ulcers, local calcium antagonists (nifedipine) and intravenous prostanoids are used. Bosentan®, an endothelin receptor antagonist, can be used long-term for the prevention of digital ulcers. Methotrexate has proven effective in the early inflammatory swelling of diffuse cutaneous systemic scleroderma, as has mycophenolic acid. Severe courses, e.g. involving the lungs, may require a **cytotoxic therapy with cyclophosphamide**. Newer therapy strategies, such as Janus kinase (JAK) inhibitors, appear promising. Rituximab is described as a rescue therapy. Gastroesophageal reflux should be treated with antacids (Di Battista et al. 2021). Patients with pulmonary arterial hypertension can rapidly deteriorate in their overall condition, even if the symptoms are mild at the time of diagnosis (Apitz and Girschick 2021). For this, there are two approved concepts

in childhood, a phosphodiesterase-5 inhibition with sildenafil or the endothelin receptor antagonist bosentan (Apitz and Girschick 2021), also in combined use.

15.8 Summary

15.8.1 Etiology

The etiology of Pia's and Klara's scleroderma autoimmune diseases is ultimately unknown. It is assumed to be a complex disorder, primarily of the humoral immune system, with the development of measurable autoantibodies, but all areas of the immune system seem to be involved. According to recent findings, signaling pathways in the area of **Interferon-α**/Type I interferon are at least involved in plasmacytoid dendritic cells (Ghoreishi et al. 2012). A monogenetic cause is not discussed in scleroderma.

15.8.2 Pathogenesis/Clinic

The complex inflammatory disorder of the skin and subcutis, including muscles, heart, vessels, and joints, ultimately leads to severe local or systemic organ disorders, up to permanent restriction of facial expressions and movement, arthritis, heart failure, kidney failure, pulmonary arterial lung disease with pulmonary insufficiency. In the overlap with SLE, all organs can ultimately be involved in the pathogenesis (Saito et al. 2021).

15.8.3 Diagnosis

In addition to a detailed medical history and clinical examination, scleroderma-associated autoantibodies are available in laboratory chemistry: antibodies against nuclear components (ANA, ENA, dsDNA) can be helpful.

15.8.4 Therapy

According to the current CARRA/EULAR recommendations, consensus-based guidelines are available for *localized scleroderma* (Zulian et al. 2019); locally or systemically applied immunosuppressants/modulators, phototherapy with UVA1 are options. Systemic immunosuppressive therapy is sensible for severe localized, or the systemically widespread severe circumscribed course (see Pia). *Systemic scleroderma* often requires measures to improve circulation, anti-inflammatory therapy including immunosuppressants, and cytotoxic drugs (Di Battista et al. 2021). Pulmonary arterial hypertension requires consistent therapy (Apitz and Girschick 2021).

15.8.5 Diagnosis

The diagnosis is primarily based on the clinical picture of the disease, it is supported in the context of classification efforts and modern laboratory diagnostics including SAA and SLE-associated autoantibodies. In childhood and adolescence, similar to adults, the diagnosis of possibly affected organs is paramount.

15.8.6 Prophylaxis

There is no prophylaxis to prevent the disease. Attention should be paid to exacerbations of pulmonary and cardiac manifestations, possibly also in the context of viral infections. Close connection to a specialized interdisciplinary center for dermatology and autoimmunity is highly desirable.

> **Conclusion**
>
> Patients with complex autoimmune diseases require an interdisciplinary diagnostic and therapeutic approach. In the case of scleroderma, this includes rheumatology, dermatology, pulmonology, and cardiology, among others. This is flanked by intensive physiotherapy and respiratory therapy, promotion of musculoskeletal fitness, and local skin care.

References

Apitz C, Girschick H (2021) Systemic sclerosis-associated pulmonary arterial hypertension in children. Cardiovasc Diagn Ther 11:1137–1143. ▶ https://doi.org/10.21037/cdt-20-901

Arkachaisri T, Vilaiyuk S, Torok KS, Medsger TA Jr (2010) Development and initial validation of the localized scleroderma skin damage index and physician global assessment of disease damage: a proof-of-concept study. Rheumatology (Oxford) 49:373–381. ▶ https://doi.org/10.1093/rheumatology/kep361

Di Battista M, Barsotti S, Orlandi M, Lepri G, Codullo V, Della Rossa A, Guiducci S, Del Galdo F (2021) One year in review 2021: systemic sclerosis. Clin Exp Rheumatol 39(Suppl 131):3–12

Ghoreishi M, Vera Kellet C, Dutz JP (2012) Type 1 IFN-induced protein MxA and plasmacytoid dendritic cells in lesions of morphea. Exp Dermatol 21:417–419. ▶ https://doi.org/10.1111/j.1600-0625.2012.01475.x

Holl-Wieden A, Klink T, Klink J, Warmuth-Metz M, Girschick HJ (2006) Linear scleroderma 'en coup de sabre' associated with cerebral and ocular vasculitis. Scand J Rheumatol 35:402–404. ▶ https://doi.org/10.1080/03009740600556126

van den Hoogen F, Khanna D, Fransen J, Johnson SR, Baron M, Tyndall A, Matucci-Cerinic M, Naden RP, Medsger TA Jr, Carreira PE, Riemekasten G, Clements PJ, Denton CP, Distler O, Allanore Y, Furst DE, Gabrielli A, Mayes MD, van Laar JM, Seibold JR, Czirjak L, Steen VD, Inanc M, Kowal-Bielecka O, Müller-Ladner U, Valentini G, Veale DJ, Vonk MC, Walker UA, Chung L, Collier DH, Csuka ME, Fessler BJ, Guiducci S, Herrick A, Hsu VM, Jimenez S, Kahaleh B, Merkel PA, Sierakowski S, Silver RM, Simms RW, Varga J, Pope JE (2013) 2013 classification criteria for systemic sclerosis: an American College of Rheumatology/European League against Rheumatism collaborative initiative. Arthritis Rheum 65:2737–2747. ▶ https://doi.org/10.1002/art.38098

Kreuter A, Krieg T, Worm M, Wenzel J, Gambichler T, Kuhn A, Aberer E, Scharffetter-Kochanek K, Hunzelmann N (2009) AWMF guideline no. 013/066. Diagnosis and therapy of circumscribed scleroderma. J Dtsch Dermatol Ges 7(Suppl 6):S1–S14. ▶ https://doi.org/10.1111/j.1610-0387.2009.07178.x

Laxer RM, Zulian F (2006) Localized scleroderma. Curr Opin Rheumatol 18:606–613. ► https://doi.org/10.1097/01.bor.0000245727.40630.c3

Li SC, Torok KS, Pope E, Dedeoglu F, Hong S, Jacobe HT, Rabinovich CE, Laxer RM, Higgins GC, Ferguson PJ, Lasky A, Baszis K, Becker M, Campillo S, Cartwright V, Cidon M, Inman CJ, Jerath R, O'Neil KM, Vora S, Zeft A, Wallace CA, Ilowite NT, Fuhlbrigge RC (2012) Development of consensus treatment plans for juvenile localized scleroderma: a roadmap toward comparative effectiveness studies in juvenile localized scleroderma. Arthritis Care Res (Hoboken) 64:1175–1185. ► https://doi.org/10.1002/acr.21687

Rabinovich CE (2011) Challenges in the diagnosis and treatment of juvenile systemic sclerosis. Nat Rev Rheumatol 7:676–680. ► https://doi.org/10.1038/nrrheum.2011.148

Saito S, Endo Y, Nishio M, Uchiyama A, Uehara A, Toki S, Yasuda M, Ishikawa O, Muro Y, Motegi SI (2021) Anti-polymyositis/Scl antibody-positive overlap syndrome of diffuse cutaneous systemic sclerosis, dermatomyositis, systemic lupus erythematosus, and antiphospholipid syndrome. J Dermatol. ► https://doi.org/10.1111/1346-8138.16219

Stevens AM, Kanaan SB, Torok KS, Medsger TA, Mayes MD, Reveille JD, Klein-Gitelman M, Reed AM, Lee T, Li SC, Henstorf G, Luu C, Aydelotte T, Nelson JL (2016) Brief report: HLA-DRB1, DQA1, and DQB1 in juvenile-onset systemic sclerosis. Arthritis Rheumatol 68:2772–2777. ► https://doi.org/10.1002/art.39765

Stevens AM, Torok KS, Li SC, Taber SF, Lu TT, Zulian F (2019) Immunopathogenesis of juvenile systemic sclerosis. Front Immunol 10:1352. ► https://doi.org/10.3389/fimmu.2019.01352

Torok KS (2012) Pediatric scleroderma: systemic or localized forms. Pediatr Clin North Am 59:381–405. ► https://doi.org/10.1016/j.pcl.2012.03.011

Torok KS, Li SC, Jacobe HM, Taber SF, Stevens AM, Zulian F, Lu TT (2019) Immunopathogenesis of pediatric localized scleroderma. Front Immunol 10:908. ► https://doi.org/10.3389/fimmu.2019.00908

Zulian F, Woo P, Athreya BH, Laxer RM, Medsger TA Jr, Lehman TJ, Cerinic MM, Martini G, Ravelli A, Russo R, Cuttica R, de Oliveira SK, Denton CP, Cozzi F, Foeldvari I, Ruperto N (2007) The Pediatric Rheumatology European Society/American College of Rheumatology/European League against Rheumatism provisional classification criteria for juvenile systemic sclerosis. Arthritis Rheum 57:203–212. ► https://doi.org/10.1002/art.22551

Zulian F, Culpo R, Sperotto F, Anton J, Avcin T, Baildam EM, Boros C, Chaitow J, Constantin T, Kasapcopur O, Feitosa K, de Oliveira S, Pilkington CA, Russo R, Toplak N, van Royen A, Saad Magalhães C, Vastert SJ, Wulffraat NM, Foeldvari I (2019) Consensus-based recommendations for the management of juvenile localised scleroderma. Ann Rheum Dis 78:1019–1024. ► https://doi.org/10.1136/annrheumdis-2018-214697

A Feverish 7-Year-Old Turkish Girl

Christiane Reiser

Contents

16.1 Medical History

A 7-year-old patient of Turkish origin is presented for the first time with a fever up to 40 °C for one day. The fever was difficult to reduce. Other symptoms included productive cough and runny nose. The initial examination findings described a good general condition, a quiet systolic murmur, and coarse crackling sounds. In the ENT area, a reddened tongue and oral mucosa as well as rhinitis were observed. Under the suspected diagnosis of an uncomplicated respiratory infection, the patient was sent home. Two days later, the patient is presented again with the same symptoms. The fever remained high up to 40 °C.

16.2 Examination Findings

Upon admission, the child is now in a reduced general condition, lethargic without significant signs of exsiccosis. The following symptoms are noticeable: bilateral reddened conjunctivae, reddened throat, **strawberry tongue**/raspberry tongue, dry lips, discreet palmar and plantar erythema, discreet exanthema on the arms and legs, cervical lymphadenopathy, rhinitis, cough (◨ Fig. 16.1).

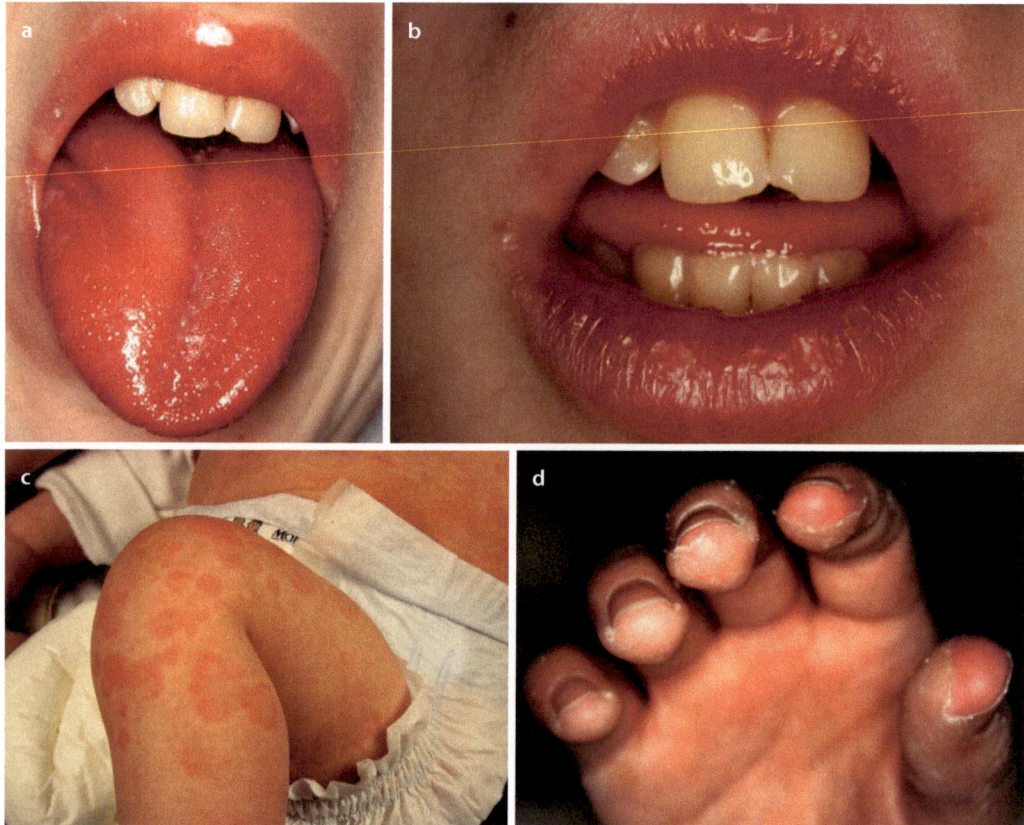

◨ **Fig. 16.1   a–d** Typical clinical findings in Kawasaki syndrome. **a, b** Lacquer lips/raspberry tongue; **c** a variant of the exanthema, here: garland-shaped, resembling erythema infectiosum; **d** skin scaling weeks after the acute stage

16

16.3 **Laboratory Values**

Laboratory values on admission: Sodium 133 mmol/l, Chloride 94 mmol/l, GOT 48 U/l, LDH 320 U/l, Albumin 3.3 g/dl, CRP 8.4 mg/dl, **ESR 39 mm/h, Ferritin 580 ng/ml.**

Blood count: Leukocytes 15,000/µl, 13% band neutrophils, 72% segmented neutrophils, 8% lymphocytes, 3% metamyelocytes.

Urine status: Leukocytes 500/µl, otherwise unremarkable.

16.4 **Educational Questions**

1. What suspected diagnosis should be considered based on the symptoms and medical history? How can a septic event be ruled out?
2. How is incomplete Kawasaki syndrome defined? What pitfalls must be considered in the diagnosis?
3. What examinations are initially or subsequently necessary to detect complications early?
4. What disease monitoring in the long term is recommended?

16.5 **Differential Diagnostic Considerations**

The differentiation of **Kawasaki syndrome (KD)** from other diseases can be challenging, especially in incomplete/atypical courses and very young children. In our case, an uncomplicated viral infection was initially assumed. With a sufficiently good general condition and short duration of illness, a blood draw was also waived or was not desired by the legal guardians. With the increasing duration of the fever and deterioration of the general condition, the need for a new presentation and further diagnostics arose. The diagnosis could thus be made in our patient on day 5.

As detailed in answers 1 and 3, the diagnosis can be challenging in individual cases. In addition to ruling out infectious causes, other inflammatory diseases can also hide behind the symptoms. In times of COVID-19, differential diagnosis must also consider a **Paediatric Inflammatory Multisystem Syndrome** (PIMS), where there are many overlaps with KD, both clinically and therapeutically.

16.6 **Further Course**

The patient was diagnosed with Kawasaki syndrome (fever, 4/5 main criteria, see Table 15.1). The initial echocardiography showed an unremarkable finding. After a single dose of immunoglobulins on day 5, the patient's fever subsided persistently. She also received acetylsalicylic acid (ASA) in the recommended dosages. The patient is assigned to risk level 1, further pediatric rheumatological and pediatric cardiological controls (after 1 week, 6 weeks, 6 months, and 12 months) were unremarkable. The therapy with ASA was discontinued after 8 weeks.

16.7 **Educational Answers**

▪ **1. What presumptive diagnosis should be considered based on the symptoms and medical history? How can a septic event be ruled out?**

The clinical findings strongly suggest the presence of Kawasaki disease (KD)/mucocutaneous lymph node syndrome (☐ Table 16.1). Important differential diagnoses include infectious diseases (various bacterial or viral pathogens, e.g., streptococci, mycoplasmas, adeno-/enteroviruses, etc.). However, the detection of a viral pathogen in particular should not directly rule out the presumptive diagnosis of Kawasaki disease, as infectious diseases can

◘ **Table 16.1** Diagnostic criteria for Kawasaki syndrome (Newburger et al. 2004): The diagnosis of KD is made in the presence of fever and 4 out of 5 criteria

5 days of therapy-resistant fever and the following criteria	
Eyes	Bilateral conjunctival injection without exudate
Mucous membrane	Redness of the oral and pharyngeal mucosa with lacquer lips, dry cracked lips, strawberry tongue
Skin	*Acute*: Edema and/or erythema of the hands and feet; *subacute*: Skin peeling of the fingers and toes, starting in the Second-Third week
	Polymorphic, mostly trunk-centered exanthema
Lymph nodes	Cervical (often unilateral) lymphadenopathy > 1.5 cm

be considered a possible trigger and are often detected. Other differential diagnoses include various inflammatory diseases, such as Stevens-Johnson syndrome, generally uncontrolled macrophage activation, or systemic JIA (Morbus Still).

Kawasaki disease is a clinical diagnosis. Laboratory diagnostics help us particularly in assessing differential diagnoses. Typical laboratory constellations in KD are as follows:

Blood count: Leukocytosis with left shift, DD septic event, therefore other values, such as procalcitonin, are rather negative in KD. Thrombocytosis: usually occurs in the course of persistent inflammation. Anemia: normocytic, as a sign of inflammation.

NT-pro-BNP: Has been identified as a parameter that can be elevated early in patients with cardiac involvement (Dahdah et al. 2009; McNeal-Davidson et al. 2012), even compared to febrile controls (Cho et al. 2011). Its promising role in the standard diagnosis of KD is being further investigated (Parthasarathy et al. 2015). In everyday life, it seems to correlate not only with cardiac stress, but also generally with the intensity of inflammation, independent of cardiac involvement.

■ **2. How is incomplete Kawasaki syndrome defined? What pitfalls must be considered in the diagnosis?**

The term "atypical" or incomplete Kawasaki syndrome encompasses the disease that is accompanied by at least 4 days of fever and *fewer* than the required four secondary criteria, so it should in principle be considered in all patients with prolonged fever and appropriate symptoms—regardless of the number. Incomplete Kawasaki syndrome should be particularly considered in infants under one year of age (see also Jakob 2016).

The diagnosis of KD is confirmed by coronary changes/aneurysms. Coronary complications often occur only after a week of illness, especially with delayed diagnosis and correspondingly late start of therapy. The ideal time to start IVIG therapy seems to be day 5—at the latest day 10 from the start of fever. Infants in the first half of life are at particularly high risk for a delayed diagnosis of KD, as their symptoms can often consist only of persistent fever and irritability. But older children also have a risk of their disease being diagnosed late. For example, sterile leukocyturia can be confused with a febrile urinary tract infection, and the rash can subsequently be confused with a drug rash. Sterile cerebrospinal fluid pleocytosis with irritability can also be "misinterpreted" as infectious meningitis, especially if antibiotic therapy has already been started. Therefore, in principle, in patients with prolonged fever, reduced general condition, and lack of response to therapies, the presence of Kawasaki syndrome should be considered from day 5 of the continua (McCrindle et al. 2017). For a detailed discussion of risk scores and stratification, we refer to the relevant textbooks on pediatric rheumatology (Dannecker and Hospach 2020). In summary, there are several risk scores that have been established for Japanese/Asian children (e.g., Kobayashi score), their transferability to European children is being discussed (e.g., Jakob et al. 2018).

- **3. What examinations are initially or subsequently necessary to detect complications early?**

Echocardiography: This is of crucial importance. If KD is suspected, the initial examination should ideally take place within the first 5–7 days, ultimately quickly, without delaying the start of therapy. Further possibly close-meshed follow-up checks are carried out depending on the findings and course.

ECG: To detect myocardial involvement, ST-segment changes and arrhythmias must be ruled out.

Sonography: Abdomen: In individual patients, gallbladder hydrops may occur. Aneurysms of the vessels originating from the aorta are rare, but are particularly described in coronary complications. Lymph nodes: Can be considered for differential diagnostic considerations and to exclude abscess formation.

Ophthalmological examination: In up to about 70% of patients, initial photophobia occurs due to conjunctivitis or uveitis (Smith et al. 1989), so an ophthalmological examination should be carried out after the

acute symptoms have subsided due to possible rare consequential damage.

Audiogram: There are some publications that describe the presence of sensorineural hearing loss in about a third of patients (Smith and Yunker 2014). Since this hearing loss can persist in some patients, an audiogram should be performed initially and after 6 weeks (Neudorf et al. 2021), to prevent restrictions in the development of children that can be caused by hearing disorders.

Cardiac catheter examination: According to the guideline (Neudorf et al. 2021), only acute myocardial ischemia is an indication for cardiac catheter examination *in the acute inflammatory phase*. In the further course, angiography is a suitable diagnostic tool especially for young children with giant aneurysms, for larger children CT angiography may also be suitable.

Cardiac MRI/(Low-dose-)CT angiography: The examinations represent good alternatives to conventional angiography, which must be performed under anesthesia and involves a high radiation exposure. Advantages of cardiac MRI are the assessability of myocardial function and distal coronary arteries. CT angiography is widely available, shows stenoses and aneurysms also in the distal coronary arteries, but has a high radiation exposure. Promising approaches exist here for low-dose CT angiography procedures (Dietz et al. 2015).

- **4. What disease monitoring in the long term is recommended?**

In the acute phase, the focus is on stabilizing the patients and ending the inflammation. The therapy recommendations for this are published, for example, in a German AWMF guideline (Neudorf et al. 2021) or also in a recommendation of the American Heart Association (Newburger et al. 2004). The latter was updated in 2017 (McCrindle et al. 2017). In the further course, the risk assessment for the individual patient is then carried out depending on the cardiac involvement. Thus, the classification into levels from 1 to 5 is carried out, with level 1 (Z-Score ≤2) describing the absence of coronary involvement and level 5 encompassing large and giant aneurysms with a Z-Score of ≥10 or absolute dilation of ≥ 8 mm. Note: The Z-Score is a mathematical size that measures the diameter of the coronary artery in relation to the body surface area and can be calculated here: ► http://parameterz.blogspot.com/2008/09/coronary-artery-z-scores.html.

16.8 Summary

16.8.1 Etiology

Kawasaki syndrome is a vasculitis of the small and medium arteries. A multifactorial event is assumed. A genetic predisposition for different therapy responses is suspected. A viral "triggering" of the disease seems possible (Rowley et al. 2008).

16.8.2 Clinic/Diagnosis

The diagnosis is made based on the criteria listed in ◻ Tab. 16.1. The diagnosis is considered certain if, in addition to the criterion of fever, at least 4 main criteria are present (Newburger et al. 2004). In this context, a detailed medical history is important, as one or more symptoms may have already disappeared at the time of admission. If only 2–3 criteria are present, a careful evaluation is needed to determine whether an incomplete Kawasaki syndrome is present. In most cases, the diagnosis is considered confirmed as soon as coronary anomalies are detected. If further appropriate findings are present (laboratory values: CRP > 3 mg/dl, anemia, thrombocytosis,

hypoalbuminemia, elevated GOT, leukocytosis, sterile leukocyturia etc.), an incomplete Kawasaki syndrome may also be present. Infants in the first half of the year of life in particular often show less than the full picture of a Kawasaki syndrome and may also have a particularly high risk of vascular and coronary anomalies due to delayed diagnosis and initiation of therapy (McCrindle et al. 2017).

In addition, a number of other symptoms can occur, which should by no means lead to the exclusion of the diagnosis. These include, among others, peribronchial infiltrates, arthralgia/arthritis, nausea/abdominal pain/vomiting/diarrhea, aseptic meningitis, and many others.

16.8.3 Diagnostic

A detailed description of the diagnostic options has already been given in question 3. In principle, the diagnosis of Kawasaki syndrome is a clinical one. Pathognomonic laboratory parameters do not exist. Typical laboratory constellations, which strongly suggest the presence of the disease, have already been discussed in question 1.

16.8.4 Therapy

Here, the therapy recommendations of the S2k guideline from 2021 (Neudorf et al. 2020, 2021) are adopted (see also ◻ Fig. 16.2): The initial therapy, which should be initiated as quickly as possible, includes a single IVIG administration (*IVIG*: Once 2 g/kg BW over 12 h) in combination with ASA (*ASA*: 30–50 mg/kg BW/day. Switch to 3–5 mg/kg BW/day after 2–3 days after defervescence). If risk factors can be identified (initial coronary involvement, age < 1 year, severe course of disease, e.g. macrophage activation syndrome, shock), *should* the initial therapy be expanded by the administration of prednisolone. In case of age > 7 years, male gender, pathological laboratory values (significantly increased inflammation parameters, liver enzyme elevation, hypoalbuminemia, anemia, hyponatremia), duration of disease until the start of therapy ≤ 4 or > 14 days *can* the administration of prednisolone be considered (Neudorf et al. 2021).

Therapy resistance: If defervescence is not achieved within 36 h after the first IVIG administration, a Second administration should then be given in combination with steroids. ASA should continue to be given at the high dose. If there is persistently no response, the therapy can be expanded to include a TNF-α blocker (e.g. infliximab), an Il-1 blocker (e.g. anakinra) or an i.v. methylprednisolone pulse over 3 days. The administration of cyclosporin A or plasmapheresis can also be considered, whereby in therapy-resistant courses, transfer to a clinic with a rheumatological and cardiological focus should be considered (Neudorf et al. 2021) (◘ Fig. 16.2).

16.8.5 **Prognosis**

Classically, the skin on the fingers and feet of the patients peels off after several weeks, starting periungually. After a few months, a Beau's line is often recognizable on the fingernails and/or toenails.

Untreated, coronary aneurysms occur in about a quarter of patients. With effective therapy options within the first 10 days from the onset of the disease, the number of these patients can be reduced to about 5% (Newburger et al. 1991; McCrindle et al. 2017).

In pregnant women with a history of KD and coronary complications, close risk management is recommended to minimize their cardiac risk.

> **Conclusion**
>
> If the disease is diagnosed and treated early, the short- and long-term outcome of the patients can be significantly improved. In persistently febrile patients who do not respond to other therapies, Kawasaki syndrome should be considered by day 5–7 at the latest.

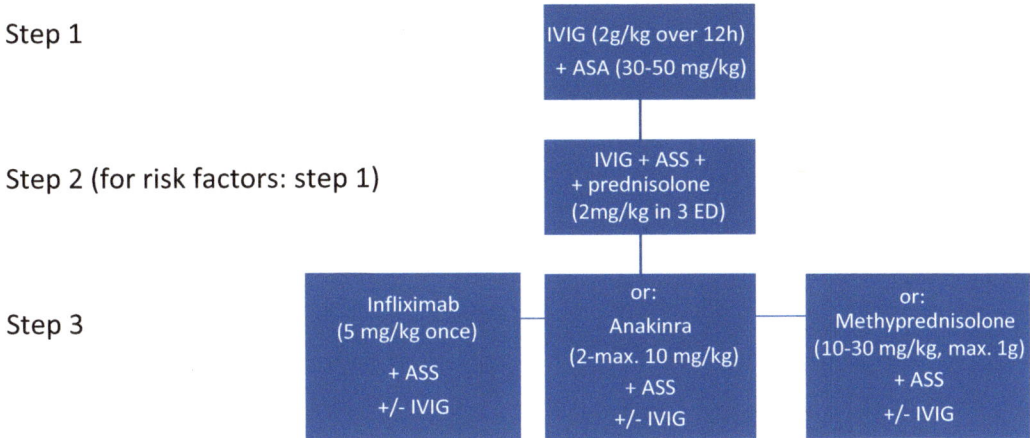

◘ **Fig. 16.2** Schematic representation of the therapy recommendations (adapted from Neudorf et al. 2020): The next therapy step is always taken if defervescence is not achieved ≥ 36 h after the end of the IVIG administration. Two IVIG administrations are considered sufficient. Therapy escalation depending on the risk factors. (See guideline)

References

Cho SY, Kim Y, Cha S-H et al (2011) Adjuvant laboratory marker of Kawasaki disease; NT-pro-BNP or hs-CRP? Ann Clin Lab Sci 41:360–363

Dahdah N, Siles A, Fournier A et al (2009) Natriuretic peptide as an adjunctive diagnostic test in the acute phase of Kawasaki disease. Pediatr Cardiol 30:810–817. ▶ https://doi.org/10.1007/s00246-009-9441-2

Dannecker G, Hospach T (2020) Kawasaki-Erkrankung. In: Wagner N, Dannecker G, Kallinich T (Eds) Pädiatrische Rheumatologie. Springer, Berlin/Heidelberg, pp 1–19

Dietz SM, Tacke CE, Kuipers IM et al (2015) Cardiovascular imaging in children and adults following Kawasaki disease. Insights Imaging 6:697–705. ▶ https://doi.org/10.1007/s13244-015-0422-0

Jakob A (2016) Kawasaki-Syndrom. Monatsschr Kinderheilkd 164:241–256. ▶ https://doi.org/10.1007/s00112-016-0048-4

Jakob A, von Kries R, Horstmann J et al (2018) Failure to predict high-risk Kawasaki disease patients in a population-based study cohort in Germany. Pediatr Infect Dis J 37:850–855. ▶ https://doi.org/10.1097/INF.0000000000001923

McCrindle BW, Rowley AH, Newburger JW et al (2017) Diagnosis, treatment, and long-term management of Kawasaki disease: a scientific statement for health professionals from the American Heart Association. Circulation 135:e927–e999. ▶ https://doi.org/10.1161/CIR.0000000000000484

McNeal-Davidson A, Fournier A, Spigelblatt L et al (2012) Value of amino-terminal pro B-natriuretic peptide in diagnosing Kawasaki disease. Pediatr Int Off J Jpn Pediatr Soc 54:627–633. ▶ https://doi.org/10.1111/j.1442-200X.2012.03609.x

Neudorf U, Jakob A, Eggert L, Hospach T (2020) S2k-Leitlinie der Deutschen Gesellschaft für Pädiatrische Kardiologie und angeborene Herzfehler e.V. ▶ https://register.awmf.org/de/leitlinien/detail/185-003

Neudorf U, Jakob A, Hospach T (2021) Kawasaki-Syndrom. Arthritis Rheum 41:358–362. ▶ https://doi.org/10.1055/a-1607-2442

Newburger JW, Takahashi M, Beiser AS et al (1991) A single intravenous infusion of gamma globulin as compared with four infusions in the treatment of acute Kawasaki syndrome. N Engl J Med 324:1633–1639. ▶ https://doi.org/10.1056/NEJM199106063242305

Newburger JW, Takahashi M, Gerber MA et al (2004) Diagnosis, treatment, and long-term management of Kawasaki disease: a statement for health professionals from the Committee on Rheumatic Fever, Endocarditis and Kawasaki Disease, Council on Cardiovascular Disease in the Young, American Heart Association. Circulation 110:2747–2771. ▶ https://doi.org/10.1161/01.CIR.0000145143.19711.78

Parthasarathy P, Agarwal A, Chawla K et al (2015) Upcoming biomarkers for the diagnosis of Kawasaki disease: a review. Clin Biochem 48:1188–1194. ▶ https://doi.org/10.1016/j.clinbiochem.2015.02.013

Rowley AH, Baker SC, Shulman ST et al (2008) RNA-containing cytoplasmic inclusion bodies in ciliated bronchial epithelium months to years after acute Kawasaki disease. PloS One 3:e1582. ▶ https://doi.org/10.1371/journal.pone.0001582

Smith KA, Yunker WK (2014) Kawasaki disease is associated with sensorineural hearing loss: a systematic review. Int J Pediatr Otorhinolaryngol 78:1216–1220. ▶ https://doi.org/10.1016/j.ijporl.2014.05.026

Smith LB, Newburger JW, Burns JC (1989) Kawasaki syndrome and the eye. Pediatr Infect Dis J 8:116–118

A Seriously Ill 15-Year-Old Girl—A Few Weeks After a Covid-19 Infection, the Fever Rises Again

Christian Huemer

Contents

17.1 Medical History

The 15-year-old girl was referred for hospital admission by her general practitioner in December 2021. The girl has had a **fever for 4 days** up to 41 °C associated with neck pain and a confluent rash emphasizing the extremities that has been present for 2 days. This led to a visit to the general practitioner and referral to the children's clinic. Inflammatory parameters carried out by the general practitioner showed a normal blood count, but a significant increase in CRP (16.8 mg/dl). An oral cephalosporin was prescribed by the general practitioner 2 days ago, but there was no sign of improvement until hospital admission. General medical history completely unremarkable, **Covid-19 infection** 4 weeks ago with a mild course (subfebrile, mild myalgia). Two other family members also had Covid infection without further sequelae. Family history unremarkable for chronic inflammatory diseases.

17.2 Examination Findings

15 $^1/_2$-year-old girl with fever (39.2 °C) in significantly reduced general condition, good nutritional status, awake, oriented and responsive on all sides. Cor: tachycardic (HR 130/min), heart sounds pure, rhythmic, unremarkable blood pressure; Pulmo vesicular on both sides, no pathological breathing sounds. Abdomen soft, no tenderness on pressure, no flank percussion pain, no defense tension. Peristalsis regularly present in all 4 quadrants. ENT findings: eardrums unremarkable on both sides, tongue heavily coated white in the front third, tonsils bland. Lymph node status: submandibular right slightly enlarged (approx. 2 cm), painless, movable lymph node. Eyes show slight conjunctivitis on both sides. Skin: macular non-itching rash, confluent lesions, blanchable, more pronounced in the area of the lower extremities. Neurological status shows no signs of meningism. Musculoskeletal status shows movement-dependent moderate arthralgia, but no evidence of synovitis.

17.3 Laboratory Values and Imaging

17.3.1 Laboratory Findings at Admission

Blood count: Leukocytes 9.8/nl, Ery 5.6 mio/ul, Hb 15 g/dl, Platelets 167/nl, differential blood count shows increased granulocytosis with slight left shift.

CRP 17 mg/dl, ESR 29 mm/h, unremarkable liver and kidney function parameters, Sodium 132 mmol/l, Chloride 94 mmol/l, LDH 284 U/l, **Ferritin 998 ng/ml**, CPK 38 U/l, **NT-proBNP 314 pg/ml (<130)**, Albumin 3.8 g/dl. Urine findings unremarkable. Coagulation findings: Quick 100%, PTT 24.9 s, Fibrinogen 594 mg/dl. Autoimmunology (ANA, ENA, dsDNA, ANCA, Rheumatoid factor, Complement factors) unremarkable. Infection serological findings (CMV, Enteroviruses, EBV): no evidence of fresh infection; Blood cultures and stool culture negative; **SARS-CoV-2 spike antibodies: 90.06 BAU/ml (<0.82)**. Pathogen direct detection (PCR panel) in nasal-pharyngeal secretions: negative.

17.3.2 Imaging

Chest X-ray unremarkable, abdominal ultrasound unremarkable. ECG and echocardiography: age-appropriate normal anatomy, tachycardia and minimal pericardial effusion are noticeable, no abnormalities in the coronary vessels.

17.4 Educational Questions

1. What differential diagnoses would you consider for this seriously ill child?
2. Do you see a connection to the anamnestic Covid-19 infection?
3. What immediate therapy would you discuss?
4. What therapeutic considerations should be taken into account, especially in the absence of controlled therapy studies in children and adolescents?

17.5 Differential Diagnostic Considerations and Educative Responses

The investigation of the highly inflammatory disease in the school child, which also presents a significant reduction in general condition, is urgent. In addition to the most important causes of infection (bacterial and viral infections), in specific histories (travel history, tampon exposure) also selected infections (e.g., malaria, toxoplasmosis, parasitic diseases, toxic shock syndrome, etc.), the differential diagnosis of a neoplastic process (leukemia, non-Hodgkin lymphoma, etc.) or an autoimmune multisystem process (collagenosis, Still's disease, systemic vasculitis, macrophage activation syndrome) is always to be worked out. After thorough examination in the clinic, laboratory, and imaging diagnostics, the girl showed no signs of a malignant process, no certain indications of collagenosis, and for an acute infection. The clear indications in the history (and laboratory) of a past **Covid-19 infection** led, after excluding the above-mentioned differential diagnoses at the time of the girl's presentation in December 2021, to consider a diagnosis that has been described worldwide in the context of the Covid-19 pandemic: **PIMS (Pediatric Inflammatory Multisystem Syndrome)**. PIMS can in individual cases phe-notypically resemble Kawasaki syndrome, the treatment recommendations in this case are accordingly based on the guidelines for the treatment of Kawasaki Syndrome with immunoglobulin therapy as the first choice of treatment. A PIMS disease without symptoms of Kawasaki syndrome would initially be treated analogously to the therapy of Kawasaki syndrome primarily with immunoglobulin therapy, followed by high-dose steroid therapy. If there are still signs of inflammation in the clinic and laboratory, an IL-1 blockade e.g., with Anakinra would be discussed (Schlapbach et al. 2021).

17.6 Further Course

Our patient presented a highly inflammatory clinical picture with fever, cutaneous, musculoskeletal, cardiac, and ocular symptoms at admission. The laboratory findings showed clearly elevated inflammatory parameters, the infectious findings showed no indications of an acute infection, but the infection serological findings clearly indicated a past Covid-19 infection. There was a moderate increase in the cardiac biomarker NT-pro-BNP, the girl was tachycardic and showed pericarditis. Due to this clinical symptomatology, the girl met the criteria of a mild PIMS with individual additional criteria of Kawasaki syndrome (conjunctivitis, exanthema, lymphadenopathy, pericarditis, see Schlapbach et al. 2021). Therefore, an initial single i.v. immunoglobulin therapy (IVIG 2 g/kg body weight single dose) supported by a low-dose aspirin therapy (3 mg/kg body weight/day p.o.) was indicated. Since febrile temperatures persisted after 48 hours and there were still mild cutaneous symptoms and tachycardia, a systemic (oral) steroid therapy (1 mg/kg body weight/day prednisolone) was administered on the 3rd day of hospital stay. A second dose of immunoglobulin was not given. As a result, rapid defervescence, normalization of inflammatory parameters by day 10 of the stay, and complete recovery by discharge on day 12. Aspirin therapy was also discontinued at discharge. Outpatient follow-up visits a few weeks after this stay showed complete remission without medication.

17.7 Summary

PIMS is a severe disease, which (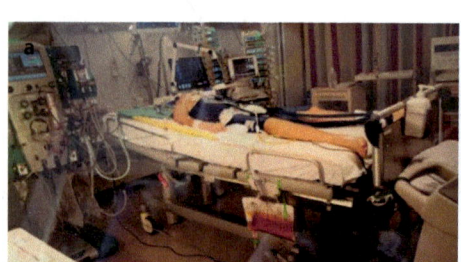 Fig. 17.1a, b) occurs as a multisystemic highly inflammatory event and has been reported worldwide in children and adolescents during the Covid-19 pandemic. It usually occurs **a few weeks after an infection with Sars-CoV-2**. The novel children's disease PIMS, first described in the UK in April 2020, does not yet have a uniform name in the professional world. The following terms are currently used synonymously:

- Pediatric Inflammatory Multisystem Syndrome (**PIMS**)
- Pediatric Inflammatory Multisystem Syndrome Temporally associated with SARS-CoV-2 (**PIMS-TS**)
- Multisystem Inflammatory Syndrome in Children (**MIS-C**)

17.7.1 Etiology and Frequency

Measured against the total coronavirus infection events among children, **PIMS is very rare**. Based on current data, it is clear that only very few infected children become ill from it. However, the exact frequency cannot be reliably quantified due to the limited data situation. Experts estimate that **one in 3000–4000 children** could be affected (Davies et al. 2020; Feldstein et al. 2020). Boys accounted for about two-thirds of the cases and are therefore more frequently affected than girls. A large part (85%) of the sick children had no pre-existing comorbidity. As the general infection events in the population increased, so did the registered PIMS cases. It is suspected that the PIMS risk depends very much on the involved virus variant. The highest risk was therefore borne by those children who were infected in the early phases of the pandemic, particularly with the wild type or the Alpha variant (Davies et al. 2020). Currently, the frequency of PIMS has drastically decreased among the Omicron variants.

17.7.2 Pathogenesis/Clinic

The main symptom of PIMS is severe **fever** that **persists for at least 2–3 days**. It usually sets in 2–8 weeks after a coronavirus infection has occurred (Goldstein et al. 2005; Carter et al. 2021).

In addition, the following symptoms may occur with PIMS:

- Vomiting, nausea, diarrhea and/or abdominal pain
- (Bilateral) Conjunctivitis

 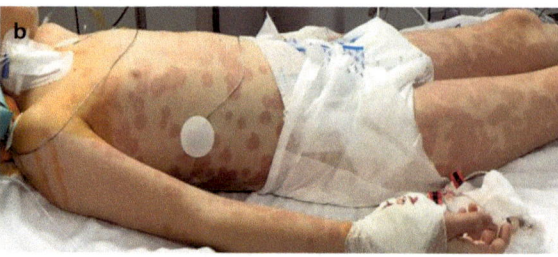

□ Fig. 17.1   a, b PIMS in clinical impression. Intensive care patient with PIMS and typical skin efflorescences in PIMS. (With kind permission of PD Dr. A. Skrabl, Medical University of Graz)

- Mucocutaneous lesions (maculopapular exanthema)
- Lymphadenopathy
- Cardiac symptoms (tachycardia, serositis, myocarditis)
- Neurological symptoms (cephalea, feeling of weakness, sensory disturbances and/or concentration difficulties)
- Hepatopathy
- Thromboses

17.7.3 Diagnosis

For the diagnosis of PIMS, physicians have defined precise characteristics that make up the inflammatory syndrome. Accordingly, it is present if the following criteria are met (so-called case definition of the World Health Organization, WHO 2020):
- Children and adolescents up to and including 19 years,
- proven or probable Sars-CoV-2 infection due to risk contacts,
- Fever for at least 3 days

and at least two of the following criteria:
- Skin rash (exanthema) or bilateral, non-purulent conjunctivitis or inflammations on the *skin* or mucous membrane,
- Low blood pressure (arterial hypotonia) or *shock,*
- Heart involvement (myocardial dysfunction), *pericarditis* (pericarditis), valvulitis or *coronary heart disease* (CHD; coronary pathologies),
- Coagulopathy,
- Acute gastrointestinal problems (diarrhea, vomiting, abdominal pain, suspected appendicitis)

and
- Abnormalities in the blood count (lymphopenia, neutrophilia)
- Increased inflammation values (increased *CRP*, increased procalcitonin, increased ESR, increased ferritin).

17.7.4 Therapy

The therapy management of PIMS requires an unconditional step-by-step interdisciplinary approach: Doctors from different pediatric subspecialties—such as infectious diseases, rheumatology, cardiology and pediatric intensive care—are primarily to be involved in order to achieve a rapid diagnosis and initiation of therapy. Many children and adolescents with PIMS meet the criteria for intensive care and should therefore be admitted to a pediatric intensive care unit where sufficient monitoring conditions exist. In addition to intensive medical care (for example, ventilation etc.), three strategies are generally applied for PIMS therapy:
- Administration of anti-inflammatory and immunomodulatory drugs,
- Administration of anticoagulant drugs (Goldenberg et al. 2020),
- Administration of accompanying medications (circulatory stabilization) (Alsaied 2021).

The immunomodulatory therapy of PIMS is based on therapy guidelines for the treatment of already established autoinflammatory syndromes and systemic vasculitides, such as the **Macrophage Activation Syndrome** and Kawasaki Syndrome. The best-practice recommendations published so far by numerous authors for the treatment of PIMS aim at a rapid anti-inflammatory treatment and achieving a rapid clinical response as well as reduction of inflammation parameters (Ouldali et al. 2021; Schlapbach et al. 2021). As initial therapy, intravenous immunoglobulin therapy (2 g/kg body weight as a single dose) and also aspirin accompanying therapy (3-5 mg/kg body weight/day p.o.) are recommended for confirmed PIMS, analogous to the therapy guidelines for Kawasaki Syndrome. If the response is insufficient or if there are clear indications for coronary artery aneurysms, high risk for IVIG resistance and very young patients (< 1 year), additional treatment with systemic steroids (prednisolone 2 mg/kg body weight/day) is recommended (Henderson et al. 2020). For PIMS patients who do not respond sufficiently to this initial therapy, the use of biologicals (Anakinra, Tocilizumab) is described in a few case reports and cohort studies (Whittaker et al. 2020; Mehta et al. 2020; Fouriki et al. 2020). In the recently available guidelines, the initiation of an initial intravenous Anakinra therapy is therefore suggested as a further therapeutic step (Schlapbach et al. 2021; Whittaker et al. 2020).

Conclusion

In children and adolescents with a multisystemic disease after a COVID-19 infection, there is an autoinflammatory process similar to a systemic JIA or Kawasaki Syndrome. Recognizing and treating this serious disease quickly based on precise medical history and clinical findings is potentially of vital interest to the affected patients.

References

Carter MJ, Shankar-Hari M, Tibby SM (2021) Paediatric inflammatory multisystem syndrome temporally-associated with SARS-CoV-2 infection: an overview. Intensive Care Med 47:90–93

Davies P, Evans C, Kanthimathinathan HK (2020) Intensive care admissions of children with paediatric inflammatory multisystem syndrome temporally associated with SARS-CoV-2 (PIMS-TS) in the UK: am multicentre observational study. Lancet Child Adolesc Health 4:669–677

Feldstein LR, Rose EB, Horwitz SM (2020) Multisystem inflammatory syndrome in U.S. children and adolescents. N Engl J Med 383:334–346

Fouriki A, Fougere Y, De Camaret C, Blanchard Rohner G, Grazioli S, Wagner N et al (2020) Case report: case series of children with multisystem inflammatory syndrome following SARS-CoV-2 infection in Switzerland. Front Pediatr 8:594127. ► https://doi.org/10.3389/fped.2020.594127

Goldenberg NA, Sochet A, Albisetti M, Biss T, Bonduel M, Jaffray J (2020) Consensus-based clinical recommendations and research priorities for anticoagulant thromboprophylaxis in children hospitalized for COVID-19-related illness. J Thromb Haemost 18:3099–3105

Goldstein B, Giroir B, Randolph A (2005) International pediatric sepsis consensus conference: definitions for sepsis and organ dysfunction in pediatrics. Pediatr Crit Care Med 6:2–8

Henderson LA, Canna SV, Friedman KG, Gorelik M, Lapidus SK, Bassiri H et al (2020) American College of Rheumatology clinical guidance for multisystem inflammatory syndrome in children associated with SARS-CoV 2 and hyperinflammation in pediatric COVID-19: version 1. Arthritis Rheumatol 72:1791–1805

Licciardi F, Pruccoli G, Denina M (2020) SARS-CoV-2-induced Kawasaki-like hyperinflammatory syndrome: a novel COVID phenotype in children. Pediatrics 146(2):e20201711. ► https://doi.org/10.1542/peds.2020-1711

Mehta P, Cron RQ, Hartwell J, Manson JJ, Tattersall RS (2020) Silencing the cytokine storm: the use of intravenous anakinra in haeomophagocytic lymphohistiocytosis of macrophage activation syndrome. Lancet Rheumatol 2:358–367

Ouldali N, Toubiana J, Antona D, Javouhey E, Madhi F, Lorrot M (2021) Association of intravenous immunoglobulins plus methylprednisolone vs immunoglobulins alone with course of fever in multisystem inflammatory syndrome in children. JAMA 325:855–864

Schlapbach LJ, Andre MC, Grazioli S, Schöbi N, Ritz N, Aebi C, Agyemn P, Albisetti M, Bailey DGN, Berger C et al (2021) Best practice recommendations for the diagnosis and management of children with pediatric inflammatory multisystem syndrome temporally associated with SARS-CoV-2 in Switzerland. Front Pediatr 9:1–14

Whittaker E, Bamford A, Kenny J, Kaforou M, Jones CE, Shah P (2020) Clinical characteristics of 58 children with a pediatric inflammatory multisystem syndrome temporally associated with SARS-CoV-2. JAMA 324:259–269

World Health Organisation (2020) Multisystem inflammatory syndromes in children and adolescents with COVID-19. ► https://www.who.Int/news-room/commentaries/detail/multisystm-inflammatory-syndrome-in-children-and-adolescents-with-covid-19. 11.12.2022

A 7-Year-Old Patient with Gastroenteritis and Petechiae

Christiane Reiser

Contents

18.1 Medical History

A 7-year-old patient was presented in the emergency room in the early evening with abdominal pain, vomiting, and diarrhea for 4 days, lack of fluid intake, and additionally isolated pinpoint "spots" on both lower legs since the morning. The parents report that the patient has also had a fever up to 39 °C for 2 days.

18.2 Examination Findings

7-year-old patient in reduced general condition and normal nutritional status, moderate dehydration. Isolated raised **hemorrhages** on both lower legs. **Pain in the left ankle** during pronation and extension, no passive movement restriction, no swelling. Abdomen soft, but universally tender to pressure. No neck stiffness, negative Lasègue sign. Blood pressure age-appropriate (◘ Fig. 18.1a, b).

18.3 Laboratory Values and Imaging

18.3.1 Initial Laboratory Values

Laboratory: Leukocytes: 12.3 G/L, CRP 1.8 mg/dl. Coagulation: Quick, PTT, fibrinogen normal. Other overview values (kidney, liver, bone) within the normal range.

ABG: pH 7.24, BE –8.

18.3.2 Imaging

Sonography of the ankles: unremarkable, no evidence of joint effusion or arthritis.

18.4 Further Course

The patient was admitted for parenteral rehydration. After a few days, there was a significant improvement in the general condition and discharge with the diagnosis of

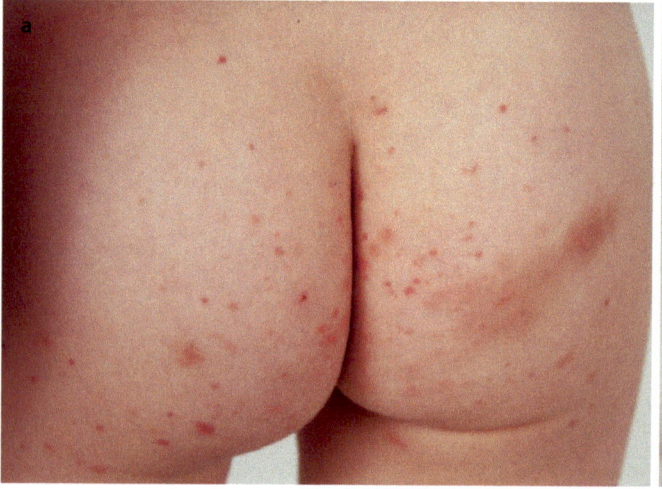

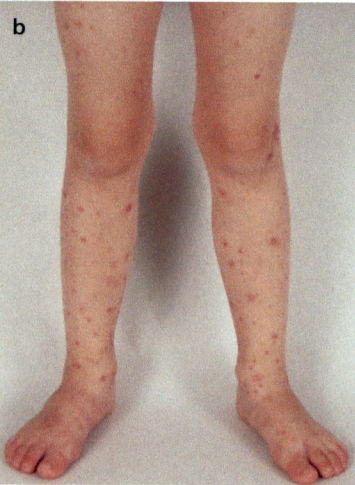

◘ **Fig. 18.1** **a, b** Skin findings of the patient. Palpable purpura on the pelvis and lower extremity

Campylobacter enteritis with accompanying vasculitis/arthralgia.

Stool diagnostics: Occult blood in stool: positive. *Stool culture:* Detection of Campylobacter jejuni.

After 4 days, the patient was readmitted. The clinical examination now showed a **palpable purpura** in the gluteal area and in the area of the lower extremity (◘ Fig. 18.1a, b), as well as **eyelid edema** and **arthritis** of the ankles. The blood pressure was 125/93 mmHg (95th percentile: 111/71)

Laboratory: *Blood count:* Leukocytes 15,300/μl, normochromic, normocytic anemia with **Hb 9.8 g/dl,** Platelets 496,000/μl. Normal values for electrolytes, liver function parameters, creatinine, complement. Iron status: Normal values for ferritin. Transferrin 193 mg/dl (normal value 200–360); Transferrin saturation 8% (normal value 18–51%). Protein 5.8 g/dl (normal value 6.4–8.3). **Albumin 2.4 g/dl** (normal value 3.5–5.2). CRP 2.0 mg/dl (normal value < 0.5)

Urine diagnostics: Urine strip: **Ketone +++,** specific gravity 1005, protein ++, erythrocytes +++++. Sediment: Leukocytes 40/μl, **Ery 703/μl.** 24-hour urine collection: Protein/creatinine ratio 1.93 g/g. Protein excretion in urine 0.71 g/24 h; 0.70 g/l.

The diagnosis of **Henoch-Schönlein purpura** (HSP) is made with involvement of the skin, joints, abdomen, and kidneys. In addition to the ACE inhibitor to control hypertension, the patient receives ibuprofen and prednisolone (1.5 mg/kg body weight/day). Under this treatment, rapid normalization of blood pressure and disappearance of eyelid edema. The gastrointestinal as well as the joint and skin symptoms completely disappear over time. A persistent microhematuria and mild proteinuria can still be detected over 4 weeks, until these also no longer occur in the following checks.

18.5 Educational Questions

1. What tentative diagnosis should be considered based on the symptoms? How do you assess the petechiae/the purpura? What differential diagnoses are you considering?
2. What criteria are used to make the diagnosis?
3. What diagnostic and therapeutic steps should be initiated? How often are checks required?
4. What is the prognosis of nephritis?

18.6 Educational Answers

▪ **1. What tentative diagnosis should be considered based on the symptoms? How do you assess the petechiae? What differential diagnoses are you considering?**

Initially, the picture of gastroenteritis is evident, with corresponding pathogen detection in the course. The patient already shows a slight acidosis with increased BE as an indication of exsiccosis. The petechiae are noticeable from the beginning, which is also important for differential diagnostic considerations, as is the painful ankle joint.

Petechiae: The causes of petechiae are diverse and can be roughly divided into 3 groups: disturbance of the platelets (number or function), disturbance of the plasmatic coagulation, and vasopathy (Elling et al. 2012). In the present case, overview values to exclude thrombocytopenia and coagulation disorder were at least inconspicuous. The most likely cause of the purpura initially appeared to be accompanying vasculitis/capillaritis. Clinically, there was no evidence of sepsis with accompanying skin hemorrhages/septic pathogen spread.

Arthralgia/Arthritis: e.g., reactive in infectious gastroenteritis. If there are indications of an acute bacterial-septic joint inflammation, further diagnostic steps must be initiated immediately.

Differential diagnostic considerations: At the initial presentation, the patient's reduced general condition was striking, which does not necessarily fit the classic presentation of HSP. Here, other causes such as sepsis, disseminated intravascular coagulation (DIC), possibly also malignancy (leukemia clarification is in the foreground) or hemolytic-uremic syndrome (HUS) must be sought using infectious disease clarification and coagulation diagnostics (Hospach and Huppertz 2013).

■ **2. What criteria are used to make the diagnosis?**

Purpura Schönlein-Henoch is usually a clinical diagnosis in pediatrics (Huppertz 2006). The international classification criteria of 2010 (Ozen et al. 2010) require as the main criterion the **Purpura**—or **Thrombocytopenia-*in*dependent petechiae**—at a classic location (lower extremity, buttock region) (◘ Fig. 18.1). The secondary criteria (at least one is required) include abdominal pain, positive histopathology with evidence of leukocytoclastic vasculitis and/or **glomerulonephritis** with IgA deposits, as well as arthritis/arthralgia and the (clinical) renal involvement.

Our patient met the required criteria for the diagnosis of HSP (palpable purpura, abdominal pain, arthralgia, mild renal involvement). Rather atypical—and therefore well compatible with the diagnosis of gastroenteritis—was the high-fever onset of the disease and the reduced general condition, which is why the differential diagnoses had to be clarified. The positive pathogen detection supported the diagnosis of Campylobacter enteritis. Possibly triggered by this infection, the skin findings and renal involvement developed into the classic picture of Purpura Schönlein-Henoch.

■ **3. What diagnostic and therapeutic steps should be initiated? How often are checks required?**

Purpura: Here, primary therapy is not necessary. A skin biopsy should only be considered after prolonged persistence and diagnostic uncertainty.

Arthritis/Arthralgia: Here, the start of therapy with NSAID is recommended (e.g., Ibuprofen 30 mg/kg body weight/day in 3 doses). Clinical follow-up checks every 2–3 days in the acute phase are recommended (Hospach and Huppertz 2013).

Gastrointestinal manifestations: The exclusion of intussusception as a complication of the disease is essential, especially in smaller children with corresponding symptoms. For the treatment of abdominal pain and gastrointestinal complications (bleeding), steroid therapy is initiated (Prednisolone 1–2 mg/kg body weight/day [possibly higher dosed] over 1–2 weeks) (Pohl 2014). These shorten the duration and intensity of abdominal pain, but have little or no influence on the development of nephritis (Dudley et al. 2013).

Kidney involvement: Here, early contact with a pediatric nephrology is recommended for coordination. A kidney biopsy is recommended for a large **proteinuria** or for impaired kidney function (Society for Pediatric Nephrology GPN et al. 2013). The therapy is interdisciplinary with a methylprednisolone pulse (max. 30 mg/kg body weight/day, max. 1 g over 3 days) followed by oral steroids in a tapering dose over 12 weeks. Depending on the severity of the nephropathy, other immunosuppressants (including cyclosporine A, mycophenolate mofetil, cyclophosphamide, etc.) may be considered.

In the case of a small proteinuria (< 2 g/g creatinine) that persists for over 6 weeks, the start of therapy with an ACE inhibitor or angiotensin II antagonist is recommended (Hospach and Klaus 2013). The

18

publication of the new S2k guideline for Purpura Schönlein-Henoch with updated recommendations is expected in 2022.

If no kidney biopsy is required and there is no arterial hypertension, it is recommended to monitor the patient once a week on an outpatient basis over the first month in case of persistent hematuria/proteinuria, then once a month for the next 5 months (Hospach and Huppertz 2013).

Uncomplicated course/checks: In the case of an uncomplicated course, outpatient checks including blood pressure, urine every 3-4 days in the first month are indicated, then once a month for another 5 months. In any form of kidney involvement, checks (also possible at home) over 5 years. Women who have had HSP have an increased risk of renewed kidney involvement during pregnancy, so pregnant women should be regularly checked for blood pressure and urine (Hospach and Huppertz 2013).

- **4. What is the prognosis of nephritis?**
Approximately half of the children with HSP develop nephritis, which usually goes along with minor micro-/hematuria and heals without consequences. In about 12% of cases, however, HSP leads to chronic courses, with 1-2% of **chronic terminal renal insufficiency** HSP is found as the cause (Calviño et al. 2001; Society for Pediatric Nephrology GPN et al. 2013).

18.7 Summary

18.7.1 Etiology

The etiology of HSP is not fully understood to this day. A connection with pathogens such as streptococci and parvoviruses or a "triggering" by medications is discussed. HSP is the most common vasculitis in childhood and affects the small vessels.

A genetic predisposition is suspected, it is already known that there is an increased occurrence in patients with familial Mediterranean fever (FMF) (Ozdogan et al. 1997). An association with certain HLA characteristics is also likely.

18.7.2 Pathophysiology

The exact pathophysiology of the disease is unclear. In principle, there are **IgA antibody complex-**deposits, which form through antigen presentations (e.g., infection-mediated). These deposits in the walls of small vessels lead to a cytokine-mediated inflammatory reaction with different effects depending on the location of the vessels (skin: palpable purpura, gastrointestinal tract: erosions/hemorrhage, kidney: e.g., proliferative glomerulonephritis) (Saulsbury 2001).

18.7.3 Diagnosis/Clinic

The presentation of Henoch-Schönlein purpura can vary greatly. The vasculitis of the skin in the form of palpable purpura, particularly of the lower extremity, is a mandatory criterion. In addition to joint involvement in the form of arthralgia/arthritis, severe, colicky abdominal pain may occur, as well as kidney involvement of varying severity in 40% of cases (Saulsbury 2007). Other gastrointestinal complications include **bleeding** and **intussusception.** In the case of groin pain, testicular involvement should be considered. Very rarely, neurological (e.g., seizures, paresis) or ocular complications (anterior uveitis) occur, which should lead to further differential diagnostic considerations.

According to the diagnostic criteria for Henoch-Schönlein purpura according to EULAR/PRINTO/PRES from 2010 (◘ Tab. 18.1), the diagnosis is considered confirmed if the main criterion is present,

◻ **Tab. 18.1** Diagnostic criteria for Henoch-Schönlein purpura according to EULAR/PRINTO/PRES. (Ozen et al. 2010)

Criteria	Explanation
Purpura (main criterion)	Mostly palpable, independent of thrombocytopenia, particularly affecting the lower extremity
Abdominal pain	Diffuse pain, acute onset, colicky
Histopathology	Typical leukocytoclastic vasculitis and/or glomerulonephritis with IgA immune complex deposits
Arthritis/Arthralgias	Arthritis: acute onset of painful joint swelling with limited mobility Arthralgia: acute onset of joint pain without swelling or limited mobility
Nephritis	Proteinuria > 0.3 g/24 h or > 30 mmol/mg albumin/creatinine ratio in morning urine Hematuria or erythrocyte casts (>5/field of view) or erythrocytes 2 + positive in urine dipstick

as well as at least one secondary criterion (sensitivity 100%, specificity 87%) (Ozen et al. 2010).

18.7.4 Diagnostics

The disease is usually a clinical diagnosis. However, further diagnostics are necessary to assess the severity of accompanying symptoms/complications. In particular, the extent of kidney involvement hardly correlates with the extrarenal symptoms (Pohl 2014).

18.7.5 Therapy

The therapy for extrarenal symptoms depends on their severity. Arthritis is treated with nonsteroidal anti-inflammatory drugs. Severe abdominal pain or gastrointestinal complications are additionally treated with steroids, as these can shorten the duration of symptoms.

18.7.6 Prognosis

In 30% of cases, there is a recurring occurrence of gastrointestinal and skin symptoms, which usually disappear completely within a few months (Saulsbury 2007). The prognosis of kidney involvement depends on the severity of the nephritis, in very rare cases (1–2%) resulting in terminal kidney failure.

Conclusion

Henoch-Schönlein purpura is essentially a benign, self-limiting disease. Regular monitoring of blood pressure and urine is necessary to detect and treat severe courses of nephritis early.

References

Calviño MC, Llorca J, García-Porrúa C et al (2001) Henoch-Schönlein purpura in children from northwestern Spain: a 20-year epidemiologic and clinical study. Medicine (Baltimore) 80:279–290. ▶ https://doi.org/10.1097/00005792-200109000-00001

Dudley J, Smith G, Llewelyn-Edwards A et al (2013) Randomised, double-blind, placebo-controlled trial to determine whether steroids reduce the incidence and severity of nephropathy in Henoch-Schonlein Purpura (HSP). Arch Dis Child 98:756–763. ▶ https://doi.org/10.1136/archdischild-2013-303642

Elling R, Hufnagel M, Henneke P (2012) Infektionsassoziierte Hautblutungen. Monatsschr Kinderheilkd 160:545–555. ▶ https://doi.org/10.1007/s00112-012-2633-5

Gesellschaft für Pädiatrische Nephrologie (GPN), Pohl M, Dittrich K et al (2013) Behandlung der Purpura-Schönlein-Henoch-Nephritis bei Kindern und Jugendlichen: Therapieempfehlungen der Gesellschaft für Pädiatrische Nephrologie (GPN). Monatsschr Kinderheilkd 161:543–553. ▶ https://doi.org/10.1007/s00112-013-2896-5

Hospach A, Huppertz HI (2013) Handlungsempfehlung nach der Leitlinie „Purpura Schönlein-Henoch". Monatsschr Kinderheilkd 161:738–739. ▶ https://doi.org/10.1007/s00112-013-2924-5

Hospach T, Klaus G (2013) Leitlinie der Gesellschaft für Kinder- und Jugendrheumatologie und der Deutschen Gesellschaft für Kinderheilkunde und Jugendmedizin. Purpura Schönlein-Henoch. AWMF-Leitline

Huppertz H-I (2006) Purpura Schönlein-Henoch. Monatsschr Kinderheilkd 154:865–871. ▶ https://doi.org/10.1007/s00112-006-1393-5

Ozdogan H, Arisoy N, Kasapçapur O et al (1997) Vasculitis in familial Mediterranean fever. J Rheumatol 24:323–327

Ozen S, Pistorio A, Iusan SM et al (2010) EULAR/PRINTO/PRES criteria for Henoch-Schönlein purpura, childhood polyarteritis nodosa, childhood Wegener granulomatosis and childhood Takayasu arteritis: Ankara 2008. Part II: Final classification criteria. Ann Rheum Dis 69:798–806. ▶ https://doi.org/10.1136/ard.2009.116657

Pohl M (2014) Purpura Schönlein-Henoch im Kindesalter. Monatsschr Kinderheilkd 162:917–925. ▶ https://doi.org/10.1007/s00112-014-3233-3

Saulsbury FT (2001) Henoch-Schönlein purpura. Curr Opin Rheumatol 13:35–40. ▶ https://doi.org/10.1097/00002281-200101000-00006

Saulsbury FT (2007) Clinical update: Henoch-Schönlein purpura. Lancet Lond Engl 369:976–978. ▶ https://doi.org/10.1016/S0140-6736(07)60474-7

An 11-Year-Old Patient After Stem Cell Transplantation with Head and Chest Pain

Christiane Reiser

Contents

The original version of the contribution was published under: Reiser C, Kurringer A, Lawitschka A, et al (2018) Takayasu arteritis of childhood after allogeneic stem cell transplantation in hyper-IgE syndrome with evidence of a NOD2 mutation. Arthritis Rheuma 38:363–366. ▶ https://doi.org/10.1055/s-0038-1675730.

19.1 Medical History

An 11-year-old boy from Chechnya presented himself during a routine check-up with increasing **chest and headaches** for several weeks. The patient was diagnosed with a **Hyper-IgE syndrome** (DOCK8 mutation. OMIM: #243700) in early childhood due to severe cutaneous inflammations, aggravated by severe stomatitis, therapy-resistant candidiasis, and chronic otitis. Since his younger sister suffered from the same disease and had been successfully stem cell transplanted, the same allogeneic stem cell transplantation (SCT) was decided for our patient. The SCT was successful, and the patient was cured of his primary disease. The immunosuppressive therapy with Cyclosporin A could be stopped 1.5 years later.

19.2 Examination Findings

No abnormalities were observed in the pediatric-internal examination findings. However, the patient was lethargic, frequently in pain, and appeared ill. The blood pressure values were normal without blood pressure difference. The pulses of the A. radialis were not documented. Due to the medical history and severe complaints, imaging was performed using echocardiography, CT, and CT angiography of the lung, MR, and MR angiography.

19.3 Laboratory Values and Imaging

19.3.1 Laboratory Values

19

CRP: 2.4 mg/dl (normal value < 0.5), ESR: 23 mm/h, unremarkable values for electrolytes, kidney and liver function parameters. Coagulation overview values unremarkable. Autoimmunology: **ANA positive**, c-ANCA not assessable, ENA negative, **Rheumatoid factor positive**.

Calprotectin in serum: 5500 ng/ml (normal up to 4137); S100A12 145 ng/ml (normal values 19–157).

19.3.2 Educational Questions—Part 1

1. What suspected diagnosis should be considered based on the symptoms and medical history?
2. With which examination do we start?

19.3.3 Imaging

In the performed diagnostics (echocardiography, MR angiography of the skull and abdomen, CT angiography of the lungs), the image of a **vasculitis of the ascending aorta and thoracic and abdominal aorta**, the superior mesenteric artery, and the bilateral parietooccipital arteries and superior parietal arteries in the sense of a **Takayasu arteritis (c-TA)** (◘ Fig. 19.1, CT angiography 4 months after diagnosis).

19.3.4 Educational Questions—Part 2

1. What are the acute and long-term therapeutic options?
2. What complications of Takayasu arteritis should be expected?
3. What disease monitoring is recommended?

19.4 Further Course

The patient was started on Rituximab therapy due to increased B-cell activity (IgG), which led to a severe allergic reaction requiring intensive care. Under **Tocilizumab**

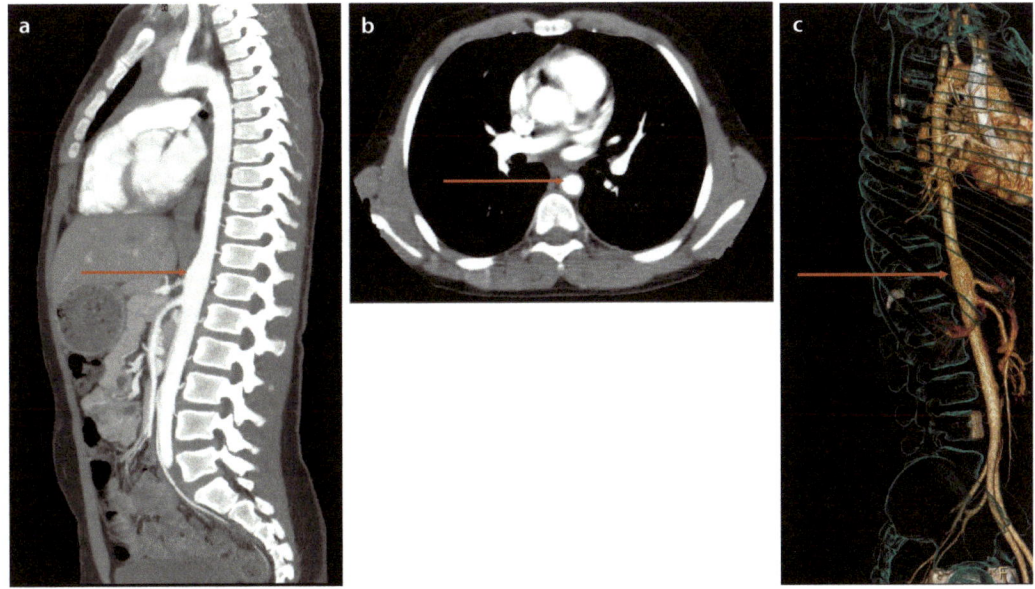

■ **Fig. 19.1   a–c Imaging studies in suspected Takayasu vasculitis. a** Sagittal MIP CT angiography: Wall-thickened thoracic aorta and superior mesenteric artery. The abdominal aorta is short-distance expanded suprarenally. **b** CT angiography axial: Circularly wall-thickened thoracic aorta. **c** CT angiography: Focally expanded suprarenal abdominal aorta. (The images were kindly provided by Primar Dr. A. Schuster, Landeskrankenhaus Bregenz. Original publication: Reiser et al. 2018 ©Thieme)

in combination with steroids (Prednisolone in varying doses, max. 1 mg/kg body weight/day), the patient was quickly symptom-free clinically, but radiologically there was a progression of vasculitic activity, so a change was made again, now to Infliximab in combination with MTX. Initially, the change was accompanied by Methylprednisolone pulse therapies (1 g/day), the oral steroids were tapered off over months. The patient now receives Infliximab (8 mg/kg body weight) every 4 weeks, MTX was discontinued due to intolerance. In the radiological follow-up examinations, no further progression of the disease was seen even after the steroid therapy was discontinued. As a complication, the patient developed arterial hypertension after long-term steroid therapy—a vasculitis-related renal artery stenosis could be ruled out.

In the meantime, we have detected a **NOD2**/CARD15 mutation in exon 4 in the patient's monocytes and his mother's, which has not been described before. Mutations in this gene have particular relevance in Crohn's disease and Early-onset Sarcoidosis (EOS) and lead to changes in NF-κB, which in turn can lead to increased secretion of interleukin-1 and interleukin-18 through regulation of the inflammasome. In our patient, there are no further clinical symptoms of Crohn's disease or EOS after allogeneic stem cell transplantation.

Furthermore, it has been reported that polymorphisms in this gene can lead to an increased occurrence of Graft-versus-Host Disease (GvHD) (Hyvärinen et al. 2017). Further investigations are to follow to further assess the clinical relevance of this finding.

19.5 Differential Diagnostic Considerations

The classic symptoms of Takayasu arteritis include pain (head/chest/abdomen), symptoms of organ/extremity hypoperfusion, blood pressure difference, and especially a **loss of pulse**.

The combination of vasculitis with B symptoms (fever, weight loss, possibly night sweats) also leads to the consideration of oncological differential diagnoses (including leukemias and lymphomas). Imaging, possibly PET-CT, provides further clarity here. Our patient did not present because of his pain, the investigation of his complaints—headaches, recurrent respiratory infections—was carried out as part of the follow-up after SCT. The initial computed tomography of the paranasal sinuses revealed a ventilation disorder and briefly directed the suspected diagnosis towards infectious issues—the patient was considered unvaccinated, immunosuppressed, and immunodeficient. The increase in complaints (especially head and chest pain) then led to further imaging.

19.6 Educative Answers

- **1. What suspected diagnosis should be considered based on the symptoms and medical history?**

The range of differential diagnoses is wide given the nonspecific symptoms. However, the severity of the complaints was striking. The narrower differential diagnostic considerations include intracerebral hemorrhage, space-occupying processes, neoplasms, affection of the esophagus/gastrointestinal tract by erosive or ulcerative changes in **Graft-versus-Host Disease** (GvHD). A chronic infection (e.g., EBV, CMV) could also explain the corresponding symptoms (Ayuk et al. 2016).

- **2. With which examination do we start?**

The answer depends on the patient's condition. Since the symptoms had been present for some time and were being investigated as part of a routine examination, it is understandable that after the usual laboratory diagnostics including coagulation parameters, an MR angiography (head, abdomen) or CT angiography of the lungs was quickly initiated.

- **3. What are the acute and long-term therapeutic options?**

The rapid, early initiation of immunosuppressive therapy is required for c-TA, but is often delayed due to the nonspecific symptoms at the beginning of the disease and the resulting delayed diagnosis. Controlled studies on the therapy of c-TA are lacking due to the rarity of the disease. Therefore, the current recommendations for the therapy of large vessel vasculitis also have low evidence (Maz et al. 2021). A systematic review, which included over 400 pediatric patients with TA, showed that the primary therapy consists of the administration of **glucocorticoids**, followed by classic DMARDs such as methotrexate, cyclophosphamide, azathioprine, and mycophenolate mofetil (Sener et al. 2021). In addition, the literature shows an increasing use of biologics, especially **TNF-α blockers**, and **Tocilizumab** (Nakaoka et al. 2020; Sener et al. 2021). After starting steroid therapy, tapering is often difficult. In the cohort of Aeschlimann (Aeschlimann et al. 2017) with 27 patients, it was shown on the one hand that flare-ups regularly occur even under continued steroid therapy. On the other hand, it was shown here that flare-ups occurred significantly less frequently under therapy with biologics (infliximab, adalimumab, tocilizumab) compared to the group of conventional immunosuppressants. According to other reports, good results were achieved in small case series with conventional immu-

19

nosuppressants, such as cyclophosphamide for induction and maintenance therapy with MTX (Ozen et al. 2007). In addition, anticoagulation with acetylsalicylic acid 2 mg/kg body weight/day, possibly in combination with a second anticoagulant (interdisciplinary consultation), can be carried out (de Graeff et al. 2019). Stem cell transplantation represents an alternative for biologic-resistant courses of autoimmune diseases, corresponding registry data are available (Laurent et al. 2020). In particular, the graft-versus-host autoimmune effect is to be used in allogeneic SCT to achieve a "re-education" of the immune system (Snowden et al. 2012). The option of autologous stem cell transplantation is discussed in the literature (Daikeler et al. 2007).

■ **4. What complications of Takayasu arteritis can be expected?**

The main complications described in the literature include arterial hypertension and myocarditis. Classic neurological complications in childhood are—analogous to our patient—headaches and dizziness; in about 20% of the affected adult TA patients, a **stroke** occurs (Hoffmann et al. 2000).

■ **5. What disease monitoring is recommended?**

The only validated score for determining clinical disease activity in vasculitis is the **PVAS** (Pediatric Vasculitis Activity Score), which, however, has deficits in large vessel vasculitis (Dolezalova et al. 2013). In clinical routine, the combination of CRP and ESR are still chosen for laboratory chemical monitoring of disease activity, although both parameters can be within the normal range despite increased disease activity, especially under therapy with tocilizumab (Tombetti et al. 2021). Interleukin-6 in serum appears to be a promising new biomarker here (note: tocilizumab naturally limits measurability), in addition, there are a number of other new biomarkers that could potentially contribute useful

parameters for measuring disease activity, such as matrix metalloproteinase (MMP)-9 and pentraxin-3 (PTX-3), but these are only conditionally available in routine diagnostics (Dagna et al. 2011; Sun et al. 2012).

Therefore, radiological diagnostics still have a very high value, especially the **MR angiography** is considered the most important examination method in pediatrics due to its good availability and lack of radiation exposure. In the representation of vascular wall irregularities, MRA is superior to conventional angiography. However, due to the high sensitivity of MRA, the degree of stenosis can be overinterpreted.

CT angiography is similar in its informative value to MRA, wall thickening and calcifications can typically be displayed. However, due to the excessive radiation exposure, it only represents a limited diagnostic option in childhood.

19.7 Summary

19.7.1 Etiology

Takayasu arteritis is an extremely rare disease in pediatric rheumatology with a total incidence in the population reported to be between 1.2–2.6/1000,000/year (Hall et al. 1985; Reinhold-Keller et al. 2005). The etiology is unclear, recently described were, in addition to the known **HLA-B52 association**, some "suspicious" HLA and non-HLA gene loci (Ortiz-Fernández et al. 2021). Also in the case described here, it remains unclear whether the vasculitis can be explained as a GvHD or has a genetic component.

19.7.2 Clinic

The clinical picture in our patient was nonspecific and in Takayasu arteritis depends on the location of the inflammation. In the present case, the upper sections of the aorta including the cerebral vessels were also affected, which explains the head and chest pain. In addition, one would expect, for example, a blood pressure difference in the arms or the absence of pulses at a wrist. Cerebral symptoms from syncope to stroke are also described. If the abdominal aorta is affected, a large number of pediatric patients develop renal hypertension. Complex further symptoms e.g. consistent with a GvHD after allogeneic SCT did not occur.

19.7.3 Diagnosis

Inflammatory values can be nonspecifically elevated, especially during flares of the disease. This is very individual. Specific autoantibodies are usually not found. Conventional angiography, CT/or especially also for follow-up examinations in children, MR angiography is the most frequently used diagnostic method for visualizing vasculitis.

19.7.4 Therapy

As already explained above and as our case shows, the therapy of Takayasu arteritis poses a challenge for the treating physicians. In addition to the immunosuppressive options discussed above, anticoagulation is also required in some cases. Rarely in pediatrics, vascular surgical procedures such as percutaneous transluminal angioplasty are performed with good results in adult medicine (Dong et al. 2019).

Conclusion

With this case, we would like to present the very rare case of Takayasu arteritis in pediatric rheumatology, which occurred after stem cell transplantation in severe hyper-IgE syndrome. In our estimation, this represents an extremely rare coincidence of two rare immunological dis-

eases. Possibly the detected mutation in the **NOD2 gene** is pathogenetically relevant and can provide further insights in the future (see also the case reports on sarcoidosis and Blau syndrome).

A fundamental challenge in the therapy of c-TA is, in addition to the selection of immunosuppressive medication, the assessment of disease activity and the resulting question of the need for escalation. Due to the rarity of the disease, randomized studies are lacking that would facilitate a standardized approach both in terms of monitoring and induction of therapy and maintenance therapy (Reiser et al. 2018).

References

Aeschlimann FA, Eng SWM, Sheikh S et al (2017) Childhood Takayasu arteritis: disease course and response to therapy. Arthritis Res Ther 19:255. ▶ https://doi.org/10.1186/s13075-017-1452-4

Ayuk F, Bug G, et al (2016) Langzeitnachsorge nach Stammzelltransplantation aus: Leitlinien zur allogenen Stammzelltransplantation von der Deutschen Arbeitsgemeinschaft für Knochenmark- und Blutstammzelltransplantation (DAG-KBT). Kapitel 11

Dagna L, Salvo F, Tiraboschi M et al (2011) Pentraxin-3 as a marker of disease activity in Takayasu arteritis. Ann Intern Med 155:425–433. ▶ https://doi.org/10.7326/0003-4819-155-7-201110040-00005

Daikeler T, Kötter I, Bocelli Tyndall C et al (2007) Haematopoietic stem cell transplantation for vasculitis including Behcet's disease and polychondritis: a retrospective analysis of patients recorded in the European Bone Marrow Transplantation and European League Against Rheumatism databases and a review of the literature. Ann Rheum Dis 66:202–207. ▶ https://doi.org/10.1136/ard.2006.056630

Dolezalova P, Price-Kuehne FE, Özen S et al (2013) Disease activity assessment in childhood vasculitis: development and preliminary validation of the Paediatric Vasculitis Activity Score (PVAS). Ann Rheum Dis 72:1628–1633. ▶ https://doi.org/10.1136/annrheumdis-2012-202111

Dong H, Chen Y, Xiong H-L et al (2019) Endovascular treatment of iliac artery stenosis caused by Takayasu arteritis: a 10-year experience. J Endovasc Ther Off J Int Soc Endovasc Spec 26:810–815. ► https://doi.org/10.1177/1526602819874474

de Graeff N, Groot N, Brogan P et al (2019) European consensus-based recommendations for the diagnosis and treatment of rare paediatric vasculitides—the SHARE initiative. Rheumatol Oxf Engl 58:656–671. ► https://doi.org/10.1093/rheumatology/key322

Hall S, Barr W, Lie JT et al (1985) Takayasu arteritis. A study of 32 North American patients. Medicine (Baltimore) 64:89–99

Hoffmann M, Corr P, Robbs J (2000) Cerebrovascular findings in Takayasu disease. J Neuroimaging Off J Am Soc Neuroimaging 10:84–90. ► https://doi.org/10.1111/jon200010284

Hyvärinen K, Ritari J, Koskela S et al (2017) Genetic polymorphism related to monocyte-macrophage function is associated with graft-versus-host disease. Sci Rep 7:15666. ► https://doi.org/10.1038/s41598-017-15915-3

Laurent C, Marjanovic Z, Ricard L et al (2020) Autologous hematopoietic stem cell transplantation with reduced-intensity conditioning regimens in refractory Takayasu arteritis: a retrospective multicenter case-series from the Autoimmune Diseases Working Party (ADWP) of the European Society for Blood and Marrow Transplantation (EBMT). Bone Marrow Transplant 55:2109–2113. ► https://doi.org/10.1038/s41409-020-0907-4

Maz M, Chung SA, Abril A et al (2021) American College of Rheumatology/Vasculitis Foundation Guideline for the management of giant cell arteritis and Takayasu arteritis. Arthritis Rheum. ► https://doi.org/10.1002/art.41774

Nakaoka Y, Isobe M, Tanaka Y et al (2020) Long-term efficacy and safety of tocilizumab in refractory Takayasu arteritis: final results of the randomized controlled phase 3 TAKT study. Rheumatol Oxf Engl 59:2427–2434. ► https://doi.org/10.1093/rheumatology/kez630

Ortiz-Fernández L, Saruhan-Direskeneli G, Alibaz-Oner F et al (2021) Identification of susceptibility loci for Takayasu arteritis through a large multi-ancestral genome-wide association study. Am J Hum Genet 108:84–99. ► https://doi.org/10.1016/j.ajhg.2020.11.014

Ozen S, Duzova A, Bakkaloglu A et al (2007) Takayasu arteritis in children: preliminary experience with cyclophosphamide induction and corticosteroids followed by methotrexate. J Pediatr 150:72–76. ► https://doi.org/10.1016/j.jpeds.2006.10.059

Reinhold-Keller E, Herlyn K, Wagner-Bastmeyer R, Gross WL (2005) Stable incidence of primary systemic vasculitides over five years: results from the German vasculitis register. Arthritis Rheum 53:93–99. ► https://doi.org/10.1002/art.20928

Reiser C, Kurringer A, Lawitschka A et al (2018) Takayasu-Arteriitis des Kindesalters nach allogener Stammzelltransplantation bei Hyper-IgE-Syndrom mit Nachweis einer NOD2-Mutation. Arthritis Rheum 38:363–366. ► https://doi.org/10.1055/s-0038-1675730

Sener S, Basaran O, Ozen S (2021) Wind of change in the treatment of childhood-onset Takayasu arteritis: a systematic review. Curr Rheumatol Rep 23:68. ► https://doi.org/10.1007/s11926-021-01032-8

Snowden JA, Saccardi R, Allez M et al (2012) Haematopoietic SCT in severe autoimmune diseases: updated guidelines of the European Group for Blood and Marrow Transplantation. Bone Marrow Transplant 47:770–790. ► https://doi.org/10.1038/bmt.2011.185

Sun Y, Ma L, Yan F et al (2012) MMP-9 and IL-6 are potential biomarkers for disease activity in Takayasu's arteritis. Int J Cardiol 156:236–238. ► https://doi.org/10.1016/j.ijcard.2012.01.035

Tombetti E, Hysa E, Mason JC et al (2021) Blood biomarkers for monitoring and prognosis of large vessel vasculitides. Curr Rheumatol Rep 23:17. ► https://doi.org/10.1007/s11926-021-00980-5

Much More than just a Blocked Nose

Annette Holl-Wieden

Contents

20.1 Medical History

Zoe, 15 9/12 years old, had been experiencing recurring frontal **headaches**, **restricted nasal breathing**, and increased **fatigue** and **lethargy** for 2 months.

Suspecting rhinosinusitis, an initial oral antibiotic treatment with Cefaclor and a treatment with decongestant nasal drops were administered, but the symptoms did not improve. Consequently, the girl was presented at an ear, nose, and throat (ENT) clinic. A computed tomography (CT) scan of the paranasal sinuses was performed, which showed a pronounced mucosal swelling of the right-sided **paranasal sinuses** (◘ Fig. 20.1). After insufficient improvement through an oral antibiotic treatment with Clarithromycin and an intravenous antibiotic treatment with Ampicillin/Sulbactam, as well as multiple doses of systemic steroids, the indication for a paranasal sinus operation was given. An infundibulotomy was performed on both sides, as well

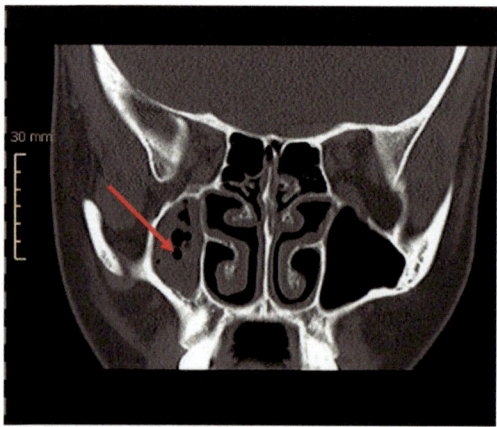

◘ **Fig. 20.1   Zoe's CT scan of the paranasal sinuses at the onset of symptoms.** It shows an almost complete shadowing of the right maxillary sinus. (With kind permission from Dr. Clemens Benoit, Institute for Diagnostic and Interventional Radiology, University Hospital Würzburg)

as a removal of the concha bullosa and an enlargement of the maxillary sinus ostia. Particularly on the right side, polypous tissue and pus could be removed from the anterior ethmoid. Histologically, an extensive **granulomatous, chronic florid inflammation** with numerous giant cells was found, and **atypical mycobacteria** were detected by PCR. Subsequently, she was referred to our clinic for further investigation. The parents reported that Zoe had been suffering from cough, subfebrile temperatures, severe fatigue, and night sweats for 2 weeks, and had lost about 3 kg in weight. No foreign travel was reported, and contact with patients with a tuberculosis infection was denied.

20.2 Examination Findings

The clinical examination showed a 15 9/12 year old girl, in a reduced general condition and very slender nutritional status. She had a pale skin color, and appeared tired. Her body weight was 37.3 kg, 4 kg below the 3rd percentile, and her body length was 159 cm, on the 20th percentile. The auscultation of the lungs revealed a slightly **weakened breath sound** on the right basolateral, no rattling sounds. The rest of the internal and neurological examination was unremarkable.

20.3 Labor Values and Imaging

20.3.1 Labor Values

The inflammation parameters were elevated, **CRP 8.2 mg/dl** (normal value 0–0.5), **ESR at room temperature 67 mm/h, at 4 °C 87 mm/h.** The blood count was unremarkable except for a slight thrombocytosis (platelets 540,000/µl, normal value 150–450,000).

The overview laboratory values, especially liver values, kidney values, uric acid, LDH, CK showed no abnormalities. Complement (C3/C4) was not reduced, the immunoglobulins (IgA, IgM and IgG) were within the normal range. A urine examination (particle count, total protein/creatinine ratio) was unremarkable.

20.3.2 Imaging

A chest X-ray showed a cavity in the lower field on the right.

An **MRI of the chest** revealed an approximately 5 cm diameter **cavity** on the right basolateral with a wall thickness of up to 1.6 cm, possibly another cavity in the right lung apex as well as additional **focal, T2-hyperintense lesions bilaterally in the lungs** and a bihilar lymphadenopathy. The written report stated: Overall, there is an urgent suspicion of tuberculosis. The MRI extended to the head and neck area showed **polypoid mucosal swellings** with fluid accumulation in the **maxillary sinuses,** in the **sphenoid sinus** and in the **ethmoidal cells** as well as the **mastoid cells** on both sides. A chest CT confirmed the findings obtained in the chest MRI (◘ Fig. 20.2).

20.4 Educational Questions

1. What suspected diagnosis should be made based on the complaints that have been present for several weeks (fatigue, headaches, impaired nasal breathing, cough, elevated temperatures, night sweats, weight loss)?
2. What suspected diagnoses are possible based on the biopsy results from the paranasal sinus mucosa and the lung imaging?
3. What therapy should be carried out?

20.5 Differential Diagnostic Considerations

Differentially, in the case of complaints lasting for weeks with fatigue, headaches, impaired nasal breathing, cough, elevated temperatures, a **rhinosinusitis,** possibly also complications such as an **intracranial abscess** and a **sinus vein thrombosis** must be considered. A cranial MRI showed polypoid mucosal swellings with fluid accumulations in the paranasal sinuses consistent with chronic rhinosinusitis, an abscess or thrombosis could be ruled out. A virus-induced rhinosinusitis is unlikely due to the long course, severe symptoms and high inflammation values. Unusual for bacterial rhinosinusitis is the non-response to several antibiotic therapies. In patients with certain pre-existing conditions such as cystic fibrosis, ciliary dysfunction or immune defects, rare pathogens such as *Pseudomonas aeruginosa* or **fungi** like *Aspergillus species* must be considered. However, there was no evidence of these pre-existing conditions in Zoe, and these pathogens were not detected in the microbiological examination. Allergies were also not known. Due to fatigue, night sweats, weight loss, elevated temperatures, a **malignant disease** such as a lymphoma must also be considered. Blood values and imaging did not give an urgent suspicion of this. The ENT doctors performed a paranasal sinus operation to improve the secretion drainage and ventilation of the paranasal sinuses. The biopsy of the paranasal sinus mucosa and the histological and microbiological examination were important. Based on the histological findings with evidence of a granulomatous inflammation and detection of atypical mycobacteria in the PCR as well as the imaging of the lungs carried out in the course with evidence of round foci and cavities, the suspicion of an infection with **Mycobacteria** posed. However, rhinosinusitis caused

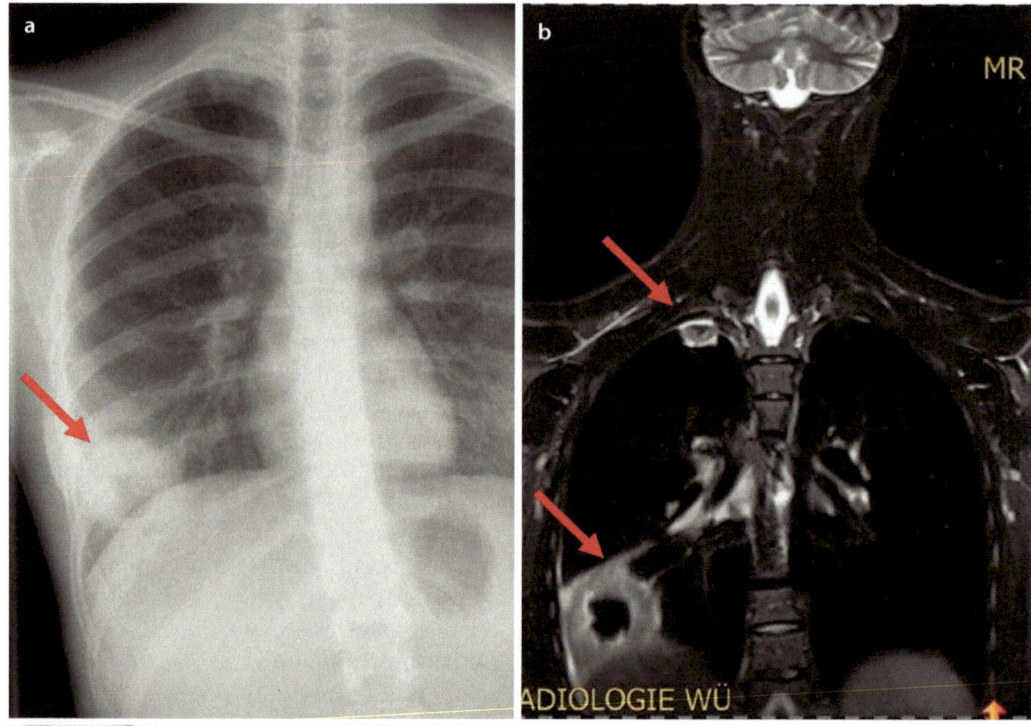

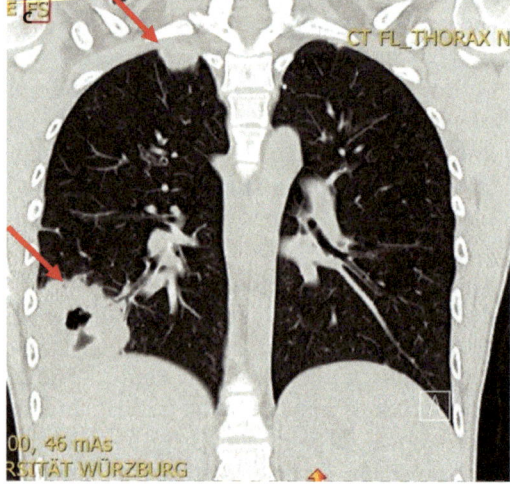

■ **Fig. 20.2   a Chest X-ray.** It shows a cavity in the lower field on the right. **b Chest MRI:** It confirms a cavity on the right basolateral, diameter approx. 5 cm, wall thickness up to 1.6 cm, and showed another cavity in the right lung apex. **c Chest CT:** It also revealed an air-filled cavity in segment VIII as well as a consolidation with a questionable cavity in the right lung apex. (With kind permission from Dr. Clemens Benoit, Institute for Diagnostic and Interventional Radiology, University Hospital Würzburg)

20

by mycobacteria is very rare. Serologically, there was no indication of a **pulmonary echinococcosis**, which must also be included in the differential diagnostic considerations given the imaging findings. In the presence of general symptoms, organ manifestations, and elevated inflammation values, the existence of a **systemic vasculitis** must also be considered. Symptoms of the upper and lower respiratory tract, the histological evidence of a granulomatous inflammation, and round foci and cavities detected in the lung imaging are suggestive of a **Granulomatosis with Polyangiitis (GPA)** (Ozen et al. 2010) (◘ Tab. 20.1). ANCA testing should be carried out as quickly as possible.

20.6 Further Course

Initially, investigations were carried out to rule out an infection with mycobacteria. A tuberculin skin test and a tuberculosis ELISpot (**Enzyme-linked Immunospot**) were negative. A **laryngo-tracheo-bronchoscopy** showed a vulnerable, erythematous altered mucosa in the right and left bronchial system, which bled easily on contact. In addition, several granulomatous, whitish changes were seen in the main bronchi. Two microbiopsies were taken from the granulomatous changes in the right main bronchus. Histologically, a chronic inflammation was found. The altered biopsy material contained no vessels, granulomas and giant cells were not detected. In the microbiological examination of the **bronchial lavage**, no acid-fast rods, no DNA of mycobacteria from the tuberculosis complex, no atypical mycobacterial DNA were detected. The mycobacterial

◘ **Tab. 20.1**   EULAR/PRINTO/PReS classification criteria for Granulomatosis with Polyangiitis (GPA). (Mod. after Ozen et al. 2010)

	Criteria	Glossary	Sensitivity (%)	Specification (%)
1.	Histopathology	Granulomatous inflammation in the wall of an artery or in the perivascular or extravascular area	54	99.6
2.	Upper respiratory tract involvement	Chronic purulent or bloody nasal discharge or recurrent epistaxis/crusts/granulomas	83	99
		Nasal septum perforation or saddle nose Chronic or recurrent sinusitis		
3.	Laryngo-Tracheo-Bronchial involvement	Subglottic, tracheal or bronchial stenoses	22	99.8
4.	Lung involvement	X-ray or CT showing the presence of nodules, caverns or solid infiltrates	78	92
5.	ANCA	ANCA positivity by immunofluorescence or by ELISA (MPO/p or PR3/c-ANCA)	93	90
6.	Renal involvement	Proteinuria > 0.3 g/24 h or > 30 mmol/mg albumin/creatinine ratio in morning urine	65	69.6
		Hematuria: > 5 erythrocytes/high power field or		
		Erythrocyte casts in urinary sediment or ≥ 2+ on strip test		
		Necrotizing Pauci-Immune Glomerulonephritis		

At least 3 of the 6 criteria must be met

culture was sterile. The *Aspergillus* antigen ELISA was also negative, *Aspergillus* DNA and *Pneumocystis jiroveci* DNA were not detectable. No growth of fungi and bacteria was seen in the culture. The investigations therefore provided no evidence of tuberculosis or an infection by atypical mycobacteria. The detection of atypical mycobacterial DNA in the biopsy of the nasal mucosa was classified as "physiological colonization".

Due to the urgent suspicion of granulomatosis with polyangiitis (GPA), the ANCAs were quickly determined. In immunofluorescence, **c-ANCA** were found (1:2560, normal value < 1:40). In the ELISA, **PR3-ANCA** were detected (PR3-ANCA 86 U/ml, normal value < 3.5 U/ml), no MPO-ANCA. The antinuclear antibodies (ANA) were negative. According to the **EULAR/PRINTO/PReS classification criteria**, the criteria for GPA were met. Three out of six criteria must be met (Ozen et al. 2010) (◖ Tab. 20.1). Although histological evidence of vasculitis was not obtained, the suspected diagnosis of GPA could thus be made. Extensive diagnostics ruled out further organ manifestations. As **remission induction**, a therapy with **glucocorticoids (GC)** and **Rituximab** was initiated. Zoe received a **methylprednisolone pulse therapy** on three consecutive days (1 g/day, corresponding to 27 mg/kg BW/day) and then a therapy with **prednisolone orally** (1 mg/kg BW/day) with gradual reduction. Rituximab was administered four times at intervals of one week (375 mg/m² BSA, corresponding to 500 mg as a single dose). In addition, a therapy with **Trimethoprim**-Sulfamethoxazole (TMS) was carried out for 3 months for the prophylaxis of **Pneumocystis jiroveci pneumonia (PJP)**. Under the therapy, there was a rapid improvement in the general condition, the patient had no more fever, no cough. The inflammation values were rapidly decreasing. However, the patient still had a strongly crusted nasal mucosa. Regular visits to the ENT clinic for nasal care with loosening of the crusts/scabs were still

necessary. In the course of time, the patient developed a **perforation of the nasal septum** as well as a sinking of the nasal bridge, a so-called **saddle nose**. As a prophylaxis against recurrence, a therapy with **MTX** was started 3 months after the last Rituximab administration. A CT thorax at this time showed a significant regression of the pulmonary lesions, the formerly large cavity in the right lower lobe now appeared as a consolidated residue. The medication with prednisolone was further reduced in the course.

6 months after diagnosis, Zoe developed a small **relapse**. The ENT examination showed continued strong crust formation, but also an increasing swelling of the nasal mucosa. A CT of the paranasal sinuses revealed a mucosal swelling of both maxillary sinuses with slight residual ventilation, a partial obstruction of the ethmoidal cells as well as a perforation of the anterior nasal septum and also new osseous discontinuities of the posterior septum parts. The inflammation values were not increased this time. For remission induction, a therapy with Rituximab and a short-term increase of prednisolone orally was carried out again. It would also have been possible to try only a sole increase of the GC. Since the patient had already developed a pronounced Cushing's symptomatology, this option was not considered for us. The therapy with prednisolone was quickly reduced in the course and ended 12 months after the initial diagnosis. Today, 2 years after the relapse, Zoe is in remission under the therapy with MTX. The saddle nose is slightly pronounced, the patient does not want to have a surgical correction.

20.7 Educational Answers

■ **1. What suspected diagnosis should be made based on the complaints that have been present for several weeks?**

Based on the complaints that have been present for several weeks (fatigue, headaches, restricted nasal breathing, cough, elevated temperatures, night sweats, weight loss), a differential diagnosis of rhinosinusitis possibly with complications such as an abscess or sinus vein thrombosis must be considered. Rhinosinusitis with rare pathogens such as *Pseudomonas aeruginosa* or fungi, as well as a malignant disease such as lymphoma, must also be ruled out. Consideration should already be given to GPA and relevant diagnostics should be carried out. This includes in particular the determination of ANCA.

- **2. What suspected diagnoses are possible based on the biopsy results from the paranasal sinus mucosa and the lung imaging?**

After receiving the biopsy results from the paranasal sinus showing evidence of a granulomatous inflammation and the lung imaging showing nodules and caverns, an infection with mycobacteria must be ruled out. The organ manifestations involving the upper and lower respiratory tract, the evidence of a granulomatous inflammation in the biopsy, and the lung imaging showing nodules and caverns make granulomatosis with polyangiitis very likely.

- **3. What therapy should be initiated?**

Once a diagnosis of GPA has been made, therapy must be initiated as quickly as possible. Initially, therapy for remission induction and then for remission maintenance must be carried out. Therapy with glucocorticoids and rituximab can be used for remission induction.

20.8 Summary

20.8.1 Background/Definition/ Classification Criteria

Systemic vasculitides comprise a group of diseases in which there are inflammations of the blood vessel walls and subsequent ischemia and necrosis of the tissue. According to the revised **Chapel-Hill-Consensus-Conference(CHCC)-nomenclature of vasculitides from 2012**, systemic vasculitides are primarily classified according to vessel size. According to this nomenclature, AAVs are defined as necrotizing vasculitides with few or no immune deposits, which mainly affect small blood vessels (i.e., capillaries, venules, arterioles, and small arteries) and are associated with the presence of **ANCA (antineutrophil cytoplasmic antibodies)** directed against **myeloperoxidase (MPO)** or **proteinase 3 (PR3)**. The AAVs include granulomatosis with polyangiitis (GPA, formerly Wegener's granulomatosis), microscopic polyangiitis (MPA), and eosinophilic granulomatosis with polyangiitis (EGPA, formerly Churg-Strauss syndrome) (Calatroni et al. 2017). The classification criteria of the **American College of Rheumatology (ACR)** for 7 systemic vasculitides in adults were developed in **1990**, including for GPA and EGPA (Calatroni et al. 2017). In 2010, the **EULAR/PRINTO/PReS classification criteria** for 4 systemic vasculitides in children, including GPA, were published (Ozen et al. 2010) (◘ Tab. 20.1). There is also the **Watts classification algorithm for AAV**, which allows patients to be classified by exclusion criteria. The European Medicines Agency (EMA) found this helpful for classifying GPA and MPA in children (Calatroni et al. 2017). Recently (2022), the **new ACR/EULAR classification criteria** for 5 systemic vasculitides, including GPA, EGPA, and MPA, were published (Robson et al. 2022; Suppiah et al. 2022; Grayson et al. 2022). The aim of classification criteria should be to form disease groups in order to conduct controlled regional studies, among other things. There are no diagnostic criteria for AAV. However, the classification criteria can be helpful for diagnosis. AAV in children is very rare. GPA is the most common form of AAV in children, followed by MPA and EGPA (Cabral et al. 2016).

20.8.2 Pathogenesis

The pathogenesis is incompletely understood. Genetic factors, environmental factors, and disturbances of the innate and acquired immune systems appear to contribute to the development of the disease (Calatroni et al. 2017).

20.8.3 Clinic

In ANCA-associated vasculitides, multiple organs are usually affected, but there are also localized forms in just one organ. The largest pediatric patient registry is the **AR-ChiVe Registry (A Registry for Children with Vasculitis).** In a study by Cabral et al., clinical findings from 183 patients with GPA and 48 patients with MPA from the AR-ChiVe Registry were examined (Cabral et al. 2016). In GPA and MPA, **general symptoms** such as fatigue, fever, weight loss were common (in GPA 88%, in MPA 85%). In GPA and MPA, kidney involvement was often found (in GPA 83%, in MPO 75%). Histopathologically, a **pauci-immune glomerulonephritis** was usually found (94%). In GPA, **lung involvement** was common, this was somewhat less common in MPO (in GPA 74%, in MPA 44%). In imaging, the most common findings in GPA were **round foci, fixed pulmonary infiltrates,** and **cavities.** For GPA, a **ENT involvement** is characteristic (in GPA 70%). In MPA, ENT involvement usually does not occur. Typical findings are recurrent nosebleeds, blocked nasal breathing, nasal crusts, nasal ulcers, sinusitis, otitis, mastoiditis, oral ulcers or granulomas, hearing disorders, **nasal septum perforations, saddle nose, subglottic tracheal stenosis.** Other findings in GPA and MPA were gastrointestinal symptoms, musculoskeletal complaints, manifestations on skin, eye, CNS and heart/vessels (Cabral et al. 2016). EGPA in children is rare. There are only a

few case reports or small case series. Like adults, children often have asthma, eosinophilia, sinusitis, nasal polyps, and lung infiltrates (Calatroni et al. 2017).

20.8.4 Diagnosis

The **inflammatory parameters** (CRP, ESR) are usually elevated. The ANCAs often provide the decisive diagnostic clue due to their high sensitivity and specificity. ANCA testing should be performed not only by immunofluorescence but also by ELISA. ANCA with a cytoplasmic pattern in immunofluorescence (**c-ANCA**) are usually **PR3-ANCA,** ANCA with a perinuclear pattern in immunofluorescence (**p-ANCA**) are usually **MPO-ANCA.** PR3-ANCA are usually associated with GPA. MPO-ANCA are more common in patients with MPA or EGPA. As in adults, there are also children with AAV who do not have ANCAs. A histological confirmation of the diagnosis by a biopsy of clinically affected organs should be sought (Calatroni et al. 2017). To assess disease activity, the pediatric vasculitis activity score (**Paediatric Vasculitis Activity Score,** PVAS) should be used. It is based on the Birmingham Vasculitis Activity Score V3 (BVAS V3) for adults and has been modified for children (Calatroni et al. 2017).

20.8.5 Therapy

AAV can progress rapidly and lead to organ-threatening or life-threatening complications within a short time. Therefore, a rapidly initiated effective therapy is crucial. There are no major randomized controlled studies for the therapy of AAV in children. The therapy is based on data from adults and also follows the recommendations for adults. There are, among others, the CanVasc recommendations, the EULAR/ERA-

EDTA recommendations, and the ACR/VF Guidelines (Mendel et al. 2021; Yates et al. 2016; Chung et al. 2021). There are now also expert recommendations for AAV in children, the **SHARE recommendations** and the **CARRA treatment protocols** (de Graeff et al. 2019; Morishita et al. 2022). The treatment of AAV is divided into the very intensive **remission induction** (duration 3–6 months) and the less intensive **remission maintenance** (duration 2–4 years). A remission induction with **cyclophosphamide** and high doses of **glucocorticoids (GC)** were long considered the gold standard of therapy for AAV. Studies conducted in adults (RITUXVAS and RAVE study) have shown that therapy with **rituximab** is not inferior to therapy with cyclophosphamide (Lee et al. 2019). Compared to cyclophosphamide, rituximab does not impair fertility and has a lower malignancy risk. According to the CARRA treatment protocols for children, rituximab is listed as an alternative to cyclophosphamide for remission induction (Morishita et al. 2022). For the duration of remission induction, therapy with **trimethoprim-sulfamethoxazole (TMS)** is recommended for the prophylaxis of *Pneumocystis jiroveci* pneumonia (PJP) and other bacterial infections (de Graeff et al. 2019). The benefit of **plasmapheresis** in severe cases, such as rapidly progressing kidney disease or severe lung bleeding, is not proven and should only be considered in individual cases with severe progression (Mendel et al. 2021). The optimal dosage and duration of GC is controversially discussed, and the dosage recommendations of GC in the various treatment recommendations are different. For **remission maintenance**, various therapy options are listed in the treatment recommendations. In the CARRA treatment protocols for children, therapy with **rituximab** or alternatively therapy with **MTX** or **azathioprine** is suggested (Morishita et al. 2022).

20.8.6 Prognosis

The prognosis depends on the severity of organ involvement. Lung involvement can be life-threatening in the case of **alveolar bleeding**. One of the most severe long-term complications is **dialysis** and **kidney transplantation** in the case of kidney involvement. Large multicenter studies are necessary to make statements about the prognosis in children (Calatroni et al. 2017).

Conclusion

Systemic vasculitides are rare. Nevertheless, they must be included in the differential diagnostic considerations in cases of unclear organ manifestations and unclearly elevated inflammation parameters. This is particularly true when multiple organs are involved, but it is also necessary when only one organ is affected. As the case shows, GPA must be considered in the case of persistent rhinosinusitis and high inflammation parameters for weeks, and appropriate diagnostics must be carried out.

References

Cabral DA, Canter DL, Muscal E, Nanda K, Wahezi DM, Spalding SJ, Twilt M, Benseler SM, Campillo S, Charuvanij S, Dancey P, Eberhard BA, Elder ME, Hersh A, Higgins GC, Huber AM, Khubchandani R, Kim S, Klein-Gitelman M, Kostik MM, Lawson EF, Lee T, Lubieniecka JM, McCurdy D, Moorthy LN, Morishita KA, Nielsen SM, O'Neil KM, Reiff A, Ristic G, Robinson AB, Sarmiento A, Shenoi S, Toth MB, Van Mater HA, Wagner-Weiner L, Weiss JE, White AJ, Yeung RS, Initiative ARINwtP (2016) Comparing presenting clinical features in 48 children with microscopic polyangiitis to 183 children who have granulomatosis with polyangiitis (Wegener's): an ARChiVe cohort study. Arthritis Rheum 68(10):2514–2526. ▶ https://doi.org/10.1002/art.39729
Calatroni M, Oliva E, Gianfreda D, Gregorini G, Allinovi M, Ramirez GA, Bozzolo EP, Monti S,

Bracaglia C, Marucci G, Bodria M, Sinico RA, Pieruzzi F, Moroni G, Pastore S, Emmi G, Esposito P, Catanoso M, Barbano G, Bonanni A, Vaglio A (2017) ANCA-associated vasculitis in childhood: recent advances. Ital J Pediatr 43(1):46. ► https://doi.org/10.1186/s13052-017-0364-x

Chung SA, Langford CA, Maz M, Abril A, Gorelik M, Guyatt G, Archer AM, Conn DL, Full KA, Grayson PC, Ibarra MF, Imundo LF, Kim S, Merkel PA, Rhee RL, Seo P, Stone JH, Sule S, Sundel RP, Vitobaldi OI, Warner A, Byram K, Dua AB, Husainat N, James KE, Kalot MA, Lin YC, Springer JM, Turgunbaev M, Villa-Forte A, Turner AS, Mustafa RA (2021) 2021 American College of Rheumatology/Vasculitis Foundation Guideline for the management of antineutrophil cytoplasmic antibody-associated vasculitis. Arthritis Rheum 73(8):1366–1383. ► https://doi.org/10.1002/art.41773

de Graeff N, Groot N, Brogan P, Ozen S, Avcin T, Bader-Meunier B, Dolezalova P, Feldman BM, Kone-Paut I, Lahdenne P, Marks SD, McCann L, Pilkington C, Ravelli A, van Royen A, Uziel Y, Vastert B, Wulffraat N, Kamphuis S, Beresford MW (2019) European consensus-based recommendations for the diagnosis and treatment of rare paediatric vasculitides – the SHARE initiative. Rheumatology (Oxford) 58(4):656–671. ► https://doi.org/10.1093/rheumatology/key322

Grayson PC, Ponte C, Suppiah R, Robson JC, Craven A, Judge A, Khalid S, Hutchings A, Luqmani RA, Watts RA, Merkel PA, Group DS (2022) 2022 American College of Rheumatology/European Alliance of Associations for Rheumatology Classification Criteria for eosinophilic granulomatosis with polyangiitis. Arthritis Rheumatol 74(3):386–392. ► https://doi.org/10.1002/art.41982

Lee JJY, Alsaleem A, Chiang GPK, Limenis E, Sontichai W, Yeung RSM, Akikusa J, Laxer RM (2019) Hallmark trials in ANCA-associated vasculitis (AAV) for the pediatric rheumatologist. Pediatr Rheumatol Online J 17(1):31. ► https://doi.org/10.1186/s12969-019-0343-4

Mendel A, Ennis D, Go E, Bakowsky V, Baldwin C, Benseler SM, Cabral DA, Carette S, Clements-Baker M, Clifford AH, Cohen Tervaert JW, Cox G, Dehghan N, Dipchand C, Dhindsa N, Famorca L, Fifi-Mah A, Garner S, Girard LP, Lessard C, Liang P, Noone D, Makhzoum JP, Milman N, Pineau CA, Reich HN, Rheaume M, Robinson DB, Rumsey DG, Towheed TE, Trudeau J, Twilt M, Yacyshyn E, Yeung RSM, Barra LB, Khalidi N, Pagnoux C (2021) CanVasc Consensus recommendations for the management of antineu-

trophil cytoplasm antibody-associated vasculitis: 2020 update. J Rheumatol 48(4):555–566. ► https://doi.org/10.3899/jrheum.200721

Morishita KA, Wagner-Weiner L, Yen EY, Sivaraman V, James KE, Gerstbacher D, Szymanski AM, O'Neil KM, Cabral DA, Childhood A, Rheumatology Research Alliance Antineutrophil Cytoplasmic Antibody-Associated Vasculitis W (2022) Consensus treatment plans for severe pediatric antineutrophil cytoplasmic antibody-associated vasculitis. Arthritis Care Res (Hoboken) 74(9):1550–1558. ► https://doi.org/10.1002/acr.24590

Ozen S, Pistorio A, Iusan SM, Bakkaloglu A, Herlin T, Brik R, Buoncompagni A, Lazar C, Bilge I, Uziel Y, Rigante D, Cantarini L, Hilario MO, Silva CA, Alegria M, Norambuena X, Belot A, Berkun Y, Estrella AI, Olivieri AN, Alpigiani MG, Rumba I, Sztajnbok F, Tambic-Bukovac L, Breda L, Al-Mayouf S, Mihaylova D, Chasnyk V, Sengler C, Klein-Gitelman M, Djeddi D, Nuno L, Pruunsild C, Brunner J, Kondi A, Pagava K, Pederzoli S, Martini A, Ruperto N, Paediatric Rheumatology International Trials O (2010) EULAR/PRINTO/PRES criteria for Henoch-Schonlein purpura, childhood polyarteritis nodosa, childhood Wegener granulomatosis and childhood Takayasu arteritis: Ankara 2008. Part II: Final classification criteria. Ann Rheum Dis 69(5):798–806. ► https://doi.org/10.1136/ard.2009.116657

Robson JC, Grayson PC, Ponte C, Suppiah R, Craven A, Judge A, Khalid S, Hutchings A, Watts RA, Merkel PA, Luqmani RA, Investigators D (2022) 2022 American College of Rheumatology/European Alliance of Associations for Rheumatology classification criteria for granulomatosis with polyangiitis. Ann Rheum Dis 81(3):315–320. ► https://doi.org/10.1136/annrheumdis-2021-221795

Suppiah R, Robson JC, Grayson PC, Ponte C, Craven A, Khalid S, Judge A, Hutchings A, Merkel PA, Luqmani RA, Watts RA, Dcvas I (2022) 2022 American College of Rheumatology/European Alliance of Associations for Rheumatology classification criteria for microscopic polyangiitis. Ann Rheum Dis 81(3):321–326. ► https://doi.org/10.1136/annrheumdis-2021-221796

Yates M, Watts RA, Bajema IM, Cid MC, Crestani B, Hauser T, Hellmich B, Holle JU, Laudien M, Little MA, Luqmani RA, Mahr A, Merkel PA, Mills J, Mooney J, Segelmark M, Tesar V, Westman K, Vaglio A, Yalcindag N, Jayne DR, Mukhtyar C (2016) EULAR/ERA-EDTA recommendations for the management of ANCA-associated vasculitis. Ann Rheum Dis 75(9):1583–1594. ► https://doi.org/10.1136/annrheumdis-2016-209133

When the Skin Turns Blue, Bleeds, and Then Turns Black

Christiane Reiser and Hermann Girschick

Contents

© The Author(s), under exclusive license to Springer-Verlag GmbH, DE, part of Springer Nature 2024
C. Huemer and H. Girschick (eds.), *Clinical Examples in Pediatric Rheumatology*,
https://doi.org/10.1007/978-3-662-68732-1_21

21.1 Medical History

Due to the complexity of various forms of vasculitis in childhood and adolescence, the following presents two patients with their history:

▪▪ Alena

For the first time at the age of 13, Alena developed a reddish, painless efflorescence on the anterior left lower leg, which repeatedly ulcerated over time (◘ Fig. 21.1a). An external skin biopsy revealed a granulomatous inflammatory reaction of the vessel walls, a conventional bacterial swab was inconspicuous, cultures for typical and atypical mycobacteria were negative. As the wound did not heal and spread laterally on the lower leg with blackish tissue necrosis (◘ Fig. 21.1b), the patient was presented for further clarification 9 months later. Unremarkable family history.

▪▪ Uwe

The 15-year-old boy was acutely presented with significant pain in his arms and legs, particularly on the right side, as well as abdominal complaints that had been present for 5 days. Already 2 weeks before, **testicular pain** had occurred, the diagnosis of right testicular torsion was made and surgical fixation was performed. Antibiotic therapy had been carried out for 9 days. The local findings on the testicle were reported to have been inconspicuous in the course. Fever was denied, as were other signs of infection.

21.2 Examination Findings

▪▪ Alena

There was a 4 × 6 cm large anterior **ulcer cruris**, marginally reddened, largely healed and scarred (◘ Fig. 21.1a), next to it the

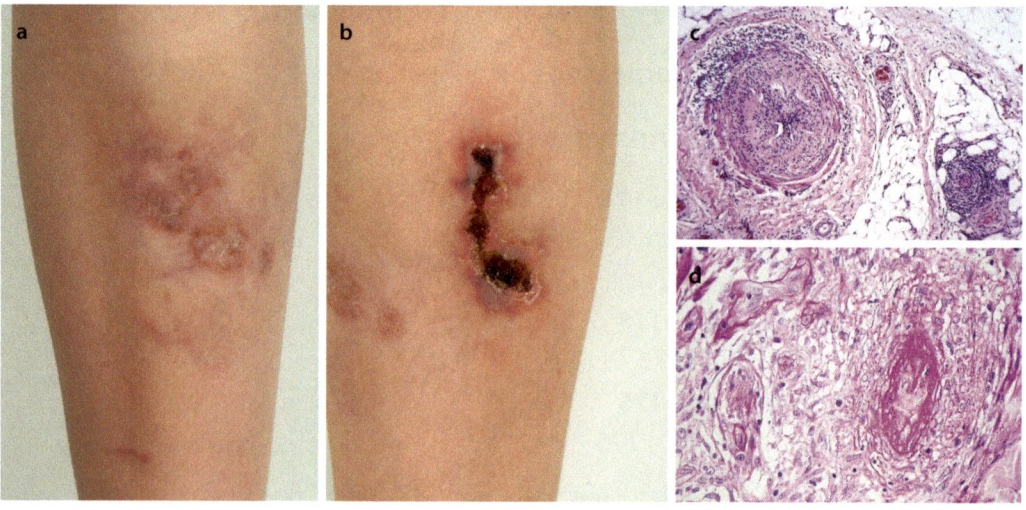

◘ **Fig. 21.1   a–d** Alena's clinic at 14 years old—almost healed granulomatous panniculitis, which flared up necrotically ulcerating laterally after another 6 months. **a** Partially healed scarred "panniculitis" on the lower leg (6 months after onset), which was repeatedly painful, reddened and swollen. **b** Another 6 months later, the lesion broke open ulcerating again laterally on the lower leg. **c** Histologically, there was arteritis of small and medium-sized arteries, which also necrotized fibrinoid **d** (Hematoxylin-Eosin 20-fold)

21

new lesion showed a blackish changed, necrotized wound base (☐ Fig. 21.1b). The rest of the pediatric internal full-body examination was unremarkable.

▪▪ Uwe

At presentation, the boy had significantly reduced muscular strength in all extremities. A myalgic picture was impressive. The skin findings were inconspicuous at this time. The pain in the area of the left lower leg, also with swelling and local tenderness, extending to the left ankle, was in the foreground. There were no indications of arthritis in the knee and ultimately also in the left upper ankle joint. Locally, there was tenderness of the M. gastrocnemius. The M. deltoid was also painful at the insertion of the acromion. Sonographically, the muscles appeared echogenic, there was no abscess formation. Even though there was no fever, the clinical suspicion of bacterial myositis was initially raised. The findings on the shoulder were initially seen separately from the lower leg. A biopsy was declined by the family at this time. Antibiotic therapy with ampicillin and imipenem intravenously was initiated, as well as anticoagulant therapy with low molecular weight heparin subcutaneously. The boy received anti-inflammatory treatment with 3 tablets of 400 mg ibuprofen per day. Under this treatment, the clinical condition initially improved hesitantly, but then significantly, the inflammation parameters were decreasing. After 2 weeks, pressure pain developed on the other, right calf. An electromyography also suggested myositis. The boy had a brief fever attack without further increase in inflammation parameters (see laboratory values in ▶ Sect. 21.3). The expansion of the clinical findings now in the sense of a systemic myositis/myopathy required a reorientation of the diagnostics/expansion also with regard to an autoimmune event.

21.3 Laboratory Values and Imaging

21.3.1 Laboratory Values

▪▪ Alena

Inflammatory parameters (ESR, ferritin, CRP, complement C3, C4) were normal, as were the blood count and overview values for liver, kidney, muscle, bone. Autoimmune diagnostics: Autoantibodies ANA, ENA, ANCA (PR3, MPO), dsDNA, cardiolipin, cryoglobulins were all negative. The fibrinogen was elevated at 4.5 g/l (< 3.5 g/l), the **D-dimers** were significantly positive at 1.9 mg/dl, with otherwise unremarkable coagulation overview values. Infection serologies for hepatitis B, HIV, leishmaniasis, bartonella, and brucella were unremarkable. A tuberculin skin test was negative.

▪▪ Uwe

Inflammatory parameters (ESR 78 mm/h, CRP 13.6 mg/dl) were elevated, the blood count was granulocytic (79%, with a total leukocyte count of 8960/ul). The CK was normal (17 U/l), a blood culture remained negative. The extension to autoimmune diagnostics revealed **ANA slightly elevated at 1:320, (MPO) c-ANCA positive**, ENA, dsDNA antibodies, p-ANCA, cardiolipin-AB were negative.

21.3.2 Imaging and Functional Tests

▪▪ Alena

The sonography of the heart, abdomen, joints, conventional X-ray examinations of the thorax, ECG, EEG, ophthalmologist including retinal reflection revealed no abnormalities.

The magnetic resonance imaging of the head was unremarkable, that of the extremities (1 year after first symptom) (◘ Fig. 21.2) with T2-weighted MRI with fat saturation (TIRM, ◘ Fig. 21.2a) and MRI angiography (T1-weighting, gadolinium administration) (◘ Fig. 21.2c) showed a regional myogenic edema. In the area of the anterior tibial compartment, there is a partial occlusion of the anterior tibial artery and a regional contrast enhancement (spider vein-like/diffuse, partial hypervascularization, ◘ Fig. 21.2c). At this point, no evidence of involvement of internal organs was found. A biopsy revealed in histology an **arteritis of small and medium-sized arteries** (◘ Fig. 21.1c), which also **fibrinoid necrotized** (◘ Fig. 21.1d). Further course in ◘ Fig. 21.3.

▪▪ Uwe

The sonography locally revealed moderately swollen muscle tissue, the increase in echogenicity was decreasing, the perfusion appeared normal. Sonographies of the abdomen, the joints, and the finger arteries were unremarkable. The conventional X-ray examination of the thorax, ECG, EEG, ophthalmologist including retinal reflection, a colonoscopy, a gastroscopy revealed no abnormalities. An MRI angiography of the kidneys was normal. A magnetic resonance imaging of the extremities (2 months after initial symptoms with T1-weighted MRI with fat saturation (◘ Fig. 21.4) and TIRM sequence (◘ Fig. 21.4b–d) showed a regional myogenic edema mainly in the left lower leg and an increased regional contrast agent uptake on the left side in the M. gastrocnemius, but also in the central vascular sheath (◘ Fig. 21.4d). Evidence of the involvement of other "internal" organs was not found. A lower leg muscle biopsy now consented with the parents revealed a lymphocytic myositis and arteritis of small and medium-sized arteries in the histology).

21.4 Educational Questions

1. What differential diagnosis do you consider for chronic ulcerating, poorly healing skin lesion with **necrotization**?
2. Are the symptoms of the two teenagers assignable to classification systems?
3. How do you design the laboratory diagnostics with the aim of analyzing the various forms of vasculitis as complex autoimmune diseases?
4. What therapeutic considerations should be taken into account, especially in the absence of controlled studies in children and adolescents?

21.5 Immunology and Classification

Vasculitic diseases are among the most complex autoimmune/autoinflammatory diseases in childhood. Certainly, every pediatrician is familiar with Henoch-Schönlein purpura as a classic and common vasculitis. Vasculitides of the musculoskeletal system or even internal organs, e.g. the CNS, are much rarer. International efforts to formulate a nomenclature for systemic vasculitides date back to 1994. The **Chapel Hill Consensus Conference** attempted at that time to achieve a classification based on reference to different vessel sizes: Thus, the subgroups *vasculitides of large vessels, medium vessels* and *small vessels* were defined. An entity defined by autoantibodies was termed *ANCA association*. The latter includes the subforms of microscopic polyangiitis, granulomatosis with polyangiitis (formerly Wegener's disease) and eosinophilic granulomatosis with polyangiitis (formerly Churg-Strauss vasculitis). The *large vessel vasculitides* include Takayasu arteritis and giant cell arteritis. Polyarteritis nodosa and Kawasaki disease are among the vasculitides of the *medium vessels*. Immune complex-mediated *small vessel vasculitides*:

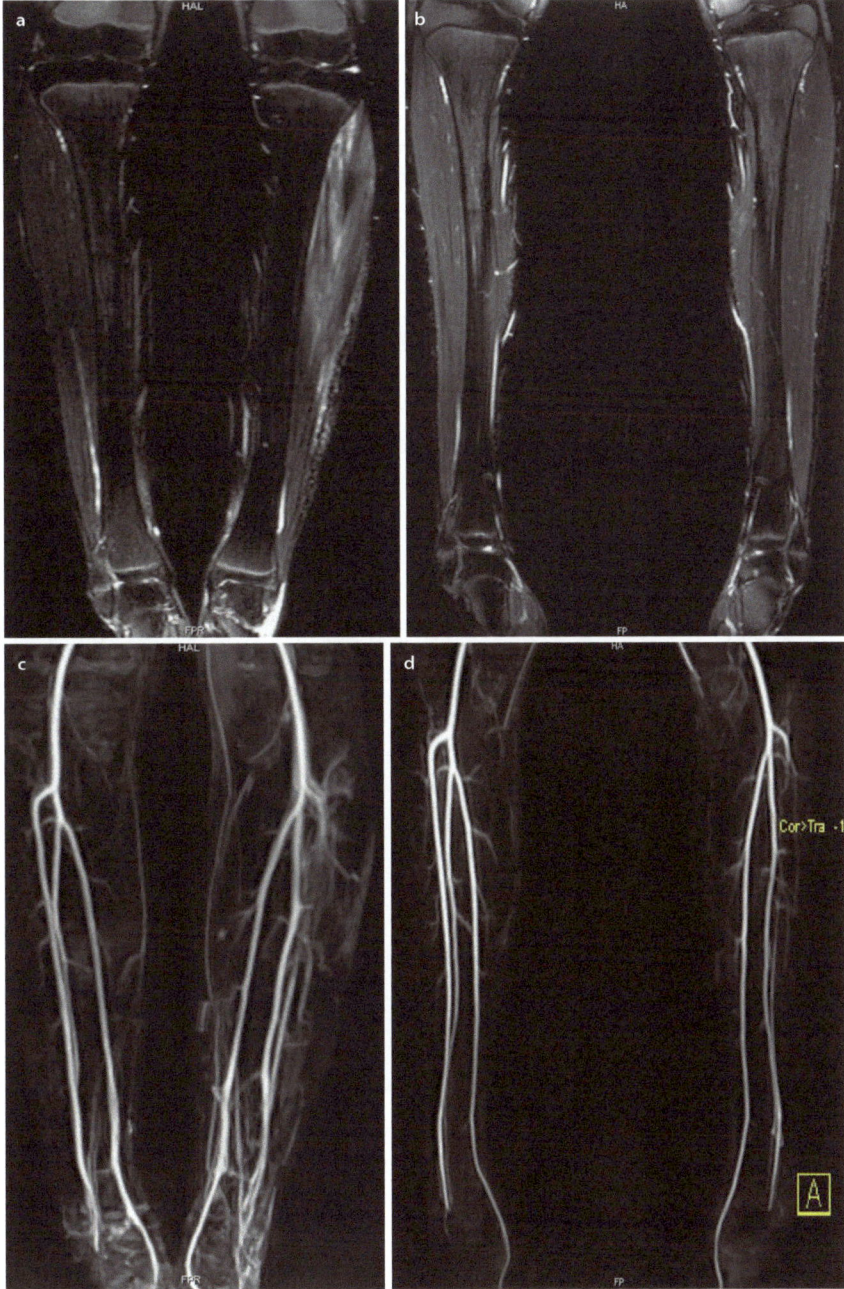

◘ Fig. 21.2   a–d Alena's imaging at diagnosis and 9 months after immunosuppressive therapy: Myositis and vasculitis, occlusion of the anterior tibial artery. **a,b** Imaging 1 year after first symptom (cf. ◘ Fig. 21.1c). T2-weighted MRI with fat saturation (TIRM). **b,d** Course another 9 months later after immunosuppressive therapy: MRI normalization, i.e., a regional myogenic edema was no longer visible. In the area of the anterior tibial compartment, there is a partial occlusion of the anterior tibial artery, which did not recanalize in the course. The regional contrast enhancement (spider vein-like, diffuse, partial hypervascularization) in **c** was no longer detectable after therapy **d**. MRI angiography (T1-weighting, gadolinium administration) and Fig. 2c,d:

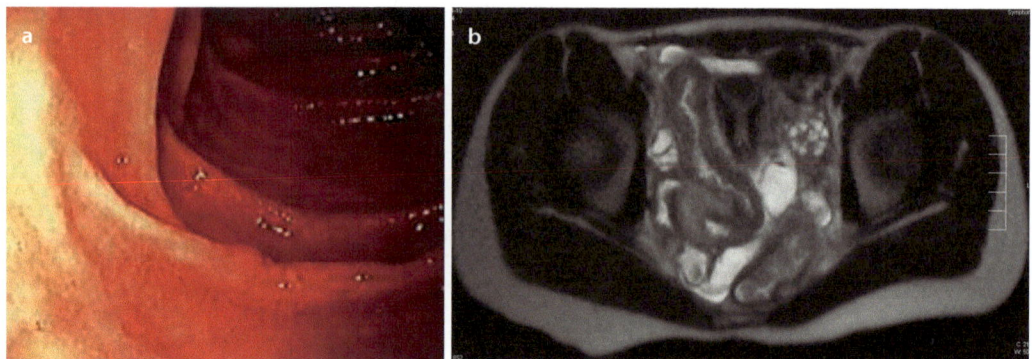

◘ Fig. 21.3 **a,b Alena's endoscopic diagnostics and MRT-Sellink 9 months after therapy initiation.** 21 months after the first cutaneous symptom, the patient developed chronic abdominal pain and lost 3 kg in weight, the skin had healed by then, the vasculitis on the leg had subsided (◘ Fig. 21.2b, d). **a** The colonoscopy showed diffuse edema, erosions, and fibrinous ulcerations. The stomach and duodenum were spared. **b** The MRT-Sellink (T2-weighting) impressively shows a terminal ileitis. (With kind permission of Prof. Dr. M. Beer, Institute for Radiology, University of Würzburg)

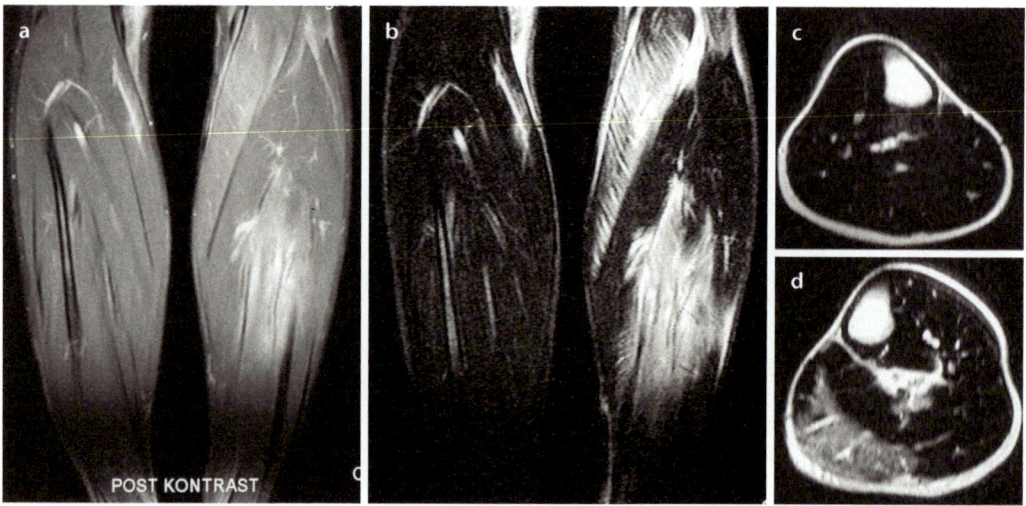

◘ Fig. 21.4 **a–d Uwe's MRI imaging at diagnosis: Myositis M. gastrocnemius and vasculitis. a,c** Initial MRI with T1 weighting and gadolinium administration **a** or T2 weighting with fat saturation (TIRM, **b–d**): A regional myogenic edema in the M. gastrocnemius, but also a clear T2 emphasis in the central vascular sheath was visible in the left calf **d**, not on the right **c**

these include IgA vasculitis, synonymous with Henoch-Schönlein purpura. Hypocomplementemic urticarial vasculitis and cryoglobulinemia vasculitis have also been associated with this (Jennette et al. 2013; Jennette 2013). This nomenclature, essentially tailored to adults, was updated in 2012 (Jennette et al. 2013; Batu and Ozen 2015). In childhood, some of these vasculitides play no role in everyday life due to their rarity or "non-occurrence". In addition to the most common variant, **Henoch-Schönlein purpura (IgA vasculitis)**, the **Kawasaki syndrome, polyarteritis nodosa, granulomatous** polyangiitis and **Takayasu arteritis** are seen in everyday life. Therefore, these entities have been specifically subjected to a new European classification consideration (with the exception of Kawasaki) and summarized into the **so-called Ankara criteria** (Batu and Ozen 2015; Ozen et al. 2006, 2010; Eleftheriou et al. 2015; Ruperto et al. 2010). The aim of this classification/division was to form as homogeneous diagnostic groups as possible in order to subject them to controlled studies on the one hand and to establish activity parameters or severity assessments on the other (Demirkaya et al. 2011; Demirkaya et al. 2012). If one compares the clinical criteria found therein with the individual subforms within the Chapel Hill nomenclature, for example, the **microscopic polyangiitis** is **not** found in the Ankara criteria. It is associated with ANCA autoantibodies, as is granulomatosis with polyangiitis. In differential diagnosis, it should be considered in our patient Uwe alongside polyarteritis nodosa. The latter shows various variants of skin involvement, myositis, peripheral neuropathy and primarily renal involvement. Thus, **hypertension**, **hematuria** and **proteinuria** are the main measurement parameters in **polyarteritis nodosa**. A **microscopic polyangiitis** can affect the kidney with a necrotizing vasculitis of small to medium-sized vessels, but also the entire respiratory tract. We discussed Uwe's synopsis, which was assessed by specialized adult rheumatologists as *microscopic polyangiitis*, also with international pediatric specialists: Here, as part of the classification efforts, a classification as *polyarteritis nodosa* was made (Ozen et al. 2004). The occurrence of testicular pain, peripheral neuropathy (Uwe's 5th finger had been intermittently numb on one side) and the histological picture of inflamed small and especially medium arteries with fibrinoid necrosis spoke for this. The presence of ANCA antibodies would, however, primarily suggest a small vessel vasculitis in the context of microscopic polyangiitis, ANCA antibodies usually do not occur in polyarteritis nodosa. Since MPA was not addressed within the Ankara criteria, this dichotomy cannot ultimately be resolved. **There are no laboratory parameters proving vasculitis or specific to subgroups.** Genetic or monogenetic causes are ultimately not sufficiently researched: An association with familial Mediterranean fever or in individual cases the detection of mutations e.g. in the adenosine deaminase-2 gene (DADA2) as well as an association with hepatitis B virus infection should be considered (Eleftheriou et al. 2015).

21.6 Further Progress

▪▪ Alena

After the diagnosis of necrotizing vasculitis of small and medium-sized arteries, an anti-inflammatory glucocorticoid therapy with methylprednisolone 20 mg/kg body weight per day was administered intravenously for 3 days. This therapy was repeated twice at intervals of 4 weeks. In parallel, the patient received intravenous hyperimmunoglobulin G. Under this treatment, the cutaneous vasculitis completely healed with scar formation. The initially elevated inflammation parameters normalized. About 9 months later (a total of 21 months after the initial cutaneous symptoms) **chronic abdominal pain** began, and a weight loss of 3 kg was reported. Endoscopic diagnostics revealed a diffuse wall edema of the colon with erosions and ulcerations (◘ Fig. 21.3a). The stomach and duodenum were spared. An MRI in Sellink technique impressively showed terminal ileitis (◘ Fig. 21.3b). According to the Chapel Hill nomenclature, Alena's vasculitis would be considered "associated with another systemic disease", specifically Crohn's disease (Jennette et al. 2013). Ultimately, the lesion would also be referred to as **pyoderma**

gangrenosum, however, the existing myositis and vasculitis of the medium-sized arteries with perfusion failure was a particularly impressive finding.

▪▪ Uwe

Oral glucocorticoid therapy (prednisolone 1 mg/kg body weight per day) initially led to rapid improvement, and the inflammation parameters also improved. However, under this medium-dose oral steroid therapy, pain in both arms and the left shoulder repeatedly occurred. The erythrocyte sedimentation rate remained elevated at 55 mm/h, and the CRP could not be reduced below 6.1 mg/dl. About 2 months after the initial manifestation of myositis, the boy's condition rapidly deteriorated, with a new onset of **livedo reticularis** which also showed erosive scabs in the forearm area (◘ Fig 21.5a–c). Histologically, the picture

in relation to the vessels was comparable to that of the first muscle biopsy. The clinical picture of polyarteritis nodosa (testicular pain, muscle pain, sensory innervation disorder of a Fifth finger, myositis and biopsy-confirmed vasculitis of small and medium vessels) was now in the foreground. Due to the particular severity of the manifestation (◘ Fig. 21.5a–c), we started a cytotoxic therapy with cyclophosphamide intravenously at 4-week intervals. A total of 14 cycles were administered. The boy's symptoms improved under this treatment, and a permanent remission was achievable (◘ Fig. 21.5d). In addition, the boy received thrombosis prophylaxis with low molecular weight heparin, an anti-inflammatory therapy with meloxicam. Supportive therapy with cotrimoxazole and amphotericin as mouth rinse was given prophylactically. The boy had significant pain issues

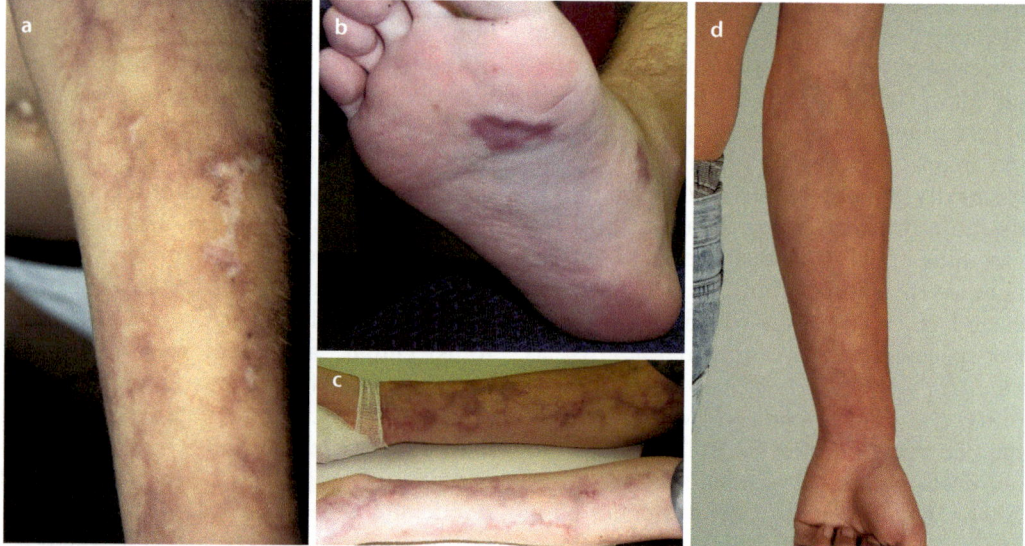

◘ **Fig. 21.5   a–d Uwe's clinic at 15 years old—Livedo racemosa, partially healed erosions/ulcers, erythema nodosum. a–c** Cutaneous findings that occurred 3 months after the myositis on the lower leg: The skin was particularly noticeable on the arms. A muscle biopsy on the lower leg had revealed myositis and vasculitis of the small and medium arteries. The diagnosis of ANCA-positive microscopic polyangiitis was initially made in the boy. The skin biopsy revealed vasculitis of the small arteries. After immunosuppressive cytotoxic cyclophosphamide therapy, a permanent remission could be achieved **d**. As part of an international classification project (Ozen J Pediatrics 2004), the symptoms were attributed to polyarteritis nodosa and was temporarily given Tramadol. ESR and CRP, as well as the blood count, were normalized after 6 months, as were the complement factors C3C and C4. No autoantibodies (ANA, c-ANCA) were measurable anymore. The boy developed a temporary hypogammaglobulinemia, most likely associated with the cytotoxic therapy. One year after the start of cyclophosphamide therapy, there was a remission of skin and muscle findings, and the laboratory parameters remained normal. A final follow-up examination after 3 years was unremarkable, a transition to adult care was initiated.

21.7 Educative Answers

- **1. What differential diagnosis do you consider for chronic ulcerating, poorly healing skin lesion with necrotization?**

One should consider bacterial or parasitic infections, possibly originating from underlying tissue structures, such as in the case of chronic bacterial osteomyelitis. Therefore, the anamnesis, e.g., the child's origin from risk areas, is of crucial importance. In Europe, one should consider diseases such as cat scratch disease, tularemia (rabbit fever), or an infection with atypical mycobacteria. In tropical areas, one should consider a mycobacterial infection with leprosy bacteria or parasitic infections such as tungiasis. On the other hand, depending on the location of the ulcer, one should consider autoimmune or autoinflammatory diseases in the broadest sense: lesions in the area of the end phalanges may be associated with a Raynaud's phenomenon, with diseases such as scleroderma or systemic lupus erythematosus being differential diagnoses. If the ulcers affect more central skin regions and underlying organ structures such as muscles or fasciae are involved, vasculitic diseases should be considered in the narrower differential diagnosis. Skin necroses that occur in the context of, for example, a chronic inflammatory bowel disease, such as pyoderma gangrenosum, are very rare in childhood, but the diagnosis had to be considered for Alena.

- **2. Can the symptoms of the two teenagers be classified in classification systems?**

The assignment within the Chapel Hill nomenclature would ultimately associate Alena with Crohn's disease as a **systemic underlying disease** (Jennette et al. 2013; Jennette 2013). Before the IBD became known, one would classify it as a **vasculitis of the medium vessels**, e.g., polyarteritis nodosa, or as a **vasculitis involving small vessels** possibly in the context of an immune complex vasculitis. ANCA antibodies were not noticeable in Alena. Within the Eular/Printo/PReS/Ankara classification, Alena's disease would ultimately not be clearly assignable (Ozen et al. 2010). The limitation can be seen in the focus of the Ankara criteria from 2008 on the more common vasculitis variants in childhood.

Uwe's disease can indeed be assigned in the two currently valid classification efforts: Due to the involvement of medium and small arteries, polyarteritis nodosa, which usually does not go along with ANCA antibodies, should be considered. The clinical description of a polyarteritis nodosa in adolescence involving skin (livedo reticularis), muscle (myalgia and myositis), neuropathy (sensory disturbance of the 5th finger), testicular pain would be very much in line with Uwe's clinical picture (Ozen et al. 2006). But here too, the observed association with ANCA antibodies would rather be an exclusion criterion. A pure cutaneous form of polyarteritis, as described by Ozen, is certainly not present in Uwe. This brings the focus to the **ANCA-associated microscopic polyangiitis,** which was favored by internal vasculitis specialists as a diagnosis for Uwe (Mukhtyar et al. 2009). However, a common pulmonary or glomerular involvement did not occur in our patient. A final assignment cannot be made unequivocally.

- **3. How do you design the laboratory diagnostics with the aim of analyzing the various forms of vasculitis as complex autoimmune diseases?**

For the assignment to individual vasculitis entities, the most important thing is the biopsy/histological representation of vascular inflammation of different sizes, granulomatous processes, the involvement of **basal membranes** or IgA deposition, and the co-involvement/deposition of complement components. An association with systemic diseases from the area of **systemic lupus, rheumatoid arthritis, sarcoidosis, Behçet's disease** should be attempted with matching autoantibody patterns or HLA associations. The reference to ANCA antibodies is important in laboratory chemistry. Also of importance is the reference to possible infectious diseases, such as hepatitis B and C. Accompanying this is the analysis of the complement system (C3, C4, CH 50, CH 100), a coagulation analysis (including D-dimers, fibrinogen) is relevant.

- **4. What therapeutic considerations should be taken into account, especially in the absence of controlled studies in children and adolescents?**

Unfortunately, the therapy for both ANCA-associated vasculitis and polyarteritis nodosa in children and adolescents is **not** based on randomized controlled studies. **Registry analyses** and expert opinions are used for therapeutic decision-making. Certainly, the severity plays a crucial role, which is expressed by the involvement of various organ systems with tissue defects or as a deviation from laboratory parameters. Typically, glucocorticoids and a cytotoxic therapy with **cyclophosphamide** are used for acute therapy. Milder forms of vasculitis usually lead to the use of basic immu-

nosuppressive therapy with, for example, azathioprine, methotrexate, or mycophenolic acid. The use of TNF-blocking biologics or B-cell depletion (rituximab) can be attempted in patients who are difficult to treat (Eleftheriou et al. 2015). The use of plasma exchange procedures and also **hyperimmune globulin preparations** is repeatedly discussed in individual studies, but the long-term success of plasma exchange is increasingly viewed critically (Walsh et al. 2020). A good guideline is the **EULAR recommendation for the management of small and medium vessel vasculitis in adults** (Mukhtyar et al. 2009): The experts recommend oral or intravenous cyclophosphamide in combination with glucocorticoid use for remission induction. For milder forms of vasculitis, weekly subcutaneous or oral methotrexate is recommended. Supportive therapies for bladder protection and infection prophylaxis against *Pneumocystis jirovecii* are emphasized.

21.8 Summary

21.8.1 Etiology

The etiology of Alena's and Uwe's vasculitis is ultimately unknown. It is assumed to be a complex disorder of the humoral immune system with the development of measurable autoantibodies (ANCA), but all areas of the immune system seem to be involved. A monogenetic cause is discussed in rare cases of vasculitis (ADA2 deficiency, STING defect). Infections, e.g., hepatitis B or C infections, should be considered as cofactors.

21.8.2 Pathogenesis/Clinic

The complex inflammatory disorder of the skin and subcutis, including muscles, heart, vessels, and joints, ultimately leads to severe local or systemic organ disorders up to permanent restrictions such as kidney failure or pulmonary insufficiency.

21.8.3 Diagnosis

In addition to a detailed medical history and clinical examination, autoantibodies are available: **ANCA antibodies** (MPO, but also PR3). However, antibodies against nuclear components (ANA, ENA, dsDNA) and a detailed coagulation analysis are also relevant.

21.8.4 Therapy

According to the current **EULAR recommendations**, consensus-based guidelines for *vasculitis in adults* are available (Eleftheriou et al. 2015; Mukhtyar et al. 2009); systemically applied immunosuppressants or cytotoxic drugs appear sensible depending on the severity. Supportive therapy for bladder protection and prevention of atypical infections is required.

21.8.5 Diagnosis

The diagnosis is primarily based on the clinical picture, in combination with a tissue biopsy and MRI imaging including contrast medium application. It is supported by the Chapel Hill nomenclature and further classification efforts. In children and adolescents, as in adults, the diagnosis of potentially affected organs is paramount.

21.8.6 Prophylaxis

There is no prophylaxis to prevent the disease, the exception would be a vaccination against hepatitis B. A close connection to a specialized interdisciplinary center for pediatric rheumatology and autoimmunity is highly desirable.

Conclusion

Patients with complex autoimmune diseases require an interdisciplinary diagnostic and therapeutic approach. In the case of vasculitis, this includes, among others, rheumatology, dermatology, pulmonology, and cardiology. This is accompanied by intensive physiotherapy and respiratory therapy, promotion of musculoskeletal fitness, and local skin care.

References

Batu ED, Ozen S (2015) Vasculitis: do we know more to classify better? Pediatr Nephrol 30:1425–1432. ▸ https://doi.org/10.1007/s00467-014-3015-0

Demirkaya E, Luqmani R, Ayaz NA, Karaoglu A, Ozen S (2011) Time to focus on outcome assessment tools for childhood vasculitis. Pediatr Rheumatol Online J 9:29. ▸ https://doi.org/10.1186/1546-0096-9-29

Demirkaya E, Ozen S, Pistorio A, Galasso R, Ravelli A, Hasija R, Baskin E, Dressler F, Fischbach M, Garcia Consuegra J, Iagaru N, Pasic S, Scarpato S, van Rossum MA, Apaz MT, Barash J, Calcagno G, Gonzalez B, Hoppenreijs E, Ioseliani M, Mazur-Zielinska H, Vougiouka O, Wulffraat N, Luqmani R, Martini A, Ruperto N, Dolezalova P (2012) Performance of Birmingham Vasculitis Activity Score and disease extent index in childhood vasculitides. Clin Exp Rheumatol 30:S162–S168

Eleftheriou D, Batu ED, Ozen S, Brogan PA (2015) Vasculitis in children. Nephrol Dial Transplant 30(Suppl 1):i94–103. ▸ https://doi.org/10.1093/ndt/gfu393

Jennette JC (2013) Overview of the 2012 revised international Chapel Hill Consensus Conference nomenclature of vasculitides. Clin Exp Nephrol 17:603–606. ▸ https://doi.org/10.1007/s10157-013-0869-6

Jennette JC, Falk RJ, Bacon PA, Basu N, Cid MC, Ferrario F, Flores-Suarez LF, Gross WL, Guillevin L, Hagen EC, Hoffman GS, Jayne DR, Kallenberg CG, Lamprecht P, Langford CA, Luqmani RA, Mahr AD, Matteson EL, Merkel PA, Ozen S, Pusey CD, Rasmussen N, Rees AJ, Scott DG, Specks U, Stone JH, Takahashi K,

Watts RA (2013) 2012 revised International Chapel Hill Consensus Conference nomenclature of vasculitides. Arthritis Rheum 65:1–11. ▶ https://doi.org/10.1002/art.37715

Mukhtyar C, Guillevin L, Cid MC, Dasgupta B, de Groot K, Gross W, Hauser T, Hellmich B, Jayne D, Kallenberg CG, Merkel PA, Raspe H, Salvarani C, Scott DG, Stegeman C, Watts R, Westman K, Witter J, Yazici H, Luqmani R (2009) EULAR recommendations for the management of primary small and medium vessel vasculitis. Ann Rheum Dis 68:310–317. ▶ https://doi.org/10.1136/ard.2008.088096

Ozen S, Anton J, Arisoy N, Bakkaloglu A, Besbas N, Brogan P, García-Consuegra J, Dolezalova P, Dressler F, Duzova A, Ferriani VP, Hilário MO, Ibáñez-Rubio M, Kasapcopur O, Kuis W, Lehman TJ, Nemcova D, Nielsen S, Oliveira SK, Schikler K, Sztajnbok F, Terreri MT, Zulian F, Woo P (2004) Juvenile polyarteritis: results of a multicenter survey of 110 children. J Pediatr 145:517–522. ▶ https://doi.org/10.1016/j.jpeds.2004.06.046

Ozen S, Ruperto N, Dillon MJ, Bagga A, Barron K, Davin JC, Kawasaki T, Lindsley C, Petty RE, Prieur AM, Ravelli A, Woo P (2006) EULAR/PReS endorsed consensus criteria for the classification of childhood vasculitides. Ann Rheum Dis 65:936–941. ▶ https://doi.org/10.1136/ard.2005.046300

Ozen S, Pistorio A, Iusan SM, Bakkaloglu A, Herlin T, Brik R, Buoncompagni A, Lazar C, Bilge I, Uziel Y, Rigante D, Cantarini L, Hilario MO, Silva CA, Alegria M, Norambuena X, Belot A, Berkun Y, Estrella AI, Olivieri AN, Alpigiani MG, Rumba I, Sztajnbok F, Tambic-Bukovac L, Breda L, Al-Mayouf S, Mihaylova D, Chasnyk V, Sengler C, Klein-Gitelman M, Djeddi D, Nuno L, Pruunsild C, Brunner J, Kondi A, Pagava K, Pederzoli S, Martini A, Ruperto N (2010) EULAR/PRINTO/PRES criteria for Henoch-Schönlein purpura, childhood polyarteritis nodosa, childhood Wegener granulomatosis and childhood Takayasu arteritis: Ankara 2008. Part II: Final classification criteria. Ann Rheum Dis 69:798–806. ▶ https://doi.org/10.1136/ard.2009.116657

Ruperto N, Ozen S, Pistorio A, Dolezalova P, Brogan P, Cabral DA, Cuttica R, Khubchandani R, Lovell DJ, O'Neil KM, Quartier P, Ravelli A, Iusan SM, Filocamo G, Magalhães CS, Unsal E, Oliveira S, Bracaglia C, Bagga A, Stanevicha V, Manzoni SM, Pratsidou P, Lepore L, Espada G, Kone-Paut I, Zulian F, Barone P, Bircan Z, Maldonado Mdel R, Russo R, Vilca I, Tullus K, Cimaz R, Horneff G, Anton J, Garay S, Nielsen S, Barbano G, Martini A (2010) EULAR/PRINTO/PRES criteria for Henoch-Schönlein purpura, childhood polyarteritis nodosa, childhood Wegener granulomatosis and childhood Takayasu arteritis: Ankara 2008. Part I: Overall methodology and clinical characterisation. Ann Rheum Dis 69:790–797. ▶ https://doi.org/10.1136/ard.2009.116624

Walsh M, Merkel PA, Peh CA, Szpirt WM, Puéchal X, Fujimoto S, Hawley CM, Khalidi N, Floßmann O, Wald R, Girard LP, Levin A, Gregorini G, Harper L, Clark WF, Pagnoux C, Specks U, Smyth L, Tesar V, Ito-Ihara T, de Zoysa JR, Szczeklik W, Flores-Suárez LF, Carette S, Guillevin L, Pusey CD, Casian AL, Brezina B, Mazzetti A, McAlear CA, Broadhurst E, Reidlinger D, Mehta S, Ives N, Jayne DRW (2020) Plasma exchange and glucocorticoids in severe ANCA-associated vasculitis. N Engl J Med 382:622–631. ▶ https://doi.org/10.1056/NEJMoa1803537

Recurrent Mouth Ulcers

Christian Huemer

Contents

22.1 Medical History

The 12-year-old girl presents at the emergency outpatient clinic. She has been symptomatic for 4 months with recurring painful **aphthae** (as an example ◘ Fig. 22.1) in the area of the oral mucosa as well as the external genitalia. The child's presentation had already been planned 2 months ago. Due to a significant improvement in findings in the interim, the family then refrained from presenting at the rheumatology clinic. Now for 2 days, sore throat, feeling of weakness, and subfebrile temperatures. Presentation then to the pediatrician. He first identified aphthous lesions in the throat area, tonsils incidentally unremarkable. Now for the first time in the admission status also clear indications of similar lesions in the area of the external genitalia. No additional symptoms in the admission status.

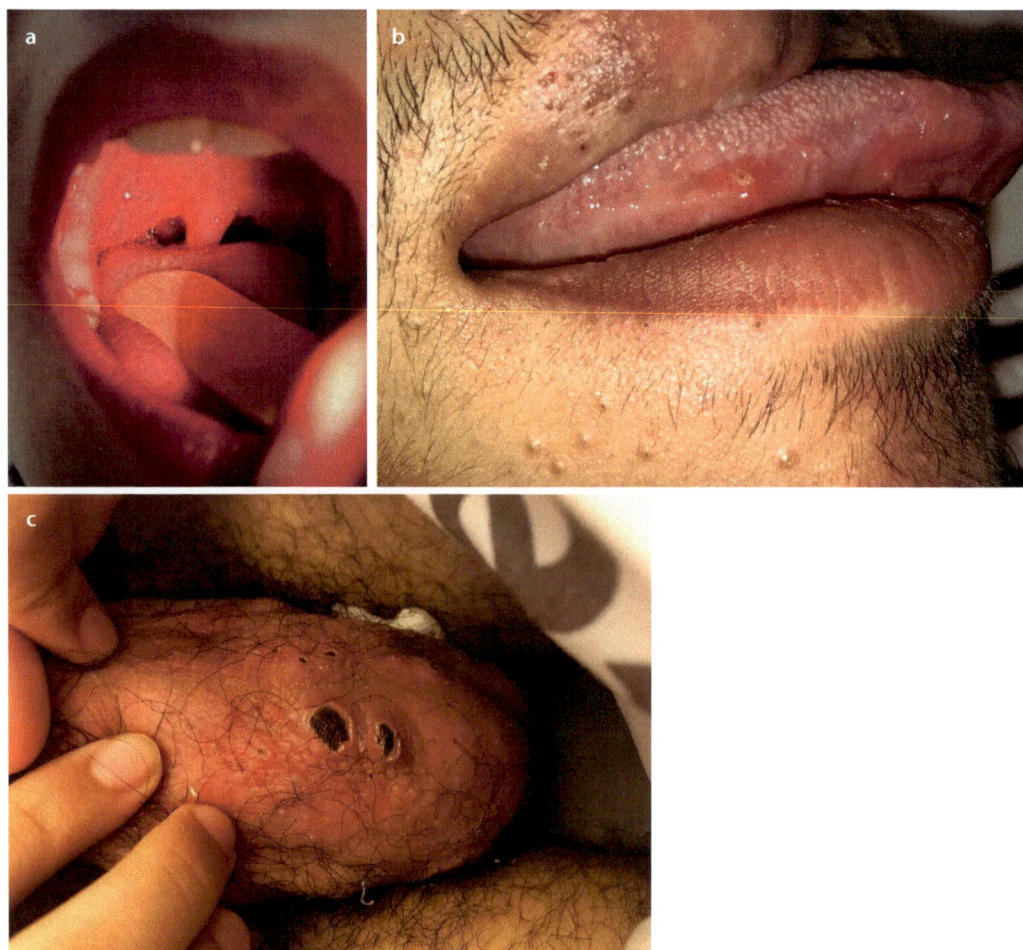

◘ **Fig. 22.1   a–c** Mucocutaneous symptoms in Behçet's disease. **a** Oral aphthae in Behçet's disease (from Hufnagel and Kallinich 2022). **b, c** Aphthae and skin lesions in the intimate area of a 16-year-old boy

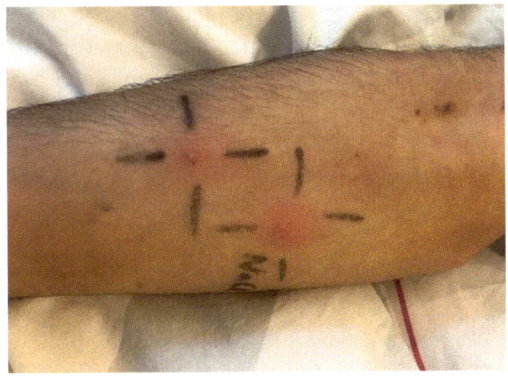

□ Fig. 22.2 Pathergy test in Behçet's disease. The figure shows a conspicuous pathergy test of a 16-year-old boy, with purely mechanical testing with needle tip and after application of NaCl 0.9%

Family history: Similar symptoms had occurred in the brother of the child's father (□ Figs. 22.1b, c and 22.2), a clear diagnosis is not remembered.

22.2 Examination Findings

12-year-old girl in slightly reduced general condition, good nutritional status, weight 36.5 kg, height 150 cm, temperature 37.5 °C. The oral mucosa shows four small aphthous changes at the back of the throat (□ Fig. 22.1) and on the inside of the lower lip, which are also pressure-sensitive. In the genital area on both sides in the area of the labia minora on the inside, an aphthae with bloody-crusty overlay on the left and right. Skin status unremarkable except for local findings. Heart: pure, rhythmic, normofrequent. Lungs: Auscultatory unremarkable findings. Abdomen: Soft, bowel sounds somewhat active, no pressure sensitivity.

22.3 Laboratory Values

Blood count, serum chemistry unremarkable, no increased inflammatory activity. Autoimmunological findings unremarkable.

22.4 Educational Questions

1. What differential diagnoses would you discuss for this primary symptomatology?
2. What further diagnostics would be useful?
3. How would you suggest an initial treatment concept?

22.5 Differential Diagnostic Considerations and Educational Answers

The *differential diagnosis* in the present case mainly concerns the clarification of the clinical symptomatology of oral and genital aphthous or ulcerative lesions. *Possible underlying infections*, e.g., herpes simplex infection, are to be definitively ruled out prior to further autoimmunological diagnostics, however, the symptom complex and the presence of a leading symptomatology with oral and genital ulcers should early raise the **suspicion of Behçet's disease**. The therapy of this disease with recurrent inflammatory character aims at *sufficient control of inflammation*, in general, symptomatic therapy is primarily indicated, further specific therapy is oriented towards other organ involvement as well as age and sex of the patient. Due to the rapid possible **eye involvement**, an ophthalmological center should also be involved very early.

22.6 Further Course

The 12-year-old girl had a **childlike Behçet's disease** with initially exclusively mucocutaneous symptoms with genital and oral aphthosis. However, 4 weeks after the initial examination, the girl also developed an **oligoarthritis** with clear palpable synovitis of a knee joint and an upper ankle joint ipsilaterally. In the further detailed examination, no further organ involvement was initially found, especially no ophthalmological involvement and gastrointestinal involvement or involvement of the nervous system. Initially, a colchicine therapy (1 mg/day p.o.) and a low-dose systemic steroid therapy (0.5 mg/kg body weight/day p.o. prednisolone) were indicated. The isolated genital and oral aphthae were additionally treated with a topical steroid therapy. After 3 months, this therapy regime provided sufficient control of the inflammation, so far no further complications have occurred in this girl, so the prognosis is considered quite good (follow-up period so far 2 years).

22.7 Summary

Behçet's disease is a rare recurrent inflammatory disease that is chronic and episodic (Hufnagel and Kallinich 2022). In attenuated forms, recurring oral and genital aphthae may remain as the only manifestation. Our case also falls into a very mild form of Behçet's disease. However, involvement of the eyes and central nervous system, as well as gastrointestinal and pulmonary symptoms, can pose threatening complications in Behçet's disease and require intensive acute

and long-term immunosuppression. Behçet's disease is classified as a vasculitis and can affect both arteries of various sizes and veins as a vasculitic peculiarity. Cutaneous symptoms in Behçet's disease resemble neutrophilic dermatoses, and overall there are parallels to autoinflammatory diseases (FMF, TRAPS). The frequency of Behçet's disease varies greatly by region, with the highest prevalence in adults in Turkey and Asia (Kotter 2004). In Europe and the USA, the rate of those affected is between 0.1 and 7.5 per 100,000.

22.7.1 Diagnosis

◘ Table 22.1 shows the diagnostic criteria of the International Study Group for Behçet's Disease based on Kallinich and Keitzer 2013.

22.7.2 Clinic

■■ Oral Aphthosis

In 97% of patients, **oral aphthae** (◘ Fig. 22.1a, b) are the first manifestation and can precede other appearances by years, especially

◘ **Tab. 22.1**   Diagnostic criteria of the International Study Group for Behçet's Disease

Recurrent oral aphthae (mandatory)	Minor, major aphthae or herpetiform aphthae recurring at least 3 times in 12 months
plus at least 2 of the following criteria:	
Recurrent genital lesions	Aphthous ulcerations or scarring
Ocular involvement	Ophthalmological diagnosis of Uveitis anterior or Uveitis posterior or vitreous infiltrates (slit lamp) or retinal vasculitis
Skin lesions	Erythema nodosum. Pseudofolliculitis or papulopustular lesions or acneiform nodules or in post-adolescent patients without steroid therapy
Positive Pathergy test (◘ Fig. 22.2)	Prick test with 20G needle (inside of forearm), read after 24–48 h

in children. These lesions do not morphologically differ from common aphthae of other origins in pediatrics, but they occur more frequently on the soft and hard palate and in the deeper pharyngeal area, as well as on the tongue. The aphthae are very painful and can be provoked by local minor traumas.

▪▪ Genital Ulcers

These occur in 60–90% of cases with significant ethnic differences, equally in children and adults. The scrotum (◘ Fig. 22.1c) and labia are predominantly affected, but the perineal and perianal region can also be involved. The ulcers are painful and often only heal after 10–30 days. Genital ulcers are more prone to scarring than oral aphthae (Kone-Paut et al. 2002).

▪▪ Other Skin Manifestations

In addition to the aphthous lesions, spontaneous pustular skin reactions, erythema nodosum, necrotizing folliculitis or acne-like lesions can occur as further cutaneous symptoms.

Pathergy phenomenon and pathergy test (◘ Fig. 22.2): The pathergy phenomenon refers to the spontaneous tendency to form pustules due to nonspecific stimuli, which can be provoked by a prick test or by intracutaneous injection of 0.1 ml isotonic saline solution. The latter reaction is referred to as a **positive pathergy test** and is a main criterion of the international classification for Behçet's disease.

▪▪ Ocular Involvement

With a frequency of about 50%, ocular involvement often stands at the center of the disease (Kone-Paut 1998; Kari et al. 2001), with ocular involvement in juvenile Behçet's disease being characterized by more frequent exacerbations. Characteristic is a usually bilateral recurring intraocular inflammation that can affect all uveal structures.

▪▪ Arthritis

This is described in up to 75% of patients and usually manifests as monoarthritis, less often as oligo- or polyarthritis.

▪▪ Gastrointestinal Symptoms

These are described in 30% of adults and are predominantly the result of mucosal ulcerations.

▪▪ Vascular Involvement

Since Behçet's disease is a systemic vasculitis, involvement of the superficial and deep veins, but also arteries, is predominantly described.

▪▪ CNS Involvement (Neuro-Behçet Disease)

In adults, CNS involvement is reported in up to 50% of cases with great variability. In pediatric case collections, up to 20% of patients with Behçet's disease with CNS symptoms are described (Uluduz 2011). In childhood, there is an increased occurrence of sinus vein thromboses with the development of possible intracranial pressure.

22.7.3 Therapy

The goal of therapy is the sufficient control of inflammation. Depending on the potentially severe organ involvement, various immunosuppressive drugs are used. See ◘ Fig. 22.3 for the therapy algorithm for the treatment of Behçet's disease (Hufnagel and Kallinich 2022, adapted from Gül 2019).

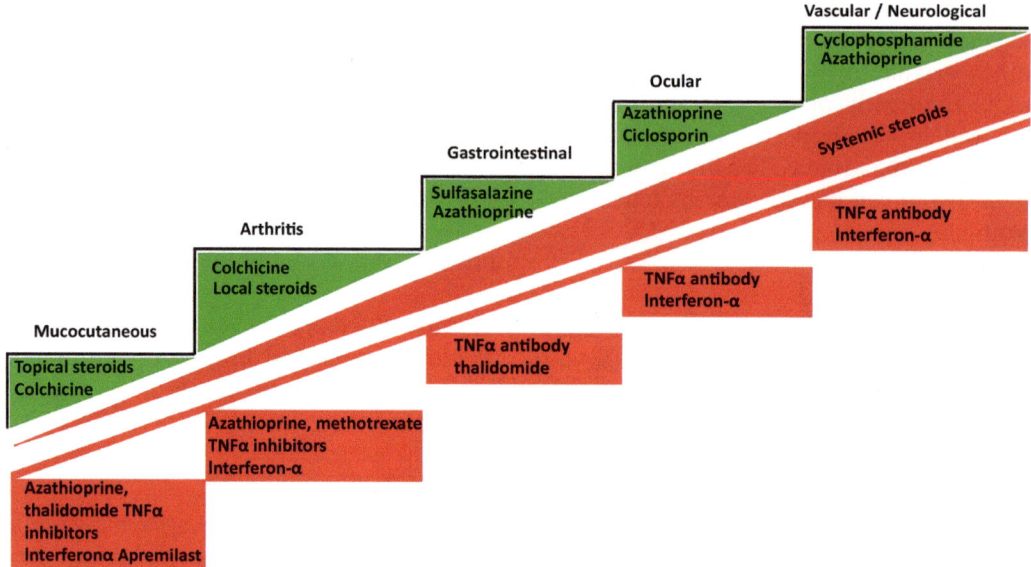

◼ Fig. 22.3 Therapy algorithm for the treatment of Behçet's disease. (From Hufnagel and Kallinich 2022, adapted from Gül 2019)

Conclusion

Behçet's disease is a serious multisystemic disease, the prognosis of which depends on rapid diagnosis. In childhood, oral and genital aphthosis as well as uveitis represent the classic diagnostic triad; it should be noted that this disease can also occur in Caucasian patients.

References

Hufnagel M, Kallinich T (2022) Morbus Behçet bei Kindern und Jugendlichen. In: Dannecker G, Kallinich T (Hrsg) Wagner N. Pädiatrische Rheumatologie, Springer, Berlin, S 665–673

Kallinich T, Keitzer R (2013) Morbus Behçet. In: Wagner N, Dannecker G (Hrsg) Pädiatrische Rheumatologie. Springer, Berlin, S 408–413

Kari JA, Shah V, Dillon MJ (2001) Behçet's disease in UK children: clinical features and treatment including thalidomide. Rheumatology (Oxford) 40:933–938

Kone- Paut I (1998) Clinical features of Behçet's disease in children: an international collaborative study of 86 cases. J Pediatr 132:721–725

Kone-Paut I, Gorchakoff-Molinas A, Weschler B, Touitou I (2002) Pediatric Behçet's disease in France. Ann Rheum Dis 61:655–656

Kotter I (2004) Behçet's disease in patients of German and Turkish origin living in Germany: a comparative analysis. J Rheumatol 31:133–139

Uluduz D (2011) Clinical characteristics of pediatric-onset neuro Behçet's disease. Neurology 77:1900–1905

A 4-Year-Old Girl with Fever Spikes and Mouth Blisters, and it Happens Every Few Weeks

Christian Huemer

Contents

23.1 Medical History

A 4-year-old girl has had a history of episodic fever outbreaks for 8 months, associated with painful oral lesions. These symptoms occur approximately every 4 weeks,
with the fever rising to 39 °C, accompanied
by painful tonsillitis. Blisters have also been
visible on the edge of the tongue and the
cheek mucosa during isolated episodes. The
child is now referred by the pediatrician, as
multiple antibiotic therapies seemed to have
no effect and the child also appears systemically ill. For about 8 weeks, there have been
isolated episodes of joint pain in the lower extremities during such fever outbreaks, which
typically occur suddenly from a state of good
health and then last about 3–5 days. Non-
steroidal anti-inflammatory drugs (Ibuprofen) seem to help, but do not bring complete
improvement. The same applies to antibiotic
therapy. General medical history unremarkable. Family medical history unremarkable.

23.2 Examination Findings

Good general and nutritional status, internal status without focal signs of inflammation. Musculoskeletal status shows no palpable synovitis or enthesopathy, but slight
arthralgia in the area of the knee joints on
both sides. ENT findings show significant
tonsillopharyngitis and two **aphthous lesions**
on the edge of the tongue, a third lesion in
the area of the gingiva (◘ Fig. 23.1). Lymph
node status shows palpable enlarged lymph
nodes subangular, otherwise unremarkable
lymph node status. Skin without abnormalities.

23.3 Laboratory Values

Blood count, differential blood count, CRP,
sedimentation rate, autoimmune findings
(ANA, rheumatoid factor, C3-, C4-comple-

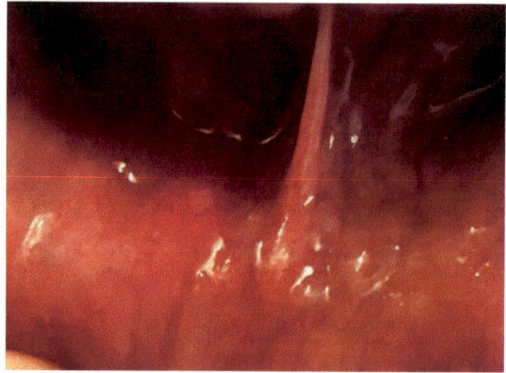

◘ **Fig. 23.1** Oral aphthae in PFAPA syndrome.
(From Lainka 2022)

ment, liver function parameters, kidney function parameters, electrolytes, immunoglobulins) unremarkable. Streptococcal antibody
findings (Anti-Streptolysin-AB, Anti-DNAse-
B-AB) unremarkable.

23.4 Educational Questions

1. What differential diagnoses should be
   discussed?
2. What further diagnostics would you
   suggest?
3. What therapies not yet tried are still
   available?

23.5 Differential Diagnostic Considerations and Educational Answers

The *differential diagnosis* for the symptoms
of recurring **tonsillitis** associated with **fever** outbreaks and **aphthous lesions** in the
oral-pharyngeal region primarily requires
the exclusion of infectious diseases such as
Herpes simplex, Adenovirus, CMV, EBV.
In a child with manifest fever outbreaks
and these symptoms, a direct pathogen detection in addition to the determination of

the laboratory chemical inflammation activity is crucial for this exclusion diagnosis. Infection serological findings in relation to the above-mentioned infectious diseases make sense in a course of several months of a disease with repeated symptoms, to document whether there is possibly a reactivation of the infection or possibly also a superinfection. In a child with 8 months of medical history, the *further diagnostics* should also consider possible underlying **immune deficiency** or autoimmune diagnoses. This has already been primarily carried out in our patient. The child has already tried a *symptomatic therapy* long-term with nonsteroidal anti-inflammatory drugs, this seemed to show no significant success, thus raising the question of an *immunomodulating therapy* (steroids?).

23.6 Further Course

In our young patient, after excluding infectious causes and insufficient response to several attempts at nonsteroidal anti-inflammatory therapy, a low-dose oral steroid therapy was tried probatorily during another fever episode associated with recurrent tonsillitis and aphthous lesions in the oral mucosa (Prednisolone 0.5 mg/kg body weight/day p.o. for up to 3 days). There was a clear immediate response to the symptoms with interruption of the fever episode and also rapid clinical improvement. The child's history, the clinical symptoms, and the rapid response to intermittent oral steroid therapy after excluding infectious diseases confirmed the **diagnosis** of a **PFAPA syndrome**. The child initially had an average of 2 to 3 fever episodes per year over a total of 2 years, which were successfully interrupted with intermittent steroid administration. Unfortunately, even after almost 2 years of conservative therapy, there was no interruption of these fever episodes, so at the age of 6, a **tonsillectomy** was indicated

in the patient. This led to a cessation of all disease symptoms. The child has since been in clinical remission and requires no further intermittent therapy.

23.7 Summary

23.7.1 Etiology

The PFAPA syndrome (**p**eriodic **f**ever, **a**phthous stomatitis, **p**haryngitis, and **a**denopathy) was first described in 1987 in 12 children, characterized by a strictly periodic fever. Due to the associated further symptoms, the same authors coined the term PFAPA syndrome (synonym Marshall syndrome) 2 years later (Marshall 1987). There are no diagnostic tests for this specific disease, the diagnosis is based on the exclusion of other diseases presenting similarly. Possibly, the PFAPA syndrome represents one of the most common periodic fever syndromes in German-speaking countries. The exact etiology is unclear, recent data suggest that an as yet undescribed, possibly infectious agent triggers activation of the complement system and the IL-1β-, IL-18-axis (Stojanov 2011; Luu 2020). The resulting immunological cascade induces, among other things, chemokines with a subsequent accumulation of T cells in the peripheral tissue (Lainka 2022).

23.7.2 Clinic

The main feature of PFAPA syndrome is the **strict periodicity** of febrile attacks. Parents often, but not always, report that they can predict the onset of a new episode in advance. The average age of onset is in the 4th year of life (Gattorno 2019). In some cases, there is a prodromal stage of marked fatigue in the child before the onset of fever, parents usually then report a sudden

23

high fever with subsequently persistently high temperatures for an average of 4 days. In about half of the patients, the fever episodes end abruptly, in the other half, the fever subsides slowly over a period of 1–2 days. Symptoms usually occur every 3–4 weeks, rarely the symptom-free intervals can also last 2–4 months. The febrile attacks are accompanied by cervical, bilateral **lymph node swelling** (88%), chills (80%), a sometimes exudative **pharyngitis** (72%) without pathogen detection, relatively painless **aphthae** in the oral mucosa (70%), headaches (60%), moderately pronounced abdominal complaints (49%). During the course, the accompanying symptoms can change, between the attacks the child is symptom-free (Foersvoll 2013; Thomas 1999; Wurster 2011). Laboratory chemical examinations show a moderate leukocytosis with a left shift, accelerated ESR, and increased CRP.

23.7.3 Diagnosis

The diagnosis of PFAPA syndrome is based on the clinical presentation, the diagnosis can only be made after excluding other diseases. Here relevant are FMF, cyclic neutropenia, or TRAPS in addition to infectious diseases.

23.7.4 Therapy

The therapy for PFAPA syndrome consists of nonsteroidal anti-rheumatic therapy (e.g., ibuprofen). In 75% of patients, an early, possibly 1 or 2-time administration of prednisolone 1–2 mg/kg body weight and dose results in a dramatic improvement in symptoms with a complete absence of fever (Gattorno 2019). The other symptoms are influenced to varying degrees by this therapy, the least of which is aphthous stomatitis.

23.7.5 Prognosis

It is noteworthy that the regular interruption of attacks by prednisolone may possibly reduce the frequency between individual episodes (Krol et al. 2013; Manthiram et al. 2017). Tonsillectomy with and without adenotomy leads to a high remission rate (91–100% depending on the publication) in PFAPA even in the long term. Differences in outcome after surgery can be explained by heterogeneous populations and inclusion criteria (Foersvoll 2013; Luu 2020; Feder 2010). Thus, this treatment option represents a further option after appropriate risk assessment.

Conclusion

PFAPA syndrome is probably one of the most common periodic fever syndromes in German-speaking countries and should be included in the differential diagnosis in cases of recurring fever episodes associated with tonsillitis, pharyngitis, and other symptoms. This is especially important to avoid too frequent antibiotic therapies in children with this syndrome; also, the discussion of tonsillectomy, which makes sense in this case, can achieve the chance of lasting remission with a clear diagnosis of PFAPA syndrome.

References

Feder HM (2010) A clinical review of 105 patients with PFAPA. Acta Paediatr 102:187–192

Foersvoll J (2013) Incidence, clinical characteristics and outcome in Norwegian children with periodic fever, aphthous stomatitis, pharyngitis and cervical adenitis syndrome: a population-based study. Acta Paediatr 102:187–192

Gattorno M (2019) Classification criteria for autoinflammatory recurrent fevers. Ann Rheum Dis 78:1025–1032

Krol P et al (2013) PFAPA syndrome: clinical characteristics and treatment outcomes in a large single centre cohort. Clin Exp Rheumatol 31:980–987

Lainka E (2022) PFAPA bei Kindern und Jugendlichen. In: Dannecker G, Kallinich T (Hrsg) Wagner N. Pädiatrische Rheumatologie, Springer, Berlin/Heidelberg, S 803–807

Luu I (2020) Immune dysregulation in the tonsillar microenvironment of periodic fever, aphthous stomatitis, pharyngitis, adenitis (PFAPA) syndrome. J Clin Immunol 40(1):179–190

Manthiram K et al (2017) Childhood arthritis and rheumatololgy research allicance (CARRA) PFAPA subcommittee. Physicians' perspectives on the diagnosis and management of periodic fever, aphthous stomatitis, pharyngitis, and cervical adenitis (PFAPA) syndrome. Rheumatol Int 37:883–889

Marshall GS (1987) Syndrome of periodic fever, pharyngitis and aphthous stomatitis. J Pediatr 110:43–46

Stojanov S (2011) Periodic fever, aphthous stomatitis, pharyngitis, and adenitis (PFAPA) is a disorder of innate immunity and Th1-activation responsive to IL-1 blockade. Proc Natl Acad Sci U S A 108:7148–7153

Thomas KT (1999) Periodic fever syndrome in children. J Pediatr 135:15–21

Wurster VM (2011) Long-term follow-up of children with periodic fever, aphthous stomatitis, pharyngitis, and cervical adenitis syndrome. J Pediatr 159:958–964

When the Infant Doesn't Thrive Because He has a Fever

Christiane Reiser

Contents

24.1 Medical History

A mother of Turkish origin presented her 10-month-old infant to her pediatrician because the introduction of supplementary feeding and pureed food was not going well and the child was repeatedly vomiting. Therefore, the mother was fully breastfeeding the child. Two months earlier, the child had been hospitalized for bronchiolitis. During this presentation, the pediatrician noticed a "percentile kink" and a lack of thriving. The presentation at the children's clinic was now to be made to clarify the recurrent vomiting in the case of poor thriving. Anamnestically, the mother reported that the child occasionally felt "warm" and also had a fever. The mother interpreted this as part of "normal" infections, as her older children attended kindergarten.

Birth measurements: Weight: 3570 g (56th percentile); Height 52 cm (53rd percentile), spontaneous delivery after 40+2 weeks of gestation. Unremarkable pregnancy and birth. Vaccination status according to plan.

Family History: Parents consanguineous, first and second degree cousin (common grandfather). Two older siblings, 6 and 3 years old, both healthy. Parents healthy. No kidney diseases in the family, no rheumatic diseases, no **familial Mediterranean fever** (FMF) known.

24.2 Examination Findings

10-month-old female infant in good general condition, slender nutritional status (Weight: 7400 g, 7th percentile; Height: 71 cm, 30th percentile), Vital parameters: Temperature 38.1 °C, otherwise unremarkable. Pediatric examination findings unremarkable, including joint status, skin, mucous membranes, abdomen, neurology. ENT: Tonsils hyperplastic, reddened, left eardrum slightly reddened.

24.3 Laboratory Values and Imaging

24.3.1 Initial Laboratory Values

Laboratory: Leukocytes: 7900/μl, CRP 1.5 mg/dl. Coagulation: Quick, PTT, Fibrinogen normal. Other overview values (kidney, liver, bone) within normal range. Tissue transglutaminase and gliadin antibodies (IgA) negative. BGA: pH 7.39, BE –4.

24.3.2 Imaging

Abdominal sonography: unremarkable

24.3.3 Educational Questions— Part 1

1. How do we explain the (recurrent?) fever and the failure to thrive in the patient? Is further clarification—possibly also expensive genetics—already indicated here?

24.4 Further Course

The patient was admitted to the hospital for clarification of the failure to thrive. Comprehensive diagnostics were carried out, in addition to the exclusion of metabolic diseases and immune defects (immunoglobulins, vaccination titers, FACS analysis of lymphocytes), the cardiac and neurological aspects were also examined, which did not reveal any relevant pathological findings. The renewed rheumatological laboratory diagnostics then showed the following findings:

Blood count: Leukocytes 12,200/μl, Hb 10.8 g/dl, Platelets 203,000/μl. Normal values for electrolytes, liver function parameters, creatinine, complement.

Serum Amyloid A (SAA): 64 g/l (normal value <10), CRP 1.48 mg/dl (normal value < 0.5), **Calprotectin/S100A8/A9 in serum: 8.3 μg/ml (normal value < 3).**

The subsequent NGS panel diagnostics for autoinflammatory diseases revealed the presence of a **homozygous M694V mutation** of the MEFV gene.

24.5 Educational Questions— Part 2

2. How is the disease treated?
3. The patient has two older siblings. Is a genetic examination also advisable for them?
4. What is the prognosis?

24.6 Educational Answers

- **1. How do we explain the (recurrent?) fever and the failure to thrive in the patient? Is further clarification—possibly also expensive genetics—already indicated here?**

The broad differential diagnostic clarification in the infant was inconspicuous. During the inpatient stay, the mother was described as routine and experienced in dealing with an infant. Repeatedly pathological were the CRP, without the child having a fever, as well as the inflammation parameters SAA, ESR and **Calprotectin/S100A8/A9** in the serum. In consanguineous parents originating from Turkey, the genetic analysis suggested the presence of an autoinflammatory syndrome, especially FMF.

In the case of a positive finding of an MEFV mutation, it is worth looking at the Infevers database, where the mutations of hereditary autoinflammatory syndromes are registered. Under ▶ ▶ https://infevers. umai-montpellier.fr/ one can view the individual variants and their possible clinical relevance/significance.

- **2. How is the disease treated?**

On the one hand, the therapy of FMF should effectively protect children from fever attacks, in order to spare them frequent phases of illness, school absences etc. In particular, however, the therapy must also effectively suppress any existing **subclinical inflammatory activity**, otherwise long-term complications such as **Amyloidosis** can occur. The effectiveness of Colchicine in the therapy of FMF and the prevention of amyloidosis has been proven for decades (Zemer et al. 1974, 1986) and is used as standard. In the application, the narrow therapeutic range and the interactions, especially in the presence of underlying diseases, should be noted. CYP3A4 inhibitors are particularly noteworthy here in pediatric patients, as Clarithromycin is a known representative of this group. When **Colchicine and Clarithromycin** are used simultaneously—which should be avoided—a dose adjustment must be made to avoid intoxications (Diesinger and Schriever 2017).

In a small proportion of patients, however, the use of IL-1 blockade may be necessary due to uncontrollable side effects/intolerances or lack of effectiveness. Approved in Germany and Austria for FMF are Anakinra (Ben-Zvi et al. 2017) and Canakinumab (De Benedetti et al. 2018). The EULAR recommendations for the therapy of FMF were published in 2016 (Ozen et al. 2016).

- **3. The patient has two older siblings. Is a genetic examination also advisable for them?**

FMF was described until this millennium as an autosomal homozygous inherited disease, so that in the case of two healthy parents—as in our case—it must be assumed that both parents are carriers and the children have a 25% risk of suffering from FMF homozygously. In addition, a "**gene dose-effect relationship**" is now assumed (Kallinich et al. 2017), according to which two pathogenic variants in a patient can generally lead to a severe course of FMF, while patients with a heterozygously inherited variant often do not or only mildly fall ill. However, in these patients, subclinical inflammatory activity is often detectable (Kallinich 2020). In our family with the detection of a certainly pathogenic homozygous mutation in the index patient, the genetic examination of the two older sibling children is certainly advisable, even if they "still" have no symptoms. In the case of the M694V variant described here, which is associated with an increased risk of amyloidosis, monitoring of subclinical inflammatory activity in asymptomatic genetically affected individuals is recommended (Ozen et al. 2016).

- **4. What is the prognosis?**

The disease requires lifelong therapy. In principle, the colchicine therapy is effective, if it fails or is intolerant, additional effective therapy options are available by means of IL-1 blockade. Amyloidosis represents the severe long-term complication in these patients and is associated with increased mortality, so therapeutic efforts as well as sensitizing the patients should have a high priority.

24.7 Summary

24.7.1 Etiology

FMF is a rare autoinflammatory disease that particularly affects ethnic groups from the Mediterranean region, especially people of Jewish, Turkish, Armenian or Arab origin are affected, with sometimes very high heterozygote frequencies (Daniels et al. 1995).

24.7.2 Pathophysiology

FMF is based on a MEFV mutation on chromosome 16 (The International FMF Consortium 1997; French FMF Consor-

tium 1997). The gene product is **pyrin**, which is involved in the activation process of the NLRP3- inflammasome. The ultimate activation of **caspase-1** leads, among other things, to cytokine activation. A detailed presentation of the pathophysiological mechanisms of the disease can be found in (Kallinich 2020). An informative compilation can be found in ▢ Fig. 24.1 (from Kallinich et al. 2020).

24.7.3 Diagnosis/Clinic

Classically, FMF is accompanied by a fever spike over 1–3 days, often associated with abdominal pain and/or arthritis. The episode is usually very uniform within individuals and can be announced by prodromes, such as constipation (more common in older adolescents and adults). Especially in (small) childhood, fever may be the only symptom. The classic symptoms besides fever include:

Abdominal pain: caused by peritonitis, the most common accompanying symptom besides fever.

Arthritis: noticeably swollen, overheated, painful joints, usually of the lower extremity (▢ Fig. 24.2).

Skin: erysipelas-like exanthema (▢ Fig. 24.3).

Thorax: Often unilateral thoracic pain occurs as a sign of pleuritis.

Other rarer manifestations: mostly unilateral testicular pain due to inflammation of the tunica vaginalis; myalgia, also protracted febrile myalgia.

Classification criteria exist, which were created in the name of PRINTO/PReS and the Eurofever Register, see ▢ Tab. 24.1.

24.7.4 Diagnostics

Initial diagnostics have already been reported. Important for follow-up checks is the detection of (subclinical) inflammatory

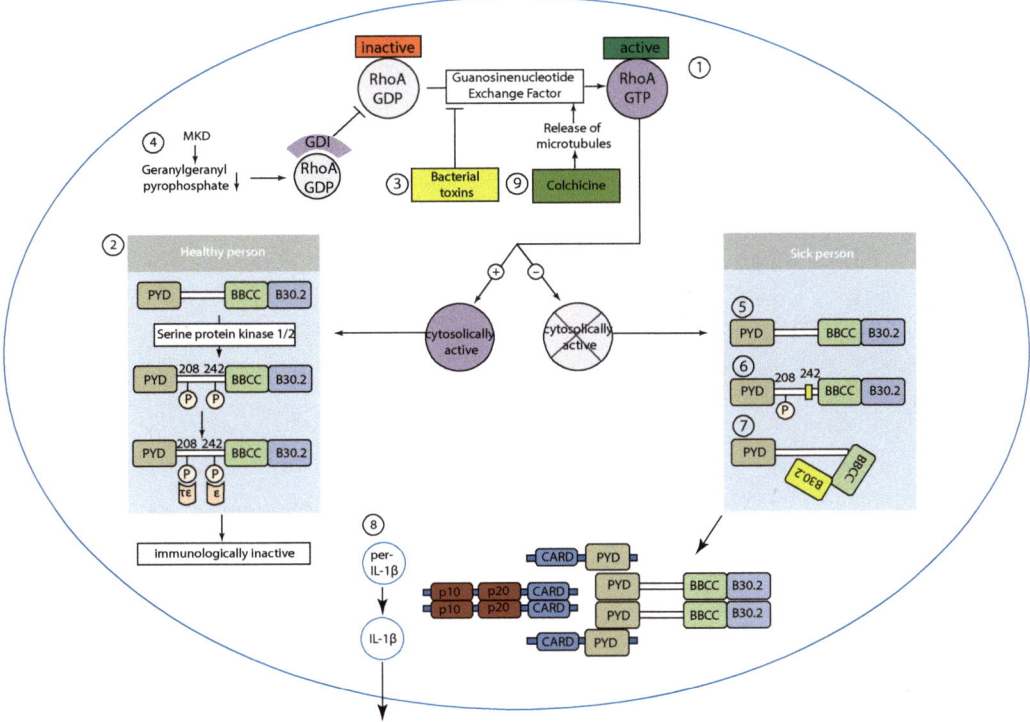

☐ **Fig. 24.1** Physiological activation of the pyrin inflammasome and its role in the pathophysiology of different diseases. Activated Rho-GTPases phosphorylate the pyrin molecule at the serine amino acids 208 and 242 through activations of the protein kinases PKN1/2 (*1*). This allows binding of the two chaperone isoforms 14-3-3ε and 14-3-3τ, which in turn keeps the pyrin inflammasome in an inactive state (*2*). Toxins of gram-positive bacteria, such as TcdB and C3 from *Clostridium difficile*, prevent the activation of the Rho-GTPases; the proinflammatory reaction proceeds unhindered under these circumstances (*3*). In HIDS (Hyper-Ig[Immunoglobulin] D Syndrome)/MKD (Mevalonate Kinase Deficiency), there is a lack of metabolic products of cholesterol synthesis (e.g., geranylgeranyl pyrophosphate). This leads via intermediate steps to a lack of activation of the Rho-GTPases (*4*). Accordingly, the pyrin inflammasome is activated under the following conditions: **a**) in the absence of activated Rho-GTPases, e.g., due to an infection with toxin-producing bacteria or a lack of metabolic products of cholesterol synthesis (*5*); **b**) in the presence of pyrin-associated autoinflammation with neutrophilic dermatosis (PAAND). Here, mutations prevent phosphorylation of the serines (*6*); **c**) in the presence of FMF (Familial Mediterranean Fever). It is suspected that mutations in the B30.2 domain prevent phosphorylation of positions 208 and 242 by changing the pyrin structure (*7*). Under these circumstances, the pyrin inflammasome is activated with subsequent cytokine processing (*8*). Colchicine leads to the release of the RhoA activator "Guanine nucleotide exchange factor" (GEF)-H1 from the microtubules. This is an essential factor for the activation of the Rho-GTPases. Abbreviations in the scheme: *BBCC* B-Box Zinc Finger Domain Coiled-coiled Domain, *GDI* "Guanine diphosphate dissociation inhibitor", *GDP* "Guanine diphosphate", *GTP* "Guanine triphosphate", *MKD* Mevalonate Kinase Deficiency, *PKN* "Serine/threonine-protein kinase N1", *PYD* Pyrin, *Rho* "Ras homologue". (From Kallinich et al. 2020, with kind permission of Springer Publishing)

activity, especially of SAA and S100A8/A9. These parameters should—in addition to the standard values—be routinely collected at patient control appointments. Especially with (highly) pathogenic variants (e.g., the mutations M694V, V726A, M680I, M694I), a target for SAA of less than 10 mg/l should be aimed for.

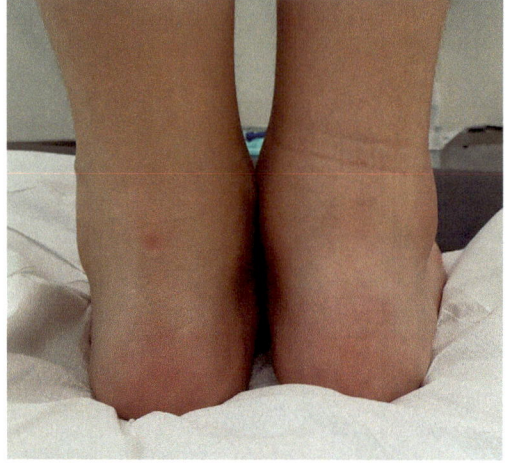

◻ Fig. 24.2 Painful arthritis of the right ankle with swelling in FMF

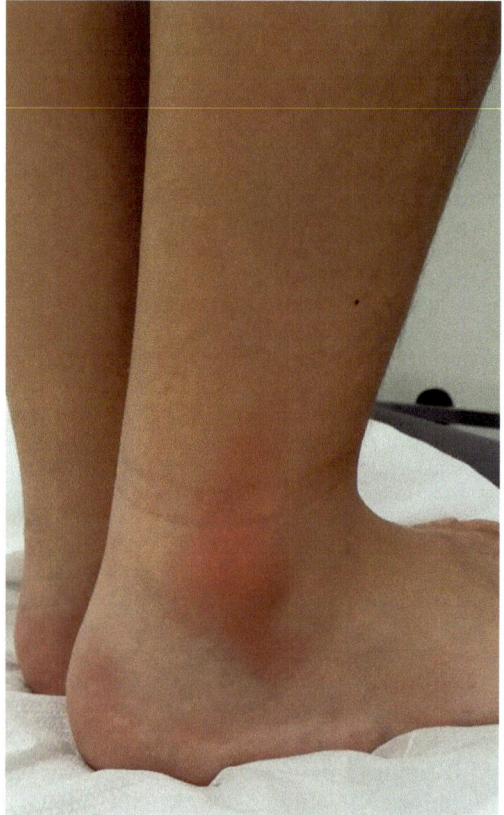

◻ Fig. 24.3 Erysipelas-like exanthema in FMF

◻ Tab. 24.1   Classification criteria of PRINTO/PReS Eurofever. (After Gattorno et al. 2019)

Confirmed genotype is present	Confirmed genotype is not present
and at least one other criterion:	and at least two other criteria:
Duration of fever 1–3 days Arthritis Pleuritic pain Abdominal pain	

24.7.5 Therapy

The first-line therapeutic is **Colchicine**. This is initially dosed according to age, not weight, starting with a dose of max. 0.5 mg/day in early childhood. The dose is then increased depending on age, response, and tolerability to max. 2–2.5 mg/day (in adolescents). To achieve better tolerability, the dose can possibly be split. Avoiding lactose-containing products can also improve tolerability, as lactose intolerance is more common in these patients (Fradkin et al. 1995). Patients with so-called **Colchicine resistance** or intolerance may need therapy expansion to Anakinra or Canakinumab (Rilonacept is also approved, but *not in Europe*). The definition of colchicine resistance is not yet clearly defined internationally (Kallinich et al. 2019): Possible components for this are persistent inflammation, several episodes per year (EULAR criteria: 1 episode/month over 6 months), amyloidosis, in which therapy expansion should be made (Ozen et al. 2016).

24.7.6 Prognosis

Provided that the disease activity is well controlled and the disease burden can be minimized, a good prognosis of the disease can be expected. It is worth mentioning that the selective advantage that the heterozygotes had in the past in the specific population groups led to a resistance against *Yersinia pestis* (Park et al. 2020).

Conclusion

Through lifelong therapy that well controls the inflammation in the body, FMF, as the most common hereditary autoinflammatory disease, is well manageable in most affected individuals.

References

Ben-Zvi I, Kukuy O, Giat E et al (2017) Anakinra for colchicine-resistant familial Mediterranean fever: a randomized, double-blind, placebo-controlled trial. Arthritis Rheumatol 69:854–862

Daniels M, Shohat T, Brenner-Ullman A, Shohat M (1995) Familial Mediterranean fever: high gene frequency among the non-Ashkenazic and Ashkenazic Jewish populations in Israel. Am J Med Genet 55:311–314

De Benedetti F, Gattorno M, Anton J et al (2018) Canakinumab for the treatment of autoinflammatory recurrent fever syndromes. N Engl J Med 378:1908–1919. ▶ https://doi.org/10.1056/NEJMoa1706314

Diesinger C, Schriever J (2017) Colchicin – gut informieren, vorsichtig dosieren. Bull Arzneimittelsich 4:15–23

Fradkin A, Yahav J, Zemer D, Jonas A (1995) Colchicine-induced lactose malabsorption in patients with familial Mediterranean fever. Isr J Med Sci 31:616–620

French FMF Consortium (1997) A candidate gene for familial Mediterranean fever. Nat Genet 17:25–31. ▶ https://doi.org/10.1038/ng0997-25

Gattorno M, Hofer M, Federici S et al (2019) Classification criteria for autoinflammatory recurrent fevers. Ann Rheum Dis 78:1025–1032. ▶ https://doi.org/10.1136/annrheumdis-2019-215048

Kallinich T (2020) FMF bei Kindern und Jugendlichen. In: Wagner N, Dannecker G, Kallinich T (Hrsg) Pädiatrische Rheumatologie. Springer, Berlin/Heidelberg, S 1–15

Kallinich T, Orak B, Wittkowski H (2017) [Role of genetics in familial Mediterranean fever]. Z Rheumatol 76:303–312. ▶ https://doi.org/10.1007/s00393-017-0265-9

Kallinich T, Blank N, Braun T et al (2019) Evidenzbasierte Therapieempfehlungen für das familiäre Mittelmeerfieber. Z Für Rheumatol 78:91–101. ▶ https://doi.org/10.1007/s00393-018-0588-1

Kallinich T, Hinze C, Wittkowski H (2020) Classification of autoinflammatory diseases based on pathophysiological mechanisms. Z Rheumatol 79:624–638. ▶ https://doi.org/10.1007/s00393-020-00794-3

Ozen S, Demirkaya E, Erer B et al (2016) EULAR recommendations for the management of familial Mediterranean fever. Ann Rheum Dis 75:644–651

Park YH, Remmers EF, Lee W et al (2020) Ancient familial Mediterranean fever mutations in human pyrin and resistance to Yersinia pestis. Nat Immunol 21:857–867. ▶ https://doi.org/10.1038/s41590-020-0705-6

The International FMF Consortium (1997) Ancient missense mutations in a new member of the RoRet gene family are likely to cause familial Mediterranean fever. Cell 90:797–807. ▶ https://doi.org/10.1016/s0092-8674(00)80539-5

Zemer D, Revach M, Pras M et al (1974) A controlled trial of colchicine in preventing attacks of familial Mediterranean fever. N Engl J Med 291:932–934. ▶ https://doi.org/10.1056/NEJM197410312911803

Zemer D, Pras M, Sohar E et al (1986) Colchicine in the prevention and treatment of the amyloidosis of familial Mediterranean fever. N Engl J Med 314:1001–1005. ▶ https://doi.org/10.1056/NEJM198604173141601

When Cold Causes Rash and Many Complaints

Annette Holl-Wieden

Contents

C. Huemer and H. Girschick (eds.), *Clinical Examples in Pediatric Rheumatology*,
https://doi.org/10.1007/978-3-662-68732-1_25

25.1 Medical History

▪▪ Leon

Leon, 9 years old, had been experiencing recurrent **urticarial rash** on his face, trunk, and limbs **after exposure to cold** for several months. He also had **pain in both ankles**, headaches, increased **fatigue**, and occasional **fever**. The symptoms occurred once every 2 weeks and lasted 2 days. The boy had been experiencing recurrent urticarial rashes lasting a few hours after exposure to cold since he was 3 months old (▪ Fig. 25.1). At the age of 2 ½ years, he had a severe episode of illness, also after prolonged exposure to cold, with rash, pain and swelling of the ankles and wrists, and fever. The symptoms lasted 3 days. The mother always tried to avoid exposing the child to cold by dressing him in warm

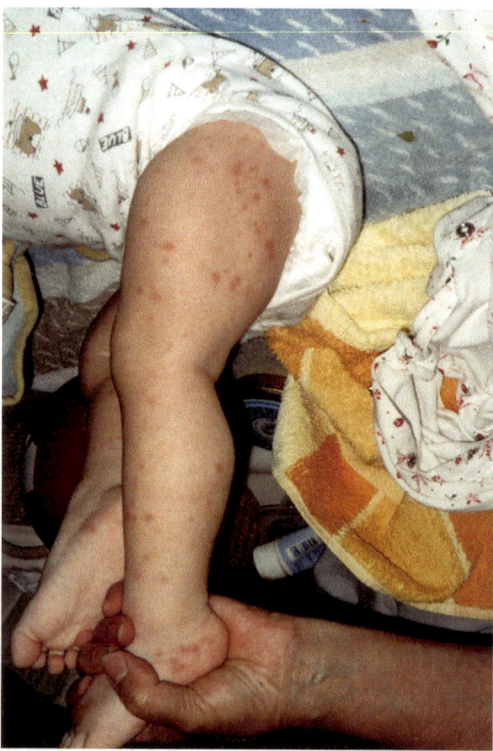

▪ Fig. 25.1   Leon at the age of 3 months with macular, partly urticarial rash

clothes. The symptoms were more pronounced in autumn and winter. New to the symptoms was the boy's strong feeling of illness and the frequency of the symptoms. Many independent activities such as outdoor soccer training in the cold season could no longer be carried out. In addition, Leon had many school absences. The boy's father, the father's brother, and the father's mother had similar symptoms. They were suspected of having a "cold allergy".

▪▪ Linus

Linus was first presented to our clinic at the age of 14 10/12 years, the family had only been living in Germany for 3 months. The boy had been experiencing recurrent fine-spotted, partly **urticarial rashes** on his arms and legs since he was 6 weeks old. The boy was fully breastfed at that time. Initially, food allergies were suspected. Various elimination diets of the mother and also weaning at the age of 9 months did not improve the situation. At the age of 12 months, it was noticed that the rash increased after exposure to cold. Shortly after exposure to cold, rashes appeared all over the body, sometimes with swelling in the face, hands, and feet. The rashes were painful to touch. At the age of 1 ½ years, Linus developed recurrent **pain and swelling of the knee joints**, and later also pain and swelling of the ankle joints, finger joints, wrist joints, and elbow joints. Later, these joint complaints were constantly present. At the age of 3 years, a prominence of the kneecaps was noticed. Then there were recurrent **fever episodes** . The boy increasingly suffered from **headaches, learning and concentration difficulties**. At the age of 11 years, the symptoms worsened. Linus constantly had headaches, joint pain, rashes, often fever. The complaints increased after cold exposure , but were also constantly present without it. Attending school was no longer possible. No one in the family had similar symptoms.

25.2 **Investigation**

▪▪ Leon

The investigation during a disease flare-up showed a **urticarial exanthem** on the trunk and trunk-proximal extremities. The exanthem was not painful and did not itch. The rest of the internal medical examination, especially the bone and joint status, was unremarkable.

▪▪ Linus

At the initial presentation, Linus had a fever around 40 °C and a maculopapular, partly urticarial **exanthem** on his face and extremities (◘ Fig. 25.2) after exposure to cold. He had a **polyarthritis** with arthritis of the finger joints (MCP I on both sides, IP I on both sides, PIP II–V on both sides, DIP II–V on both sides) (◘ Fig. 25.2d), the elbow joints, the knee joints, ankle joints and arthritis of several toe joints (PIP II and IV on both sides). Notable was a strong **bony swelling of many joints**, especially the elbow joints (◘ Fig. 25.2). The left forearm was noticeably shortened compared to the right. A prominent forehead was noticeable. Linus was noticeably small and delicate for his age. With a body length of 140 cm, he was 14 cm **below the 3rd percentile**, with a body weight of 30 kg, 10 kg below the 3rd percentile. The head circumference was 55 cm, which is on the 25th–50th percentile.

25.3 **Laboratory Values and Imaging**

25.3.1 **Laboratory Values**

▪▪ Leon

The inflammation parameters were elevated, **CRP 1.71 mg/dl** (normal value 0–0.5), **ESR 22 mm/h, Serum-Amyloid A148 mg/l** (normal value < 10). The blood count and differential blood count were unremarkable, the overview laboratory values (including liver and kidney values) showed no abnormalities. The urine status was also unremarkable.

▪▪ Linus

In Linus too, the inflammation parameters were elevated, **CRP 7.24 mg/dl** (normal value 0–0.5), **ESR 50 mm/h, Serum-Amyloid A 190 mg/l** (normal value < 10), **S100A8/A9**-proteins 50,700 ng/ml (normal value < 2940). The blood count showed a slight **leukocytosis of 14,400/μl,** (normal value 4500–13,000) with a **neutrophilia of 74.8%** (normal value 40–61.5) as well as a hypochromic microcytic anemia, **Hb 10.3 g/dl** (normal value 13–16), **MCV 67.9 fl** (normal value 78–95), **MCH 20.2 pg** (normal value 25–35). The overview laboratory values were unremarkable, as was the urine status. A cerebrospinal fluid examination showed an increase in cell count, **leukocytes 36/mm^3** (normal value 0–4), of which 65% were segmented. Glucose, protein, albumin, IgG were within the normal range. The **cerebrospinal fluid opening pressure** was elevated at **31 mmHg** (normal value 5–15). The cerebrospinal fluid culture was sterile. The cerebrospinal fluid findings thus indicated aseptic granulocytic meningitis with increased cerebrospinal fluid pressure.

25.3.2 **Imaging and Further Investigations**

▪▪ Leon

An eye examination and an ENT examination with hearing test were unremarkable. The further diagnostic imaging (including ECG, echocardiography, abdominal ultrasound) revealed no abnormal findings.

▪▪ Linus

In Linus, the eye examination showed strong abnormalities. A **keratopathy** (lipid-like deposits in the cornea) was found more on the right than on the left, a

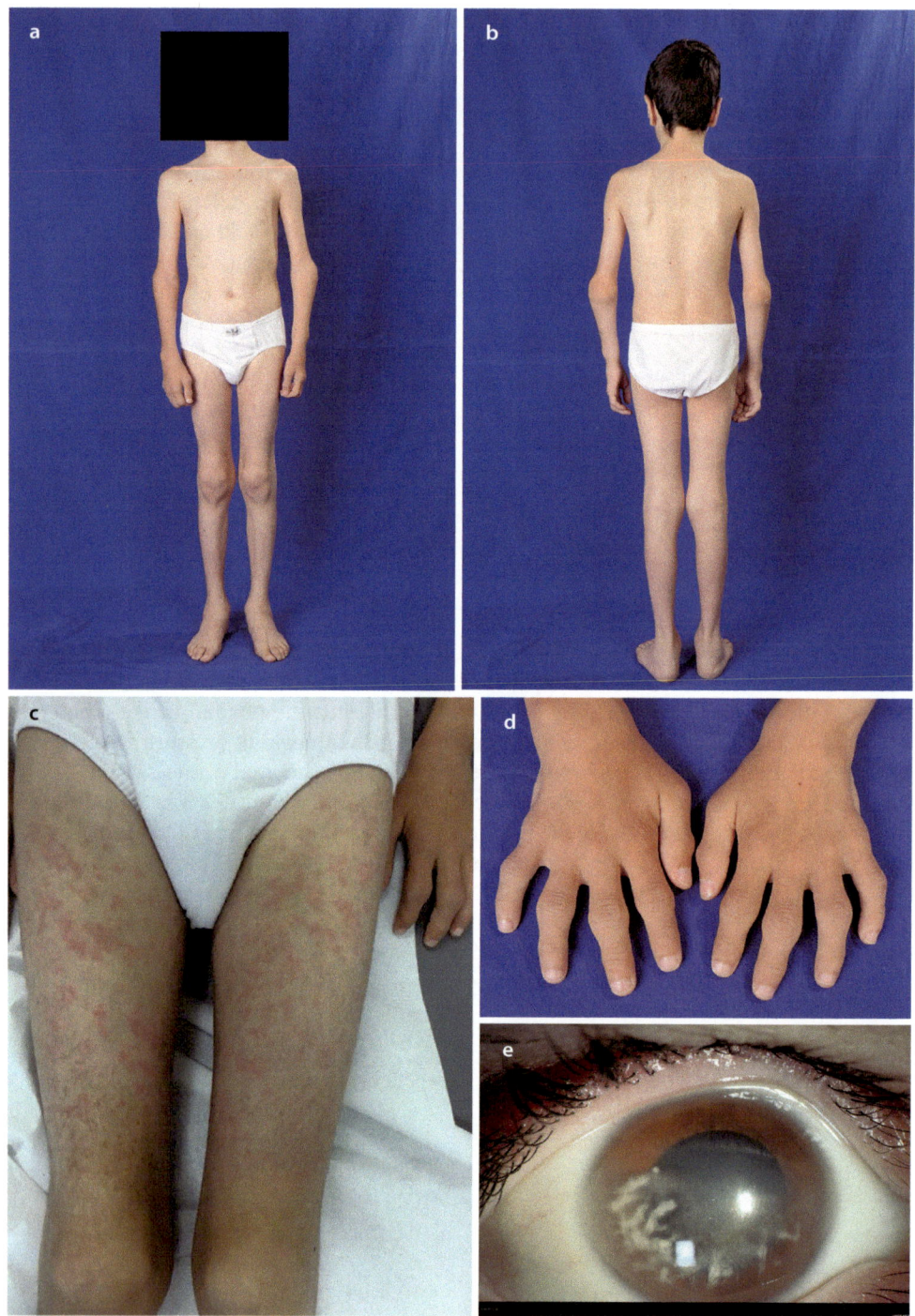

Fig. 25.2 a,b General dystrophy, bony swellings of the elbow joints, arthritis of the ankle joints with swellings and blurred ankle contours. **c** Macular, partly urticarial exanthem. **d** Arthritis MCP I on both sides, IP I on both sides, PIP II–V on both sides and DIP II–V on both sides. **e** Keratopathy. (Lipid-like deposits in the cornea)

pronounced **optic nerve papillary swelling** more on the right than on the left, and a strong reduction in visual acuity, visual acuity right 0.4, left 0.6 (■ Fig. 25.2e). An ENT examination with hearing test revealed a **sensorineural hearing loss, especially in the high-frequency range** (■ Fig. 25.3). An X-ray of the left elbow joint showed a bulbous distal humerus and a subluxation position in the humeroradial joint, an X-ray of the left forearm showed a swelling of the distal shortened ulna and an ulnar deviation of the distal radius (■ Fig. 25.4). A cranial MRI showed a normal finding appropriate for the age.

25.4 Educational Questions

1. What suspected diagnosis should be made for Leon based on the described complaints of recurrent urticarial exanthems, arthralgia, headaches, fatigue, fever triggered by cold exposure, and high inflammation parameters?
2. What diagnosis should be made for Linus based on the urticarial exanthems, arthritis, fever, exacerbated by cold exposure, the high inflammation parameters, but also the skeletal changes and cerebral involvement?

3. Should therapy be carried out in the patients? Which one?

25.5 Differential Diagnostic Considerations

■■ Leon

In the boy's relatives, there was a suspicion of a **"cold allergy",** which is generally understood to be the acquired form of cold urticaria. This is a possible cause for recurrent urticarial exanthems after cold exposure. However, patients usually also have mucosal edema, a flush, respiratory symptoms, and tachycardia. Arthralgia, fever, and high inflammation parameters are not found. The disease also does not show a familial accumulation. In our patient, the diagnosis of the acquired form of cold urticaria could therefore rather be excluded. The recurrent disease episodes with high inflammation parameters suggested a hereditary autoinflammatory disease, a so-called hereditary periodic "fever syndrome". Cold as a trigger of the disease episodes, the urticarial exanthem, the arthralgia, and the fatigue spoke for a **Cryopyrin-associated periodic syndrome**(CAPS), specifically the mildest form of CAPS, the **familial cold-induced**

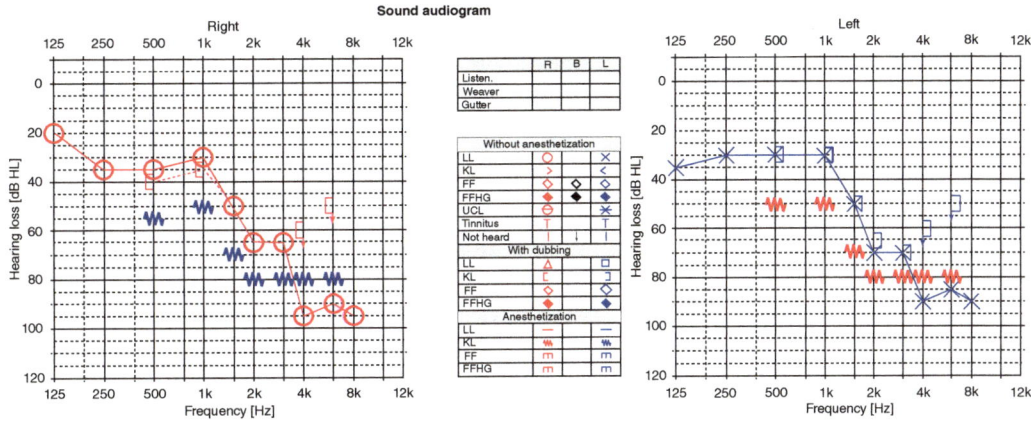

■ **Fig. 25.3** Linus' hearing test. Diagnosis of sensorineural hearing loss in the high-frequency range

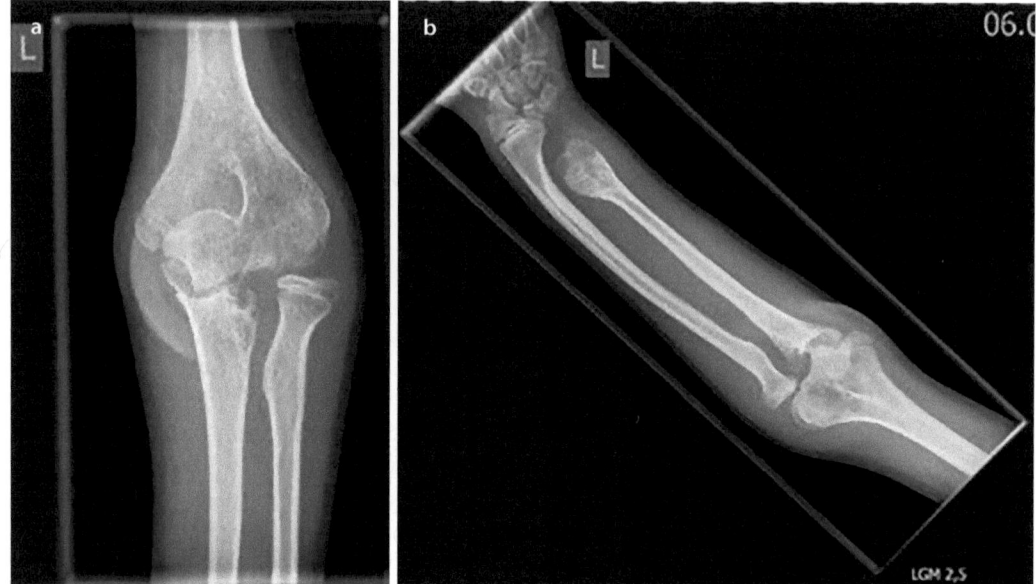

Fig. 25.4 **a,b** Conventional radiology of Linus' left arm. **a** Subluxation position in the humeroradial joint. Bulbous distal humerus. Cystic subcortical lesions in the area of the incisura radialis ulnae. Subchondral demineralization at the epicondylus radialis and the radius epiphysis. **b** Swelling of the distal shortened ulna, ulnar deviation of the distal radius, swelling of the distal humerus. (With kind permission from Dr. Clemens Benoit, Institute for Diagnostic and Interventional Radiology, University Hospital Würzburg)

autoinflammatory syndrome 1(FCAS1). The clinical suspected diagnosis must be genetically confirmed. In addition to the classic FCAS (FCAS 1), there are hereditary autoinflammatory diseases with similar symptoms, in which a mutation in another gene is present, e.g., familial cold urticaria type 2 due to mutation in the NLRP12 gene, familial cold urticaria type 3 due to mutation in the PLCG2 gene, or familial cold urticaria type 4 due to mutation in the NLRC4 gene. For the genetic examination, an **autoinflammation panel** based on a **next-generation sequencing-**approach is recommended, which includes these diseases.

▪▪ Linus

For Linus, the history and findings were indicative of a CAPS.

Initially, he had recurrent disease episodes with urticarial exanthems, joint complaints, triggered by cold, similar to the first patient. Inflammation parameters were not determined in the first years. The early onset at 6 weeks, the bony swellings of the joints, the cerebral involvement with aseptic meningitis, and subsequently learning and concentration disorders suggested the most severe form of the disease, the **NOMID/CINCAsyndrome (Neonatal Onset Multisystem Inflammatory Disease/Chronic Infantile Neurological and Articular Syndrome).** In NOMID/CINCA, the family history, as in our patient, is often negative, as there are usually sporadic new mutations.

25.6 Further Course

▪▪ Leon

A genetic examination was carried out using an **autoinflammation panel**. A **mutation in theNLRP3gene** was found, which is classified as pathogenic. The diagnosis of a cryopyrin-associated periodic syndrome (CAPS) could thus be made. There was no evidence of amyloidosis. Medication with **Canakinumab** (2 mg/kg body weight s.c. every 8 weeks) was started. Canakinumab is a human monoclonal antibody that binds and inactivates interleukin-1β. Another drug for interleukin-1 blockade was not approved at that time. Relatives of Leon were also diagnosed with CAPS through genetic testing and therapy with interleukin-1 blockade drugs was initiated. Leon has not had any severe disease flares since. However, if the administration of Canakinumab was delayed due to illness etc., the boy occasionally observed a rash after cold exposure again, and there was also an increase in inflammation parameters. Leon has now been in remission for several years under medication with Canakinumab.

▪▪ Linus

In Linus, a genetic examination for the classic hereditary periodic fever syndromes (FMF, TRAPS, HIDS, CAPS) was initiated at the age of 5 in his home country. A mutation in the NLRP3 gene was found, which was classified as pathogenic. The diagnosis of CAPS was made. Treatment attempts were made with NSAIDs, glucocorticoids, and colchicine. This did not lead to any improvement. After presentation in our clinic at the age of 14 10/12 years, the diagnosis of CAPS, subtype NOMID/CINCA, was confirmed. The examinations revealed no evidence of amyloidosis. Therapy with **Anakinra** was started. Anakinra is an interleukin-1 receptor antagonist that is administered subcutaneously once a day. Initially, the therapy was given at a dosage of 2 mg/kg body weight/day and increased to 2.7 mg/kg body weight/day corresponding to 100 mg/day. There was prompt improvement after the start of therapy. Fever, rashes, and headaches no longer occurred. The inflammation values normalized. In the course of time, the arthritis also im-

proved. After 1 1/2 years, however, MTX was added to the therapy due to persistent arthritis, especially of the left elbow joint. Remission of the arthritis was achieved, the therapy with MTX was stopped after 2 ½ years. However, the bony swelling of the left elbow joint was progressive, and the bending of the forearm also increased somewhat. The inner ear hearing loss did not improve. Hearing aids were provided. 1 year after the start of therapy with Anakinra, the cerebrospinal fluid examination was unremarkable. The learning disorders improved, Linus was later able to complete his planned school graduation and start training. The good **catch-up growth** for body length and body weight was also pleasing. At the age of 18, the body length was 167 cm on the 3rd–10th percentile, the body weight was 56 kg on the 10th–25th percentile. The patient increasingly had strong local reactions to Anakinra and increasing fear of the daily injections. We therefore recently decided to switch therapy to Canakinumab. A dose increase from Canakinumab 150 mg s.c. every 4 weeks to Canakinumab 300 mg s.c. every 4 weeks was necessary. Under this, Linus has no complaints and the inflammation parameters are not elevated.

25.7 Educative Answers

- **1. What suspected diagnosis should be made for Leon based on the described complaints?**

The recurring disease flares with high inflammation parameters suggest a hereditary periodic "fever syndrome". Cold as a trigger of disease flares, urticarial rashes and arthralgia but also headaches and fatigue, as in Leon, are consistent with a cryopyrin-associated periodic syndrome (CAPS). The suspected diagnosis must be genetically confirmed. However, there are also other hereditary autoinflammatory diseases with similar symptoms that must be ruled out by genetic testing.

- **What diagnosis should be made for Linus based on the symptoms?**

Recurring urticarial rashes, arthritis, fever, triggered/exacerbated by cold exposure, high inflammation parameters, but also bony changes and cerebral involvement, as in Linus, suggest a cryopyrin-associated periodic syndrome, specifically the most severe form, a NOMID/CINCA disease.

- **Should therapy be carried out in the patients? Which one?**

In the patients, therapy with a drug for interleukin-1 blockade should be started to prevent disease flares, improve symptoms, and especially in patient 2 to prevent sequelae such as **amyloidosis**.

25.8 Summary

25.8.1 Etiology/Pathogenesis

The Cryopyrin-associated periodic syndromes (CAPS) belong to the hereditary autoinflammatory diseases, the so-called hereditary periodic "fever syndromes". In these diseases, there are recurring episodes of inflammation, often fever with manifestation in various organs. CAPS is usually inherited in an autosomal dominant manner, somatic mosaics have been described. There is a heterozygous **mutation in the NLRP3 gene**. This encodes the NLRP3 protein/Cryopyrin. In granulocytes and monocytes, the NLRP3 protein forms a multiprotein complex with other proteins, the NLRP3 inflammasome. The inflammasome activates Caspase 1. This cleaves Pro-Interleukin-1β (pro-IL-1β) into biologically active IL-1β. IL-1β activates Nuclear factor kB (NFkB) and leads to the production of further proinflammatory cy-

tokines. In CAPS, the **NLRP3 protein** is altered, leading to enhanced activation and increased production of IL-1β (Welzel and Kuemmerle-Deschner 2021).

25.8.2 Clinic

CAPS includes 3 forms with varying degrees of severity, with some continuous transition.

1. Mild form: FCAS (familial cold-induced autoinflammatory syndrome)
2. Moderate form: MWS (Muckle-Wells Syndrome)
3. Severe form: NOMID/CINCA (Neonatal Onset Multisystem Inflammatory Disease/Chronic Infantile Neurological and Articular Syndrome)

Disease flares can be triggered by cold, stress, infections, trauma, and sleep deprivation. The disease flares last from 30 min to about 72 h. FCAS usually begins in the first months of life. Cold is the typical trigger for a disease flare. The patients have **urticarial exanthema, myalgia/arthralgia, conjunctivitis**, and possibly **fever**. In **MWS**, the onset of the disease can be in early childhood, but also in adulthood. The patients have disease flares with symptoms similar to FCAS. In addition to myalgia and arthralgia, arthritis can also occur, in addition to conjunctivitis, there can also be **episcleritis** or **papilledema**. Unlike FCAS, the patients have **inner ear hearing loss,** initially often only in the high-frequency range. In NOMID/CINCA, patients usually become ill postnatally or in the first weeks of life. Unlike FCAS and MWS, NOMID/CINCA has persistent inflammation. Characteristic is an **arthropathy** with excessive growth of the patella and epiphyses of the long tubular bones, size difference of the extremities, contractures. There is usually a chronic sterile meningitis with possible consequences such as **increased intracranial pressure,brain atrophy** and **developmental disorders** such as cerebral palsy. The amyloidosis risk is low in FCAS, higher in MWS and high in NOMID/ CINCA (Welzel and Kuemmerle-Deschner 2021).

25.8.3 Diagnosis

The diagnosis of CAPS is made clinically and confirmed genetically. Inflammatory parameters are particularly elevated during disease flare-ups. Characteristic are leukocytosis, neutrophilia, thrombocytosis, anemia, an increase in ESR, CRP, serum amyloid A (SAA) and **S100A8/A9 proteins.Serum amyloid A** is an important parameter to recognize subclinical inflammation and the risk of developing amyloidosis. The S100A8/A9 proteins are considered sensitive biomarkers for disease activity and help monitor inflammation and response to therapy (Welzel and Kuemmerle-Deschner 2021; Wittkowski et al. 2011). Other diseases with recurrent systemic inflammation such as autoimmune diseases, malignant diseases etc. must be ruled out. Important are further examinations such as hearing tests, eye examinations, possibly cranial MRI, cerebrospinal fluid examination and imaging of joints. A genetic examination should then be carried out to confirm the diagnosis. However, there are patients in whom no germline mutation is found despite a strong suspicion of CAPS. The presence of **somatic mutations(mosaics)** should then be considered and appropriate examinations carried out (Tanaka et al. 2011; Welzel and Kuemmerle-Deschner 2021). In addition, **variants of uncertain significance (VUS)** in the NLRP3 gene are often found. For CAPS, diagnostic and classification criteria have been developed (Gattorno et al. 2019; Kuemmerle-Deschner et al. 2017). The diagnostic criteria for CAPS do *not* include genetic confirmation and can be helpful when genetic testing is not available or is negative. A diagnosis of CAPS can be made if the inflammation values (CRP, SAA) are high and at least 2 of the following 6 symptoms/findings are present: urticarial rash, cold- or stress-induced disease flare-ups, chronic aseptic meningitis, sensorineural hearing loss, musculoskeletal complaints (arthralgia, arthritis, myalgia), skeletal abnormalities (overgrowth of the epiphyses, frontal bossing) (Kuemmerle-Deschner et al. 2017). The classification criteria include clinical criteria and genetic findings. They can be helpful in making a diagnosis, especially when variants of uncertain significance are present (Gattorno et al. 2019).

25.8.4 Therapy

Treatment goals are to suppress the systemic inflammatory response, prevent organ damage, improve functionality and quality of life (Hansmann et al. 2020; Welzel and Kuemmerle-Deschner 2021). The ProKind initiative of the GKJR has formulated treatment recommendations that follow a Treat-to-Target therapy approach. Interleukin-1 blockade drugs are used. The efficacy and safety of Anakinra, an Interleukin-1 receptor antagonist, and Canakinumab, a human monoclonal antibody against Interleukin-1β, have been demonstrated in several studies (Goldbach-Mansky et al. 2006; Kuemmerle-Deschner et al. 2011; Lachmann et al. 2009; Walker et al. 2021). NSAIDs can be helpful for pain and fever. Especially in milder forms of CAPS, protection from cold (warm clothing) can be helpful to prevent flare-ups (Welzel and Kuemmerle-Deschner 2021).

25

Conclusion

In cases of recurrent disease flare-ups with elevated inflammation values during the flare-up or even between flare-ups, a monogenetic autoinflammatory disease, a hereditary recurrent "fever syndrome" should be considered. Cold or stress as triggers of the **disease flare-ups,urticarial rashes, musculoskeletal complaints, eye inflammations (conjunctivitis, episcleritis, uveitis)**, but also **central nervous symptoms,hearing loss** as well as **skeletal changes** should make one think of CAPS.

References

Gattorno M, Hofer M, Federici S, Vanoni F, Bovis F, Aksentijevich I, Anton J, Arostegui JI, Barron K, Ben-Cherit E, Brogan PA, Cantarini L, Ceccherini I, De Benedetti F, Dedeoglu F, Demirkaya E, Frenkel J, Goldbach-Mansky R, Gul A, Hentgen V, Hoffman H, Kallinich T, Kone-Paut I, Kuemmerle-Deschner J, Lachmann HJ, Laxer RM, Livneh A, Obici L, Ozen S, Rowczenio D, Russo R, Shinar Y, Simon A, Toplak N, Touitou I, Uziel Y, van Gijn M, Foell D, Garassino C, Kastner D, Martini A, Sormani MP, Ruperto N, Eurofever R, the Paediatric Rheumatology International Trials O (2019) Classification criteria for autoinflammatory recurrent fevers. Ann Rheum Dis 78(8):1025–1032. ▶ https://doi.org/10.1136/annrheumdis-2019-215048

Goldbach-Mansky R, Dailey NJ, Canna SW, Gelabert A, Jones J, Rubin BI, Kim HJ, Brewer C, Zalewski C, Wiggs E, Hill S, Turner ML, Karp BI, Aksentijevich I, Pucino F, Penzak SR, Haverkamp MH, Stein L, Adams BS, Moore TL, Fuhlbrigge RC, Shaham B, Jarvis JN, O'Neil K, Vehe RK, Beitz LO, Gardner G, Hannan WP, Warren RW, Horn W, Cole JL, Paul SM, Hawkins PN, Pham TH, Snyder C, Wesley RA, Hoffmann SC, Holland SM, Butman JA, Kastner DL (2006) Neonatal-onset multisystem inflammatory disease responsive to interleukin-1beta inhibition. N Engl J Med 355(6):581–592. ▶ https://doi.org/10.1056/NEJMoa055137

Hansmann S, Lainka E, Horneff G, Holzinger D, Rieber N, Jansson AF, Rosen-Wolff A, Erbis G, Prelog M, Brunner J, Benseler SM, Kuemmerle-Deschner JB (2020) Consensus protocols for the diagnosis and management of the hereditary autoinflammatory syndromes CAPS, TRAPS and MKD/HIDS: a German PRO-KIND initiative. Pediatr Rheumatol Online J 18(1):17. ▶ https://doi.org/10.1186/s12969-020-0409-3

Kuemmerle-Deschner JB, Tyrrell PN, Koetter I, Wittkowski H, Bialkowski A, Tzaribachev N, Lohse P, Koitchev A, Deuter C, Foell D, Benseler SM (2011) Efficacy and safety of anakinra therapy in pediatric and adult patients with the autoinflammatory Muckle-Wells syndrome. Arthritis Rheum 63(3):840–849. ▶ https://doi.org/10.1002/art.30149

Kuemmerle-Deschner JB, Ozen S, Tyrrell PN, Kone-Paut I, Goldbach-Mansky R, Lachmann H, Blank N, Hoffman HM, Weissbarth-Riedel E, Hugle B, Kallinich T, Gattorno M, Gul A, Ter Haar N, Oswald M, Dedeoglu F, Cantarini L, Benseler SM (2017) Diagnostic criteria for cryopyrin-associated periodic syndrome (CAPS). Ann Rheum Dis 76(6):942–947. ▶ https://doi.org/10.1136/annrheumdis-2016-209686

Lachmann HJ, Kone-Paut I, Kuemmerle-Deschner JB, Leslie KS, Hachulla E, Quartier P, Gitton X, Widmer A, Patel N, Hawkins PN, Canakinumab in CSG (2009) Use of canakinumab in the cryopyrin-associated periodic syndrome. N Engl J Med 360(23):2416–2425. ▶ https://doi.org/10.1056/NEJMoa0810787

Tanaka N, Izawa K, Saito MK, Sakuma M, Oshima K, Ohara O, Nishikomori R, Morimoto T, Kambe N, Goldbach-Mansky R, Aksentijevich I, de Saint BG, Neven B, van Gijn M, Frenkel J, Arostegui JI, Yague J, Merino R, Ibanez M, Pontillo A, Takada H, Imagawa T, Kawai T, Yasumi T, Nakahata T, Heike T (2011) High incidence of NLRP3 somatic mosaicism in patients with chronic infantile neurologic, cutaneous, articular syndrome: results of an International Multicenter Collaborative Study. Arthritis Rheum 63(11):3625–3632. ▶ https://doi.org/10.1002/art.30512

Walker UA, Tilson HH, Hawkins PN, Poll TV, Noviello S, Levy J, Vritzali E, Hoffman HM, Kuemmerle-Deschner JB, Investigators CDS (2021) Long-term safety and effectiveness of canakinumab therapy in patients with cryopyrin-associated periodic syndrome: results from the beta-Confident Registry. RMD Open 7(2). ▶ https://doi.org/10.1136/rmdopen-2021-001663

Welzel T, Kuemmerle-Deschner JB (2021) Diagnosis and management of the cryopyrin-associated periodic syndromes (CAPS): What do we know today? J Clin Med 10(1). ▶ https://doi.org/10.3390/jcm10010128

Wittkowski H, Kuemmerle-Deschner JB, Austermann J, Holzinger D, Goldbach-Mansky R, Gramlich K, Lohse P, Jung T, Roth J, Benseler SM, Foell D (2011) MRP8 and MRP14, phagocyte-specific danger signals, are sensitive biomarkers of disease activity in cryopyrin-associated periodic syndromes. Ann Rheum Dis 70(12):2075–2081. ▶ https://doi.org/10.1136/ard.2011.152496

The Muscle Taut and Abdominal Pain

Hermann Girschick and Henner Morbach

Contents

26.1 Medical History

In the course of preoperative diagnostics, a 16-year-old adolescent girl was found to have an elevated CRP of 7.6 mg/dl and an accelerated ESR of 93 mm/h. She reported episodes of thigh pain, which were accompanied by redness of the regional skin, the muscles appeared hardened and painful there (◗ Fig. 26.1). Occasionally, she observed a mild swelling of regional joints. These symptoms lasted about 1 week. Over the years, she was able to describe about 10 episodes per year. Other symptoms, especially elevated body temperature or fever, are denied, but occasional conjunctivitis and eyelid swelling are noted. In the family history, the mother reported chronic abdominal pain due to gallstone colic/cholecystitis and a chronic inflammatory bowel disease that has not yet been further described. She also had an elevated ESR of 85 mm/h. Other family members were not affected or noticeable in terms of chronic inflammation.

26.2 Examination Findings

Pediatrically, a delayed puberty development was noted (at presentation Tanner stage B2, pH 1), her menarche had not yet

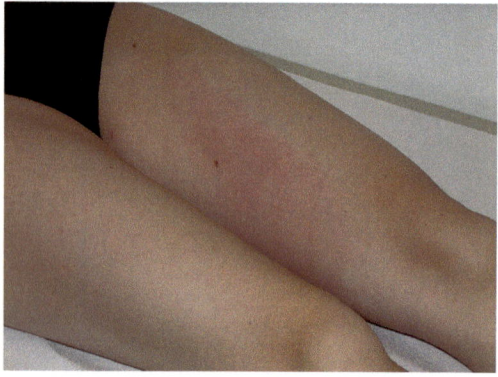

◗ **Fig. 26.1 Erythematous rash and regional myositis in TRAPS syndrome.** The image shows the painful thigh muscles with the episodic skin redness, which led to further diagnostic efforts

occurred. Compared to her parents, she was relatively short (20th percentile) and her body weight had been considered delicate for years (2 kg below the 3rd percentile). Outside of the reported attacks, the girl appeared asymptomatic except for her physical developmental delay, the whole body examination findings revealed no abnormalities, especially not on joints, tendons, and mucous membranes. Abdominally no pressure pain, no space-occupying lesion, and also no abnormalities in bowel movements.

26.3 Laboratory Values and Imaging

26.3.1 Laboratory Values

During the episodic flare, high inflammation parameters were found with leukocytosis 14,570/μl (63% granulocytes), thrombocytosis (732,000/μl), **microcytic (MCV 67 fl), hypochromic (MCH 20.3 pg) anemia (Hb 9.6 g/dl),** reticulocytes 9 ‰, CRP moderately elevated at 7.6 mg/l, the **ESR was significantly accelerated at consistently >90 mm/h, SAA of 736 mg/dl** (normal <10 mg/dl). Ferritin was not elevated at 70 ng/ml. There were no indications of an immune defect. There was a normal distribution of immunoglobulins IgG, IgA, IgM. Autoantibodies against nuclear structures were not detectable (ANA, ENA, dsDNA). ANCA, the antiphospholipid cardiolipin, and rheumatoid factors-IgM were negative. The **fibrinogen** was significantly elevated at **649 mg/dl** (180–350 mg/dl) with otherwise unremarkable coagulation. Thyroid values were normal. Infection serology: negative for EBV, streptococci, borrelia, mycoplasma, adenoviruses, parvovirus B19. Tuberculin skin test was negative. A blood culture remained negative during the flare. An endocrinological evaluation revealed an almost prepubertal status, no evidence of thyroid or growth hormone disorder.

26.3.2 Imaging

Imaging examinations with chest X-ray, abdominal ultrasound, echocardiography, MRI of the abdomen after Sellink, of the head, a bone scintigraphy, and a gastroscopy were all not indicative. A colonoscopy showed no macroscopic inflammation of the colon, but histologically there was an inflammatory, nonspecific **colitis** with lymphofollicular hyperplasia.

An ophthalmological examination including funduscopy was normal. The bone age of the left hand according to Greulich and Pyle was determined to be 13 years.

26.4 Educational Questions

1. What suspected diagnosis should be considered due to the episodic pain attacks with myositis and exanthema, without fever, only occasional polyarthralgia, and high inflammation parameters during the flare?
2. Can a prioritization of possible differential diagnoses be carried out?
3. How should the mother's history be classified: undifferentiated IBD also in the daughter?
4. What therapeutic steps could be considered in addition to symptomatic NSAIDs?

26.5 Differential Diagnostic Considerations

At the time of presentation, knowledge about autoinflammatory syndromes was still limited (2005), especially since there were no episodic or prolonged fever reactions in the patient and her mother (Drenth and van der Meer 2001). However, since there was a recurring inflammation prob-lem with erythematous rash, myositis, and polyarthralgia, as well as high inflammation parameters, **autoinflammatory-rheumatic diseases**s were ultimately included in the analysis. Generally, an oncological underlying disease, especially a leukemia from the myeloid series, was also considered in the differential diagnosis. However, the peripheral blood count analysis was normal, and a bone marrow puncture in the patient showed a reactive activation/increase of plasma cells, but was otherwise unremarkable.

Hereditary periodic autoinflammatory syndromes, which were then still called "fever syndromes", were included in the differential diagnosis, and a single gene sequencing was performed in relation to the following syndromes (Panel studies based on Next-generation-sequencing[NGS] technology were not yet available): **familial Mediterranean fever** (FMF, OMIM 249100), **Hyper-IgD**-and-periodic-fever syndrome (HIDS, OMIM 260920), Tumor necrosis factor receptor-associated periodic syndrome (**TRAPS**; OMIM 142680) and Cryopyrin-associated periodic syndrome (**CAPS**; OMIM191900, 120100, 607115) (Drenth and van der Meer 2001; Simon and van der Meer 2007; Krainer et al. 2020)

Also classified as autoinflammatory diseases would be, for example, a Crohn's disease. Since a colonic/histological inflammation was detectable, a genetic examination of risk alleles associated with chronic inflammatory bowel diseases using NGS panel diagnostics would be included in today's view. Specifically, mutations in the area of the NOD2 gene (CARD 15) would be of interest.

The diagnosis of TRAPS was confirmed by a genetic analysis of the patient and her mother. A T-to-C nucleotide exchange in exon 2 was detected, leading to a Y20H exchange.

26.6 Educational Answers

- **1. What tentative diagnosis should be considered based on the episodic pain attacks with myositis and exanthema, without fever, only occasional polyarthralgia and high inflammation parameters during the flare?**

Of the differential diagnoses considered for autoinflammatory syndromes, TRAPS with migrating, centrifugal erythemas associated with myalgias was conceptually the most likely underlying disease, even though fever was absent as a symptom. At that time, TRAPS manifestation **without** fever was not yet common.

- **2. Can a prioritization of possible differential diagnoses be carried out?**

Since the patient was of Caucasian descent, a **familial Mediterranean fever** seemed rather unlikely, as did the typical abdominal peritonitic manifestation clinically. Also, in relation to the **Hyper-IgD syndrome**, rash, arthralgia and myalgia should be considered, thus in the narrower choice. Cold-induced urticaria variants (**CAPS**) seemed rather excludable based on the patient's history. The DNA sequencing of exons 2,3, 4,6 of the TNFRSF1A gene on chromosome 12, which encodes the extracellular 55-kD receptor of TNF, revealed a change from tyrosine to histidine (Y20H) at the amino acid position 20 in exon 2.

- **3. How should the mother's history be classified: undifferentiated IBD also in the daughter?**

The genetic analysis subsequently in the mother revealed the identical mutation. Therefore, the prioritized diagnosis of TRAPS was ultimately also made in the mother. TRAPS usually follows a familial **autosomal dominant** inheritance pattern as in our family. On the other hand, the mutation can also occur as a spontaneous mutation. Ultimately, based on the daughter's findings, the IBD diagnosis in her mother was revised and the conventional basic therapy for Crohn's disease was gradually discontinued.

- **4. What therapeutic steps could be considered in addition to symptomatic NSAIDs?**

Since the TRAPS disease occurs in flares, one could consider retreating to an attack-related therapy in cases of moderate severity: e.g. the use of oral naproxen and an oral glucocorticoid therapy (0.2–0.5 mg/kg body weight prednisolone for a duration of 2 days) has generally shown good efficacy in our patient. However, since a chronic inflammation was conceptually assumed, the therapy with **Etanercept** was started after the diagnosis of TRAPS. This is a dimeric molecule that links the 70kDa-TNF-α-receptor subunits with the Fc portion of human IgG. This "soluble" TNF receptor is used as a catcher for the TNF molecule. The therapy dose corresponded to that in juvenile idiopathic arthritis (0.4 mg/kg body weight s.c. twice a week). Under this therapy, the patient benefited significantly, there was a rapid weight gain and a significant puberty development spurt. The hitherto monthly **myositis** episodes decreased significantly in frequency, an attenuated, limited flare was noticeable once a year under this therapy in the following years. We analyzed the effectiveness of the anti-TNF-α therapy not only based on conventional inflammation parameters, but also through serum concentrations of various pro-inflammatory and anti-inflammatory cytokines.

26.7 Further Progress

In the *further course*, after about 3 years, the frequency of flare-ups increased significantly despite consistent and continuous Naproxen and Etanercept therapy. An increase in Etanercept therapy did not bring about any significant change. An increased use of glucocorticoids did not seem appropriate. Therefore, another anti-inflammatory concept, an **Interleukin-1β blockade**, was discussed and initiated. A pathophysiological outlook is permitted here: Initially, it was assumed that some of the TNF receptor mutations affect the physiological extracellularly localized protease cleavage site. The idea was that a modification of this cleavage site prevents receptor-bound TNF-α from being removed from the cell surface (**"receptor shedding"**), and thus the inflammatory signal into the cell is not interrupted (Drenth and van der Meer 2001). However, it turned out that for a large part of the TRAPS patients, this was not the case for the mutation locations in the receptor. To this day, it is discussed as a possible further pathophysiology that mutated receptors have difficulties reaching the cellular surface, and may therefore accumulate in the endoplasmic reticulum. It is suspected that this can lead to a reaction against unfolded proteins (**"unfolded protein response"**). This may possibly lead to disturbances/stress in the endoplasmic reticulum, release reactive oxygen species, subsequently resulting in increased **Interleukin-1β production** (Simon and van der Meer 2007; Kul Cinar et al. 2022).

Among other things, based on these considerations, there are indications from individual case studies and a few controlled studies that the direct blockade of Interleukin-1β can have a positive therapeutic effect on TRAPS (La Torre et al. 2015). Recommendations for the management of TRAPS have been internationally coordinated (Gattorno et al. 2017; De Benedetti et al. 2018). Approval from American and European authorities for the use of Canakinumab is available. After 10 years of clinically successful Canakinumab therapy, the affected patient started a family, became successfully pregnant, and gave birth to a healthy child.

26.8 Summary

26.8.1 Etiology

At the time of diagnosis, the absence of the symptom "fever" in fever syndromes was conceptually rather unknown. However, due to the chronicity and relapsing course, an extended diagnostic including genetics for autoinflammatory syndromes was sensible. This led to the detection of a pathological mutation in the TNF receptor, and the diagnosis of TRAPS could be made (Morbach et al. 2009; Morbach et al. 2013).

26.8.2 Pathogenesis/Clinic

The TNF receptor-1-associated periodic syndrome TRAPS is the most common **autosomal-dominant inherited** autoinflammatory disease (Drenth and van der Meer 2001). It is characterized by repeated fever attacks, episodes of abdominal pain, synovial joint inflammation, migratory erythema based on regional muscle inflammation, often also **periorbital inflammation** including conjunctivitis. The inflammation episodes usually last several days and can last up to several weeks. Phenotypically, the severity varies. TRAPS is caused by mutations in the TNFRSF1A gene, which encodes the membrane-bound TNF receptor 1 (TNFR1) with an intra- and extracellular portion. The receptor can contribute to cell activation and also apoptosis via the NF-κB signaling pathway after binding of TNF-α (Drenth and van der Meer 2001).

26.8.3 Diagnosis

Based on the clinic of chronic, episodic inflammation, blood count, differential blood count, CRP, ESR, ferritin and, if available, S100A8A9 proteins should be examined in the laboratory. For differential diagnostic assessment of a possible lupus disease, an

ANA titer is certainly sensible in a first step. In the case of an arthritic component, a rheumatoid factor IgM, ACPA antibodies may be considered. Genetic diagnostics are nowadays certainly examined on the basis of an **NGS platform and panel diagnostics**. Possibly, Sanger-based sequencing may be additionally required to confirm gene variations. In rare cases, a somatic mutation in TRAPS patients may also be relevant, in which case a so-called **Deep Sequencing** based on NGS can be helpful. Infectiously, tuberculosis must be ruled out, as well as a chronic EBV infection. In individual cases, an extended view may be relevant in the case of fever of unknown origin. However, the classic episodic course rather speaks against a genuine Central European infectious disease.

26.8.4 Therapy

Therapeutically, a positive effect with symptomatic NSAID and glucocorticoid therapy is possible. As a long-term therapy, an interleukin-1 blockade with Canakinumab is approved (Grimwood et al. 2015; Lachmann et al. 2014; Krainer et al. 2020; La Torre et al. 2015; Papa et al. 2021).

26.8.5 Diagnosis

Autosomal-dominant inherited autoinflammatory syndrome: Tumor necrosis factor receptor-associated periodic syndrome (TRAPS, OMIM 142680) (Lachmann et al. 2014; Morbach et al. 2009).

26.8.6 Prophylaxis

Unknown.

Conclusion

Next-generation sequencing concepts including so-called autoinflammation panels enable a targeted diagnosis of monogenetic autoinflammatory diseases and support a pathogenesis-based, targeted immunological basic therapy, specifically in our patient a TNF-α and subsequently an interleukin-1β blockade.

References

De Benedetti F, Gattorno M, Anton J, Ben-Chetrit E, Frenkel J, Hoffman HM, Koné-Paut I, Lachmann HJ, Ozen S, Simon A, Zeft A, Calvo Penades I, Moutschen M, Quartier P, Kasapcopur O, Shcherbina A, Hofer M, Hashkes PJ, Van der Hilst J, Hara R, Bujan-Rivas S, Constantin T, Gul A, Livneh A, Brogan P, Cattalini M, Obici L, Lheritier K, Speziale A, Junge G (2018) Canakinumab for the treatment of autoinflammatory recurrent fever syndromes. N Engl J Med 378:1908–1919. ► https://doi.org/10.1056/NEJMoa1706314

Drenth JP, van der Meer JW (2001) Hereditary periodic fever. N Engl J Med 345:1748–1757. ► https://doi.org/10.1056/NEJMra010200

Gattorno M, Obici L, Cattalini M, Tormey V, Abrams K, Davis N, Speziale A, Bhansali SG, Martini A, Lachmann HJ (2017) Canakinumab treatment for patients with active recurrent or chronic TNF receptor-associated periodic syndrome (TRAPS): an open-label, phase II study. Ann Rheum Dis 76:173–178. ► https://doi.org/10.1136/annrheumdis-2015-209031

Grimwood C, Despert V, Jeru I, Hentgen V (2015) On-demand treatment with anakinra: a treatment option for selected TRAPS patients. Rheumatology (Oxford) 54:1749–1751. ► https://doi.org/10.1093/rheumatology/kev111

Krainer J, Siebenhandl S, Weinhäusel A (2020) Systemic autoinflammatory diseases. J Autoimmun 109:102421. ► https://doi.org/10.1016/j.jaut.2020.102421

Kul Cinar O, Putland A, Wynne K, Eleftheriou D, Brogan PA (2022) Hereditary systemic autoinflammatory diseases: therapeutic stratification. Front Pediatr 10:867679. ► https://doi.org/10.3389/fped.2022.867679

La Torre F, Muratore M, Vitale A, Moramarco F, Quarta L, Cantarini L (2015) Canakinumab efficacy and long-term tocilizumab administration in tumor necrosis factor receptor-associated periodic syndrome (TRAPS). Rheumatol Int 35:1943–1947. ► https://doi.org/10.1007/s00296-015-3305-2

Lachmann HJ, Papa R, Gerhold K, Obici L, Touitou I, Cantarini L, Frenkel J, Anton J, Kone-Paut I, Cattalini M, Bader-Meunier B, Insalaco A, Hentgen V, Merino R, Modesto C, Toplak N, Berendes R, Ozen S, Cimaz R, Jansson A, Brogan PA, Hawkins PN, Ruperto N, Martini A, Woo P, Gattorno M (2014) The phenotype of TNF receptor-associated autoinflammatory syndrome (TRAPS) at presentation: a series of 158 cases from the Eurofever/EUROTRAPS international registry. Ann Rheum Dis 73:2160–2167. ► https://doi.org/10.1136/annrheumdis-2013-204184

Morbach H, Richl P, Stojanov S, Lohse P, Girschick HJ (2009) Tumor necrosis factor receptor 1-associated periodic syndrome without fever: cytokine profile before and during etanercept treatment. Rheumatol Int 30:207–212. ► https://doi.org/10.1007/s00296-009-0937-0

Morbach H, Hedrich CM, Beer M, Girschick HJ (2013) Autoinflammatory bone disorders. Clin Immunol 147:185–196. ► https://doi.org/10.1016/j.clim.2012.12.012

Papa R, Lane T, Minden K, Touitou I, Cantarini L, Cattalini M, Obici L, Jansson AF, Belot A, Frenkel J, Anton J, Wolska-Kusnierz B, Berendes R, Remesal A, Jelusic M, Hoppenreijs E, Espada G, Nikishina I, Maggio MC, Bovis F, Masini M, Youngstein T, Rezk T, Papadopoulou C, Brogan PA, Hawkins PN, Woo P, Ruperto N, Gattorno M, Lachmann HJ (2021) INSAID variant classification and Eurofever criteria guide optimal treatment strategy in patients with TRAPS: data from the Eurofever registry. J Allergy Clin Immunol Pract 9:783–791.e784. ► https://doi.org/10.1016/j.jaip.2020.10.053

Simon A, van der Meer JW (2007) Pathogenesis of familial periodic fever syndromes or hereditary autoinflammatory syndromes. Am J Physiol Regul Integr Comp Physiol 292:R86–R98. ► https://doi.org/10.1152/ajpregu.00504.2006

Is Every Early Childhood Polyarthritis with Uveitis also a JIA?

Moritz Klaas and Hermann Girschick

Contents

27.1 Medical History

The 8-year-old Karla is presented for assessment in our clinic. It is reported that she had a brownish-scaly eczema in infancy, which showed granulomatous changes in a sample. While these skin manifestations receded, Karla developed severe, symmetrical **polyarthritis** mainly of the peripheral joints with involvement of the **tendon sheaths** as well as increased fatigue and weight stagnation in early childhood. Notably, there was a significant increase in inflammatory parameters in the absence of fever. The treatment was complex. Frequent changes of conventional and biological basic therapeutics (methotrexate, tocilizumab and etanercept were used) as well as the repeated use of intravenous glucocorticoid pulse therapies were necessary to control the relapsing, "rheumatoid factor-negative" polyarthritis.

27.2 Examination Findings

Karla is a school-aged child with age-appropriate development and a delicate physique (weight and height 3rd–10th percentile). She had flexion contractures of the fingers and toes, as well as cystic tendon swellings in the area of the back of the hand and dorsal midfoot (◘ Fig. 27.1a, c). There was active **arthritis** and **tendinitis** of the left upper ankle joint, the left knee joint, the metacarpophalangeal joints 2 and 3 on both sides, as well as in the area of the peroneal compartment and toe flexors on both sides. As a result of repeated steroid injections, local adipose tissue atrophies were seen on the back of the foot and hand (◘ Fig. 27.1a). The rest of the pediatric-internal examination, the inspection of the eyes and the integument were unremarkable.

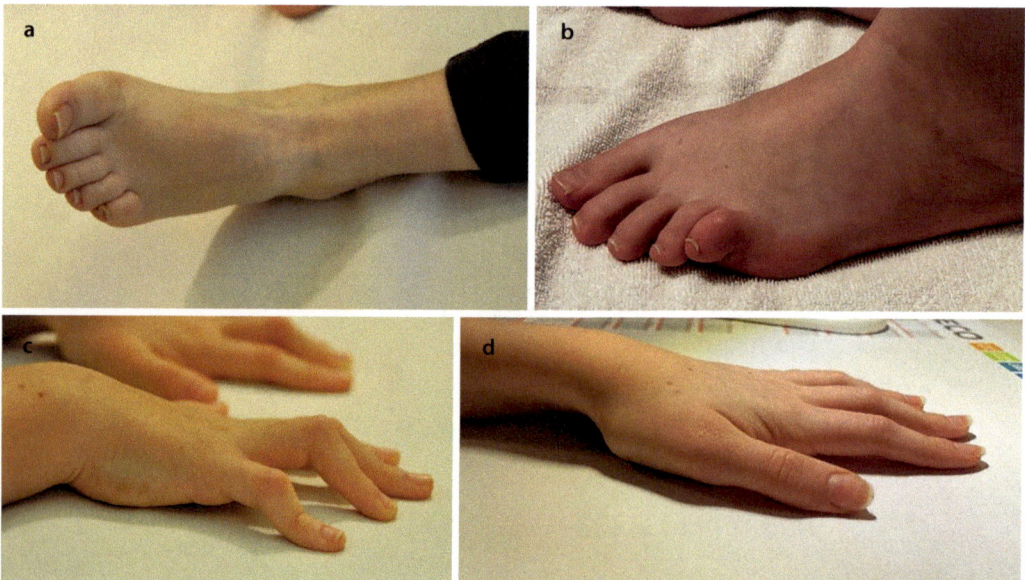

◘ **Fig. 27.1 a–d** Photos of Karla's hands and feet at the ages of 8 and 14. There is a doughy "boggy synovitis" along the extensor tendons of the back of the foot, also of the hand, a polyarthritis with flexion contractures of the PIP finger joints as well as a "side aspect" of adipose tissue atrophy after steroid injection into the upper ankle joint (**a, c**). The synovitis of the hand and foot joints/polyarthritis is no longer detectable 6 years later (**a, b**), in the course regressive flexion contractures (**c, d**) of the fingers and toes. (With kind permission from the family)

27.3 Labor Values and Imaging

27.3.1 Laboratory Values

The laboratory analysis showed a strong activation of the acute-phase proteins **C-reactive protein (102 mg/l [reference value: <5])** and **Serum Amyloid A (518 mg/l [<6.4])**. The Calprotectin in serum (**Protein S100 A8/9**) was also significantly increased at **32,000 ng/ml (<2940)**. The previously measured blood count changes with microcytic anemia as well as leuko- and thrombocytosis **(hemoglobin 7.5 g/dl [10.2–12.7], MCV 62 fl [71–84], leukocytes 16.1 G/l [4.8–13.2], platelets 675 G/l [189–394])** were now normalized. In the area of the adaptive immune system, a previously noticeable hypergammaglobulinemia had almost normalized (**Immunoglobulin G 16.3 g/l [7–15.5], previously 27 g/l**). Previously elevated ANA autoantibodies (without detection of ds-DNA antibodies) at 1:640 (< 1: 80) were now no longer detectable. Rheumatoid factor-IgM and HLA-B27 were negative.

27.3.2 Imaging

Sonographically, arthritis was confirmed in the area of the left upper ankle joint, the left knee joint, and a significant tendon sheath inflammation in the area of the peroneal compartment and the toe flexors on both sides, as well as a perifocal soft tissue swelling of the right thumb base joint. The sonography of the abdomen was age-appropriate. In the whole-body MRI examination, moderate effusions could be detected in the right hip joint, both knee and upper ankle joints (◘ Fig. 27.2). There was no bone involvement.

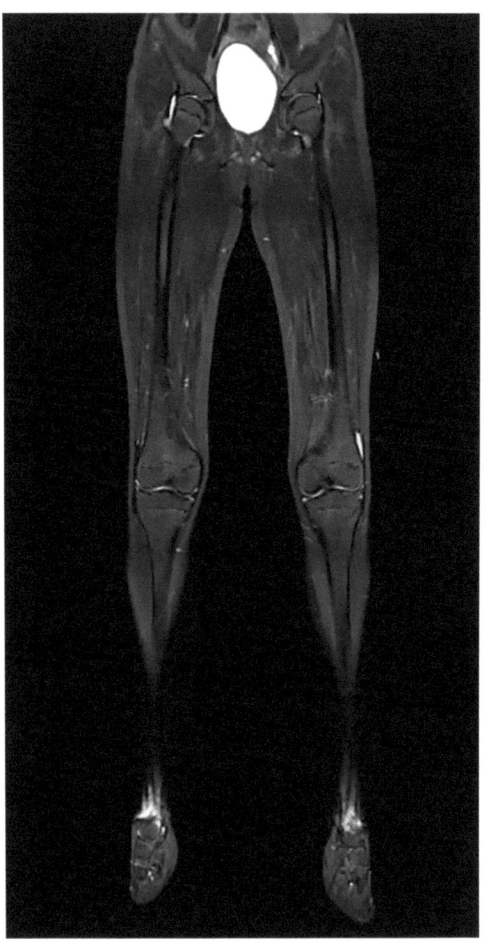

◘ **Fig. 27.2** Half-body MRI (strongly T2-weighted, fat-suppressed, TIRM) of Karla at the age of 8 years. Moderate effusions in the right hip joint, left knee joint, and in the upper ankle joints on both sides were visible in the context of arthritis. Osteomyelitis was not detectable. (With kind permission from Prof. Dr. J. Wagner, Institute for Radiology and Interventional Therapy, Vivantes Klinikum im Friedrichshain, Berlin)

27.4 Educational Questions

1. What suspected diagnosis should be considered in the case of granulomatous skin disease and polyarthritis?

2. Can a prioritization of possible differential diagnoses be carried out?
3. What medicinal approaches can be considered?
4. What other complication should be strictly monitored in the course?

27.5 Differential Diagnostic Considerations

Karla has a relapsing multisystemic disease involving skin, tendons, and joints. The disease began early in childhood and shows a strong activation of the **innate immune system**, which, in addition to the increased acute-phase proteins, also led to a general deterioration of the child's condition with increased fatigue and weight loss. The diagnosis of juvenile idiopathic arthritis JIA requires, in addition to manifestation before the age of 16 and chronic progression, the exclusion of other causes (Petty et al. 1998). In particular, the differentiation from so-called autoinflammatory syndromes often proves to be particularly difficult.

A special form of JIA, which often begins in early childhood, initially affects the skin, has high inflammation parameters, and can progress into a polyarthritic course, is the systemic form of JIA, also known as Still's disease. Even though no disease-causing gene mutations have been defined so far, this form is now classified as an autoinflammatory disease, which is also reflected in the medical treatment. Characteristically, children with **Still's disease** develop a remitting fever lasting several weeks accompanied by a fleeting rash. Karla, on the other hand, had a **granulomatous dermatitis** and did not develop any fever problems. Thus, the diagnosis of Still's disease could be ruled out.

Another form of JIA to be discussed in differential diagnosis is enthesitis-associated arthritis (EAA), which, unlike adult spondylarthritis, mainly affects the peripheral joints and leads to tendon and tendon insertion inflammation ("enthesitis"). There are large overlaps of EAA with chronic, non-bacterial osteomyelitis, chronic inflammatory bowel diseases, and reactive arthritides. Not infrequently, the laboratory-chemically measurable inflammation "erroneously" leads to the initiation of antibiotic therapy at the beginning of the disease. Against the differential diagnosis EAA in our case was that it is usually associated with the male sex and the presence of HLA-B27 positivity. In addition, this disease often develops only in school age.

Also, **psoriasis** can "affect" skin and joints as arthritis and be associated with an increased "infection laboratory"/inflammation. If the arthritis precedes skin involvement, a positive family history, typical nail changes, and the presence of dactylitis ("sausage finger" involving several joints and tendons in the ray) serve to confirm the diagnosis. Neither joint involvement and family history nor the rapid and spontaneous improvement of the skin findings before the onset of severe arthritis suggested this differential diagnosis for Karla.

In the field of collagenoses, due to the joint involvement and temporary increase in ANA, a systemic lupus erythematosus could also be discussed. Arguments against this diagnosis included, among other things, a lack of further differentiation of the ANA values and the rather early onset of the disease. **Ultimately, the diagnosis for Karla was made by the detection of a granulomatous skin, tendon, and joint disease.**

27.6 Further Progress Including Therapy

Due to the severe course, increased fatigue, high inflammation parameters, and not least the quite pronounced *doughy* tendon involvement and finger deformities for the young age, we expanded our differential diagnostic considerations beyond JIA and included Blau syndrome, the **juvenile sarcoidosis**, in the genetic **panel analysis** of the "fever syndrome" diseases. The molecular genetic examination was carried out using panel diagnostics for autoinflammatory diseases. A disease-relevant R334Q mutation in the **NOD2 gene** was able to ultimately confirm the suspected diagnosis of Blau syndrome. In addition, a low-penetrance (V198M) mutation in the NLRP3 gene for **CAPS diseases ("cryopyrin-associated periodic syndrome")** was found.

The treatment of Blau syndrome is challenging. Glucocorticoids, TNF-α and IL-1 inhibitors are usually used as part of a combination therapy. CAPS is treated with an IL-1 blockade. With the aim of treating both mentioned diseases and at the same time keeping the unwanted drug effects of long-term glucocorticoid use as low as possible, we switched the biological basic therapy from the TNF-α-blocking etanercept to a possibly more effective autoinflammatory antibody-based IL-1 blockade with canakinumab. However, this therapy had to be stopped in the following year after the occurrence of an unclear peritonitis. Under prednisolone, colchicine, sulfasalazine, and the re-use of the previously used IL-6-inhibiting tocilizumab, the family described a stable course overall in relation to the joint complaints. However, the girl had not grown in the meantime. When trying to reduce the prednisolone dose to below 10 mg/day (about 0.3 mg/kg BW/day), a painful **erythema nodosum** recurred, and at the age of 11, for the first time, a severe posterior eye inflammation on the left with **papillitis, macular edema, and a reduction in visual acuity** to 0.3 occurred under this combination therapy.

Excursus: Uveitis

Uveitis is an inflammation of the uvea (pigment-bearing eye skin: iris, ciliary body, vitreous body, retina), which - if inadequately treated - can lead to severe visual impairment. Regular ophthalmological check-ups and early, consistent therapy are crucial in the case of a corresponding risk constellation. Children with JIA, especially with oligoarthritis and the presence of ANA, have a high risk of developing uveitis. In the group of JIA, the anterior eye segments are usually affected, the uveitis initially runs externally with few symptoms, but in the course, blindness due to cataract or involvement of posterior eye segments can also threaten. Uveitis also occurs in infectious diseases such as toxoplasmosis or herpes viruses, but also in autoinflammatory diseases such as Blau syndrome, CAPS, or Behçet's disease. In these diagnoses, the posterior eye segments are more involved. The therapy of JIA-associated uveitis (Heiligenhaus et al. 2021) is initially based on the administration of local or possibly systemic glucocorticoids and, if therapy is unsuccessful, immunomodulating/suppressing basic therapeutic drugs such as methotrexate, adalimumab, or tocilizumab.

Now it was necessary to redesign the basic therapy. Local therapy on the eye had not been primarily considered due to the posterior location of the uveitis and tocilizumab seemed not sufficiently effective overall. Methotrexate and canakinumab had not been tolerated beforehand (transaminase increase, respectively peritonitis), so after another methylprednisolone pulse treatment (10 mg/kg BW/day over 3 days i.v.) we decided on TNF-α-inhibiting antibody therapy with adalimumab **and** the use of **mycophenolate mofetil**. Fortunately, this resulted in a remission of the uveitis, an end to glucocorticoid therapy, a complete regression of inflammation parameters, and a catch-up growth of 5 cm within the next 6 months. Karla is now 14 years old, attends 9th grade, and is physically active (◘ Fig. 27.1b, d). After 2 years of clinical and laboratory chemical inactivity of the disease and an attempt at medication reduction (discontinuation of sulfasalazine and reduction of dose and interval of adalimumab), a SARS-CoV2 infection with mild COVID-19 symptoms that occurred despite 2 mRNA vaccinations led to a new flare-up of the disease with erythema nodosum and reactivation of arthritis in the area of both knee and ankle joints, which, however, could be controlled by a renewed short-term oral and systemic glucocorticoid use (methylprednisolone 20 mg/kg BW/day over 3 days i.v., then prednisolone 1 mg/kg BW/day orally, gradual reduction and discontinuation within 6 weeks) and the resumption of weight-adapted adalimumab therapy. The laboratory chemical inflammation parameters were still not elevated.

27.7   Educational Answers

- **1. What suspected diagnosis should be considered for granulomatous skin disease and polyarthritis?**

The Blau Syndrome is characterized by the triad of granulomatous dermatitis, polyarthritis, and uveitis.

- **2. Can a prioritization of possible differential diagnoses be carried out?**

The differentiation from atopic dermatitis or, for example, an atypical mycobacterial infection is possible based on the localization of organ involvement. In addition to JIA – especially enthesitis-associated arthritis – due to the early onset of the disease and the strong activation of the laboratory-measurable inflammatory parameters, autoinflammatory diseases should also be the subject of differential diagnosis. Granulomatous skin changes also occur in primary immune defects such as septic granulomatosis or in combined immune defects. The determination of differential blood count, lymphocyte subpopulations, and total immunoglobulins provided no indication for this. The determination of the oxidative burst in granulocytes was omitted.

- **3. What medicinal approaches can be considered?**

In juvenile sarcoidosis, Blau Syndrome, glucocorticoids, IL-1- or IL-6- and TNF-α-inhibiting therapies are used. A directly approved medication is not available. The indication is based on the symptoms of uveitis and or polyarthritis.

- **4. What further complication should be strictly monitored in the course?**

Uveitis is a typical manifestation of Blau Syndrome, which is often **difficult to treat** and is associated with the risk of permanent damage up to and including vision loss.

27.8   Summary

27.8.1   Etiology

Autoinflammatory diseases are characterized by an excessive activation of the innate immune system. This leads to the autonomous activation of the so-called *NLRP3 inflammasomes*, an intracellular signaling cascade, which responds to danger signals such as bacterial toxins or tissue decay with an increased production of pro-inflammatory cytokines such as IL-1, IL-6 and TNF-α. For many autoinflammatory syndromes, **monogenetic changes in the germline** within the inflammasome have now been identified and characterized, and **somatic mutations** have also been described (Autoinflammatory Alliance 2021; Invefers 2021). "Gain-of-function mutations" in the NOD2 gene in Blau syndrome and in the NLRP3 gene in cryopyrin-associated periodic syndromes (CAPS diseases) lead to an excessive production of pro-inflammatory cytokines, especially IL-1, through enhanced activation of NF-kB or caspase-1. Both diseases can be inherited in an autosomal dominant manner or occur as new mutations.

27.8.2 Pathogenesis/Clinic

The disease was first described as "juvenile sarcoidosis" by pediatrician Edward Bernard Blau and named after him. In 1985, he was able to vividly demonstrate the typical characteristics of this disease in several members of a family (Blau 1985; Wouters et al. 2014; Stoevesandt et al. 2010). Blau syndrome is characterized by the **triad of granulomatous dermatitis, polyarthritis, and uveitis**. Skin manifestations are usually the first symptom and can present polymorphically. In early childhood, a symmetrical polyarthritis with flexion contractures of the fingers and toes develops, as well as characteristic tendon swellings along the hand and ankle joints, referred to in the literature as "**boggy synovitis**". More than 4 out of 5 patients with Blau syndrome develop uveitis in the course of the disease, with the risk of severe visual impairments. Other symptoms include fever, vasculitis, and erythema nodosum. In contrast to the adult form of sarcoidosis, lung involvement is extremely rare. Histologically, **non-caseating granulomas** of the skin, tendons, and synovial joint structures are found.

CAPS encompasses a group of rare inflammatory diseases. The disease spectrum ranges from the milder familial cold urticaria, with short episodes of fever and urticaria triggered by cold, to the **Muckle-Wells syndrome** with the risk of developing **amyloidosis** or high-frequency hearing loss, to the severe, neonatal onset form "**Neonatal Onset Multisystemic Inflammatory Disease**" (NOMID/CINCA). In recent years, diagnostic criteria have been developed to identify patients with a CAPS disease more quickly and, if necessary, to initiate effective treatment with IL-1 inhibition (Kuemmerle-Deschner et al. 2017).

27.8.3 Diagnosis

The focus was on a strong activation of the innate immune system with an increase, including the clinically relevant parameters of C-reactive protein and **Serum Amyloid A**. A diagnosis of Blau syndrome was confirmed molecularly by a panel examination including several genes of autoinflammatory disease groups. The additionally discovered V198M mutation in the NLRP3 gene is considered a "low-penetrance mutation", which is found both in mild CAPS diseases and in healthy individuals (Rowczenio et al. 2013). Possible characteristics of a CAPS disease (such as cold urticaria, high-frequency hearing loss) were not present in Karla. Nevertheless, an additional pro-inflammatory effect of the found NLRP3 mutation is conceivable.

27.8.4 Therapy

The therapy of Blau syndrome is to be considered symptomatic and includes glucocorticoids, TNF-α – and IL-1 inhibitors. In Karla, various biological and conventional basic medications as well as recurrent high-dose glucocorticoids were required to stabilize the musculoskeletal involvement in particular. Severe uveitis led to a change in therapy to mycophenolate mofetil and adalimumab, which proved to be pleasingly effective in combination.

27.8.5 Diagnosis

Blau Syndrome.

27.8.6 Prophylaxis

Regular pediatric rheumatological and ophthalmological assessments are necessary to detect a recurrence of the chronic inflammation and to counteract it with medication if necessary.

Conclusion

Autoinflammatory diseases represent an important differential diagnosis to JIA and should be considered especially in cases of early onset of disease, symptoms that cannot be clearly assigned, or laboratory-chemical conspicuous inflammation. Genetic panel examinations expand the diagnostic possibilities.

References

Autoinflammatory Alliance. ▶ https://autoinflammatory.org/index.php. Zugegriffen: 16. Dez. 2021

Blau EB (1985) Familial granulomatous arthritis, iritis, and rash. J Pediatr 107(5):689–693. ▶ https://doi.org/10.1016/s0022-3476(85)80394-2

Heiligenhaus A, Minden K, Tappeiner C, Baus H, Bertram B, Deuter C, Foeldvari I, Föll D, Frosch M, Ganser G, Gaubitz M, Günther A, Heinz C, Horneff G, Huemer C, Kopp I, Lutz T, Michels H, Ness T, Neudorf U, Pleyer U, Schneider M, Schulze-Koops H, Thurau S, Zierhut M, Lehmann HW (2021) Diagnostik und antientzündliche Therapie der Uveitis bei juveniler idiopathischer Arthritis. AWMF-Registernummer: 045-012. ▶ https://www.awmf.org/leitlinien/detail/ll/045-012.html. Zugegriffen: 16. Dez. 2021

Infevers: The registry of hereditary auto-inflammatory disorders mutations. ▶ https://infevers.umai-montpellier.fr/web/. Zugegriffen: 16. Dez. 2021

Kuemmerle-Deschner JB, Ozen S, Tyrrell PN, Kone-Paut I, Goldbach-Mansky R, Lachmann H, Blank N, Hoffman HM, Weissbarth-Riedel E, Hugle B, Kallinich T, Gattorno M, Gul A, Ter Haar N, Oswald M, Dedeoglu F, Cantarini L, Benseler SM (2017) Diagnostic criteria for cryopyrin-associated periodic syndrome (CAPS). Ann Rheum Dis 76(6):942–947. ▶ https://doi.org/10.1136/annrheumdis-2016-209686

Petty RE, Southwood TR, Baum J, Bhettay E, Glass DN, Manners P, Maldonado-Cocco J, Suarez-Almazor M, Orozco-Alcala J, Prieur AM (1998) Revision of the proposed classification criteria for juvenile idiopathic arthritis: Durban, 1997. J Rheumatol 25(10):1991–1994

Rowczenio DM, Trojer H, Russell T, Baginska A, Lane T, Stewart NM, Gillmore JD, Hawkins PN, Woo P, Mikoluc B, Lachmann HJ (2013) Clinical characteristics in subjects with NLRP3 V198M diagnosed at a single UK center and a review of the literature. Arthritis Res Ther 15(1):R30. ▶ https://doi.org/10.1186/ar4171

Stoevesandt J, Morbach H, Martin TM, Zierhut M, Girschick H, Hamm H (2010) Sporadic Blau syndrome with onset of widespread granulomatous dermatitis in the newborn period. Pediatr Dermatol 27(1):69–73. ▶ https://doi.org/10.1111/j.1525-1470.2009.01060.x

Wouters CH, Maes A, Foley KP, Bertin J, Rose CD (2014) Blau syndrome, the prototypic auto-inflammatory granulomatous disease. Pediatr Rheumatol Online J 12:33. ▶ https://doi.org/10.1186/1546-0096-12-33

A 16-Year-Old Boy with the Symptom Picture of Recurring Evening Episodes of Chills As Well As Weakness and Weight Loss

Christian Huemer

Contents

28.1 Medical History

The 16-year-old boy had a complaint picture of recurring evening episodes with **fever spikes** up to 39 degrees Celsius as well as weakness and a weight loss of about 7 kg in 4 months. In the additional medical history, no clear indications for associated infections, no night sweats, one episode of epistaxis. No additional indications for organ-specific symptoms. General medical history unremarkable until the onset of these symptoms. The presentation was made via the family doctor to rule out a systemic event with recurring fever spikes and general condition deterioration as well as unclear weight loss. Shortly before the referral of the patient, the family doctor also clinically suspected a **splenomegaly** and now requests urgent clarification. Family history unremarkable, the patient comes from a Somali family, which immigrated a few years ago. The patient lives alone with his mother, the father has remained in the home country since emigration from Somalia, so far no travel activity of the patient.

28.2 Examination Findings

16-year-old darkly pigmented adolescent in good general condition, normal nutritional status, body weight 75 kg (90th–97th percentile), body length 175 cm (50th percentile), BMI 24.4 (75th–90th percentile); afebrile; Cor: pure, rhythmic heart action, no additional sounds, normofrequent; normal blood pressure 113/81 mmHg; Pulmo: without signs of dyspnea, vesicular breath sound over all lung fields, sonorous percussion sound ubiquitous. ENT findings: throat bland, oral mucosa unremarkable, tongue moist, ears easily visible, eardrums unremarkable. Skin unremarkable without edema, turgor unremarkable. Neurological status unremarkable, pupils isocor, both sides light-reactive, no meningismus. Abdo-

men: abdominal wall soft, bowel sounds active, no tenderness on pressure, renal areas free, **liver palpable 3 cross fingers from the costal arch, spleen clearly palpable**; peripheral lymph nodes not enlarged; musculoskeletal status unremarkable.

28.3 Labor Values and Imaging

28.3.1 Laboratory Values

Leukocytes 4.5/nl, Hb 11.2 g/dl, Hct 0.36%, platelets 222/nl, slight monocytosis in the differential blood count, CRP not elevated, ESR not elevated, GOT 93 U/l, GPT 37 U/l, GGT 217 U/l, alkaline phosphatase 387 U/l, LDH 307 U/l. IgG 2609 mg/dl, IgA 778 mg/dl, IgM 136 mg/dl. Electrolytes unremarkable, renal function parameters unremarkable. Iron 30 μg/dl, transferrin 279 mg/dl, ferritin 88 ng/ml. Autoimmune findings (ANA, ENA, ANCA, rheumatoid factor) unremarkable. Celiac disease screening unremarkable. Infectious findings (malaria PCR, echinococcus, schistosoma, babesia, leishmania serology) negative. Hepatitis serology (A, B and C) unremarkable. Blood cultures, stool cultures negative; urine findings unremarkable; coagulation unremarkable.

28.3.2 Imaging

The *abdominal sonography* shows a **hepato-** and **splenomegaly**. The liver shows a highly inhomogeneous sonomorphology with a kissing phenomenon to the significantly enlarged spleen (axial 17 × 7 cm). Voluminous pancreas with homogeneous parenchymal contrast and slender duct. Somewhat plump configured left adrenal gland. Kidneys on both sides without higher-grade space-occupying character. Severe luminal narrowing of the inferior vena cava in the upper abdomen and the left renal vein at the mouth area with multiple enlarged adjacent lymph nodes. The largest lymph nodes are found at the liver hilum, with a diameter of 24 mm, retrocaval with 12 mm, caudal to the right renal vein with 18 mm, paraaortic with 13 mm.

CT abdomen and thorax: Here, a 12 mm enlarged lymph node is seen right axillary, lobulated in appearance, as well as additionally enlarged, relatively hypodense lymph nodes paraesophageal with a diameter max. 17 mm. The abdomen (see ◘ Fig. 28.1a, b) shows an enlarged liver (midclavicular line 21 cm without evidence of focal lesions), mild signs of cholecystolithiasis. Liver with "kissing phenomenon" to the significantly enlarged spleen (axial 17 × 7 cm). Voluminous pancreas with homogeneous parenchymal contrast and slender ductus Wirsungianus.

In summary, extensive **abdominopelvic lymphadenopathy** with bilateral inguinal, paraesophageal as well as at the cervicothoracic transition existing lymph nodes. High suspicion of lymphoma and hepatosplenomegaly.

28.4 Educational Questions

1. What differential diagnoses are considered in this adolescent with the main symptoms of fever bouts, weight loss, pronounced abdominopelvic lymphadenopathy, and hepato- and splenomegaly?
2. What further diagnostic steps do you suggest?

28.5 Differential Diagnostic Considerations and Educative Responses

In the adolescent patient, due to the clinical symptoms and the radiological findings, there was a high degree of suspicion for an **oncological** or **infectious** systemic disease. The patient was immediately presented at a hemato-oncological center for further diagnostics. To definitively rule out lymphoma and tuberculosis, a bronchoscopy and biopsy of a mediastinal lymph node were

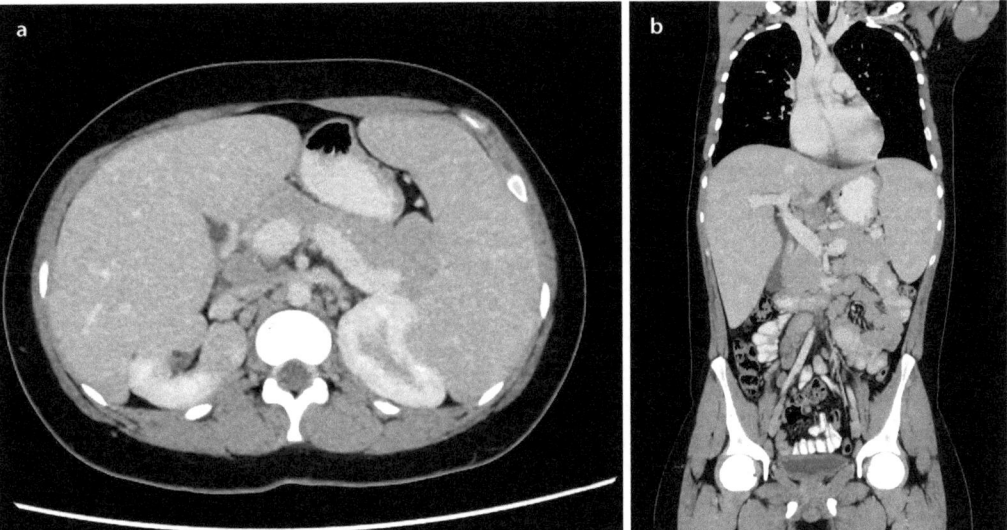

◘ **Fig. 28.1** **a**, **b** CT abdomen in sarcoidosis. Pronounced hepatosplenomegaly (liver with "kissing phenomenon" to the equally significantly enlarged spleen. Multiple enlarged intraabdominal lymphadenopathy). (With kind permission from Dr. A. Schuster, Radiological Department of the LKH Bregenz)

performed: histologically, a **granulomatous, focally necrotizing lymphadenitis** was found. The Ziehl-Neelsen stain was negative, no indication of lymphoma. Bone marrow findings and lymphocyte typing from peripheral blood were unremarkable. Due to structural abnormalities of the liver, a liver biopsy was indicated: The histological finding showed a **granulomatous hepatitis** without molecular pathological evidence of mycobacteria. Thus, with no indications of TB and lymphoma, a high degree of suspicion for a "genuine" **sarcoidosis** was established. Angiotensin converting enzyme (ACE), soluble IL-2 receptor and calcium showed no abnormalities. There were no indications for a genetic assignment to a familial, very early onset juvenile sarcoidosis/Blau syndrome (NOD2/CARD15 mutation) in the adolescent.

The patient received systemic steroid therapy (Prednisolone 1 mg/kg Kg/day p.o. for 6 weeks and additionally a basic therapy with Methotrexate (15 mg/m^2 BSA/week p.o.). Under this therapy significant regression of all described lesions and clinical remission in a follow-up period of about 1 year).

28.6 Summary

28.6.1 Etiology and Frequency

Sarcoidosis is a systemic disease characterized by the formation of immune granulomas in various organs. It is most often described in adulthood between the ages of 20 and 40. It also occurs in childhood and adolescence, but should be distinguished from the juvenile, potentially genetically inherited sarcoidosis, the Blau syndrome (Stoevesandt et al. 2010). The lungs and lymph nodes are often affected, but the disease usually follows a multisystemic course involving other organ systems. Histologically, non-caseating epithelioid cell granulomas are found. In children before the 4th

birthday, a separate course of familial sarcoidosis can often be distinguished (**Early Onset Childhood Sarcoidosis**) or a familial or sporadic juvenile systemic granulomatosis (Stoevesandt et al. 2010; Jansson and Kallinich 2022). Clinically, the child form is characterized by the triad of a granulomatous skin rash (**Granulomas**) (□ Fig. 28.2), an **Arthritis** (which can certainly be confused with a JIA) and a subsequently occurring, severe **Uveitis** (Stoevesandt et al. 2010) (□ Fig. 28.3). Symptoms often begin in the first year of life. An autosomal dominantly inherited, familial granulomatous disease of childhood (Blau syndrome) presents identically to **Early Onset**

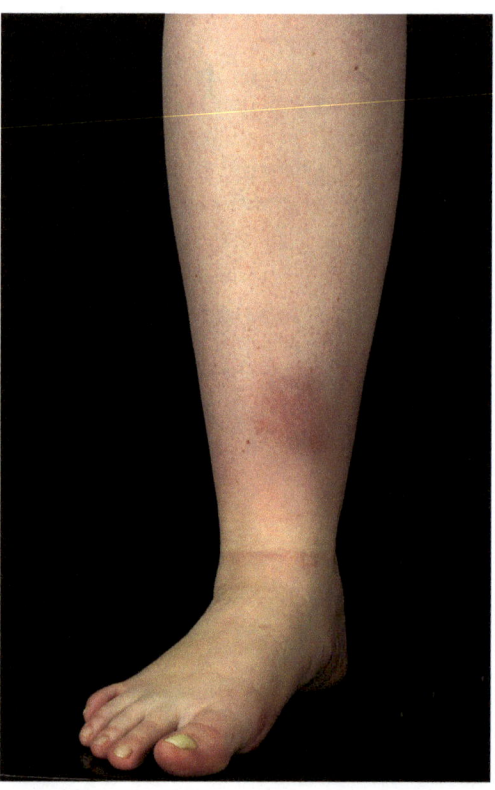

□ **Fig. 28.2** Skin finding of the "genuine" sarcoidosis in childhood and adolescence. Erythema nodosum at typical location (lower leg extensor side) in a sarcoidosis patient (not Blau syndrome). (Amschler and Seitz 2017)

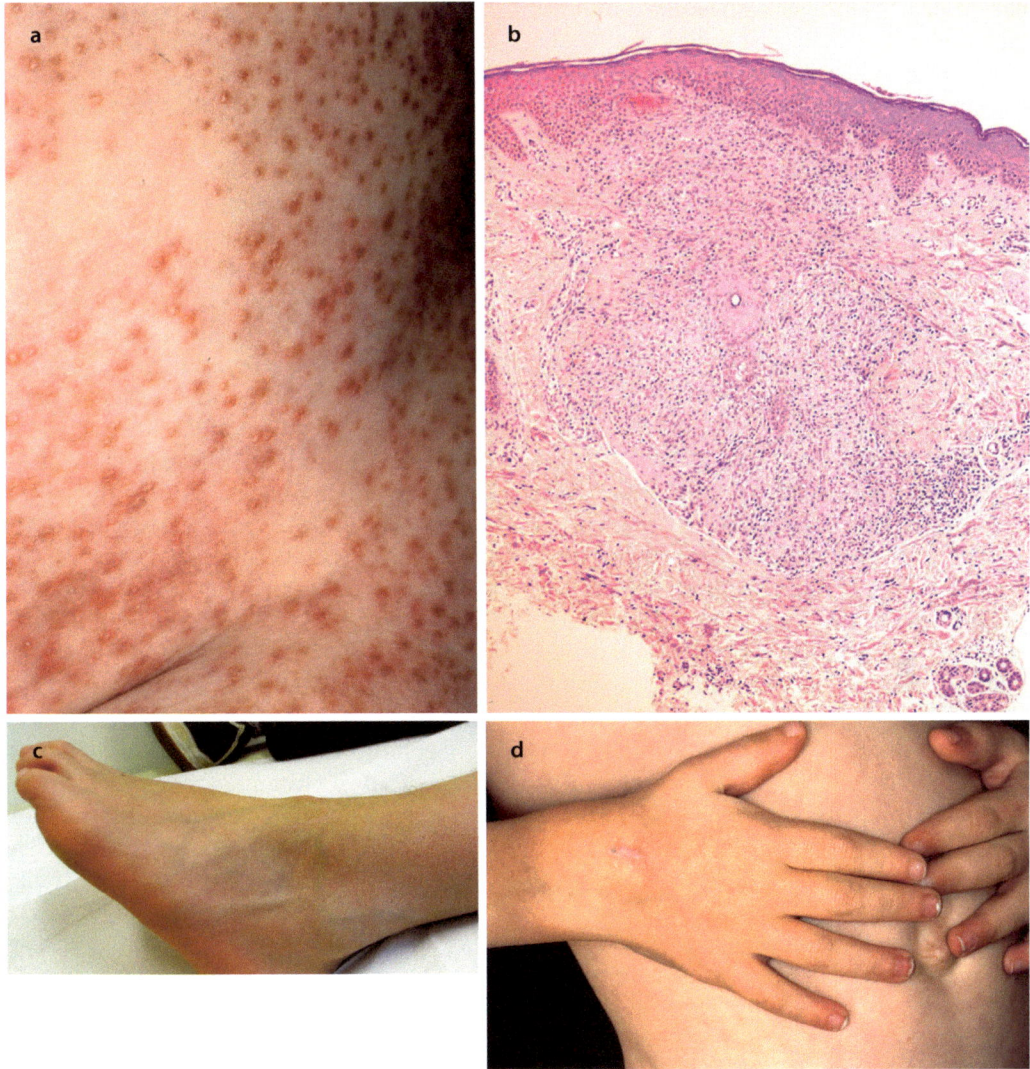

⬛ **Fig. 28.3**   **a–d** Synopsis of juvenile sarcoidosis in childhood and adolescence. **a** Juvenile sarcoidosis (Blau syndrome; NOD2 mutation) manifests with nodular skin and synovial granulomas, **b** corresponding typical histology (HE staining) in a toddler/juvenile sarcoidosis patient. **c, d** Typical are doughy tendon sheath thickening (biopsy right hand back) and joint swelling in the context of polyarthritis. (Stoevesandt et al. 2010)

Childhood Sarcoidosis, although originally fewer visceral involvements were observed in this course (Cimaz and Ansell 2002; Stoevesandt et al. 2010). The incidence of sarcoidosis in adulthood is about 4.9 per 100,000 people, which is significantly higher than in childhood. Here, the incidence is given as 0.4-0.8 per 100,000 children (Duchemann et al. 2017; Gedalia et al. 2016).

28.6.2 Pathophysiology

Many studies suggest that the pathogenesis of sarcoidosis is largely maintained by persisting pathogen-associated molecular patterns (PAMPs) of killed pathogens, which trigger an excessive immunological response (Valeyre et al. 2014). For example, in patients with sarcoidosis, various studies have shown a significant enrichment of proteins derived from myco- and propionibacteria, but inorganic substances such as silica, aluminum, and dusts are also associated with the pathogenesis of sarcoidosis (Newman and Newman 2012).

28.6.3 Clinic

The clinical symptoms of sarcoidosis have been described in only a few existing cohort studies as mainly manifesting the following symptoms: general symptoms, fever and weight loss as leading symptoms, as well as varying degrees of involvement of the lungs, eyes, skin, lymph nodes, and joints. Regardless of age, the majority of patients show involvement of multiple organs. This underlines that sarcoidosis also represents a systemic disease in childhood.

▪▪ Pulmonary Involvement

Pulmonary involvement is a common manifestation of sarcoidosis in childhood, usually presenting with a persistent dry cough, about half of all children show respiratory symptoms and abnormalities in chest X-rays (Nathan et al. 2015).

▪▪ Lymph Nodes

In addition to intrathoracic lymphadenopathy, peripheral lymphadenopathy and hepatosplenomegaly are often observed in children with sarcoidosis. The lymph nodes are usually firm, non-painful, and movable.

▪▪ Ocular Involvement

All sections of the eye can be affected by an intraocular inflammation (Uveitis). The most common form in childhood is **anterior uveitis**. Uveitis is also a typical manifestation in childhood, which often occurs initially and often represents a difficult to treat manifestation of childhood sarcoidosis (Gedalia et al. 2016).

▪▪ Cutaneous Involvement

Skin involvement in sarcoidosis is divided into specific lesions with evidence of granulomas in the skin biopsy and non-specific lesions with histological evidence of reactive changes. The presentation of chronic sarcoidosis in adulthood is very diverse. In childhood, small nodular disseminated, subcutaneous nodular and scar sarcoidosis are mainly distinguished. An Erythema nodosum (◘ Fig. 28.2) is also described in the spectrum of cutaneous symptoms of sarcoidosis (Hoffmann et al. 2004; Amschler 2017).

▪▪ Joint Involvement

Arthritis is observed in up to 30% of cases with childhood sarcoidosis, often multiple joints of the extremities are affected. The distinction from JIA is sometimes not possible. Particularly noticeable are doughy swellings of the tendon sheaths ("bulky synovitis") (Stoevesandt et al. 2010; Gedalia et al. 2016) (◘ Fig. 28.3).

▪▪ Other Organs

Involvement of the parotid can occasionally also be observed in childhood. In contrast to adulthood, involvement of the nervous system in childhood is rare (Nathan et al. 2015).

Another rare manifestation of childhood sarcoidosis is renal involvement (Wang et al. 2019).

28.6.4 Diagnosis

Even in adulthood, there are no binding criteria for the diagnosis of sarcoidosis.

In the case of a justified clinical or radiological suspicion, the disease marker ACE should be determined. A biopsy can provide evidence of non-caseating granulomas. Due to the lack of diagnostic criteria, it is essential to initially exclude other diseases and also during the course.

Laboratory diagnostics: Children with sarcoidosis usually show signs of a moderate inflammatory reaction, so many patients can demonstrate a moderate acceleration of the ESR, an inflammation-related anemia, and often a hypergammaglobulinemia. The angiotensin converting enzyme (ACE) is often not elevated in childhood in juvenile sarcoidosis (Chopra et al. 2016). There is consensus that the determination of ACE as the sole diagnostic test has insufficient specificity, however, a significant increase in ACE can support the suspicion of pulmonary involvement in sarcoidosis. In three pediatric cohorts, ACE was elevated in more than half of the patients.

Biopsy: Due to the manifold presentation, the histological evidence of non-caseating epithelioid cell granulomas plays a central role in the confirmation of diagnosis (◘ Fig. 28.3).

28.6.5 Therapy

Evidence-based data for children do not exist. The treatment is fundamentally anti-inflammatory and aims to prevent or treat organ damage. As first-line therapy, a systemic steroid therapy (prednisolone 1-2 mg/kg body weight/day) and an intravenous steroid therapy over 3 days are used in most cohorts (Nathan et al. 2019; Nunes et al. 2019).

As second-line therapies, methotrexate, azathioprine, mycophenolate mofetil, and also TNF-α-blocking drugs were investigated in several randomized controlled studies in case of insufficient response to steroid therapy (Stoevesandt et al. 2010; Culver and Judson 2019; James and Baughman 2018; Klaas et al. 2020).

28.6.6 Prognosis

Data regarding the prognosis of children with sarcoidosis were collected particularly in the context of a long-term observation of a Danish cohort, here a complete remission was shown in 78% of the cases at the average age of 28 years.

> **Conclusion**
>
> Juvenile sarcoidosis should fundamentally be included in the differential diagnosis of unclear multisystemic, inflammatory diseases of the child, especially in the case of unclear pulmonary, cutaneous, ocular, musculoskeletal symptoms associated with fever and lymphadenopathy. A particularly impressive doughy synovitis may be clinically indicative.

References

Amschler K, Seitz CS (2017) Kutane Manifestationen bei Sarkoidose. Z Rheumatol 76:382–390

Chopra A, Kalkanis A, Judson MA (2016) Biomarkers in sarcoidosis. Expert Rev Clin Immunol 12:1191–1208

Cimaz R, Ansell BM (2002) Sarcoidosis in the pediatric age. Clin Exp Rheumatol 20:231–237

Culver DA, Judson MA (2019) New advances in the management of pulmonary sarcoidosis. BMJ 15553:367

Duchemann B, Annesi-Maesano I, Jacobe de Neurois C, Sanyal S, Brillet PY, Brauner M, Kambouchner M, Huynh S, Naccache JM, Borie R et al (2017) Prevalence and incidence of interstitial lung diseases in a multi-ethnic county of Greater Paris. Eur Respir J 50:1602419

Gedalia A, Khan TA, Shetty AK, Dimitriades VR, Espinoza LR (2016) Childhood sarcoidosis: Louisiana experience. Clin Rheumatol 35:1879–1884

Hoffmann AL, Milman N, Byg KE (2004) Childhood sarcoisosi in Denmark 1979-1994: incidence, clinical features and laboratory results at presentation in 48 children. Acta Paediatr 93:30–36

James WE, Baughman R (2018) Treatment of sarcoidosis: grading the evidence. Expert Rev Clin Pharmacol 11:677–687

Jansson A, Kallinich T (2022) Sarkoidose bei Kindern und Jugendlichen. In: Dannecker G, Kallinich T (Hrsg) Wagner N. Pädiatrische Rheumatologie Springer, Berlin/Heidelberg, S 707–721

Klaas M, Nimtz-Talaska A, Trauzeddel R, Haselbusch D, Girschick HJ (2020) Ein Kind mit Polyarthritis, erhöhten Entzündungsparametern und Mutationen im NOD2- und NLRP3-Gen. Arthritis Rheum 38:56–58

Nathan N, Marcelo P, Houdouin V, Epaud R, de Blic J, Valeyre D, Houzel A, Busson PF, Corvol H, Deschildre A, Clement A (2015) Lung sarcoidosis in children: update on disease expression and management. Thorax 70:537–542

Newman KL, Newman LS (2012) Occupational causes of sarcoidosis. Curr Opin Allergy Clin Immunol 12:145–150

Nunes H, Jeny F, Bouvry D, Uzunhan Y, Valeyre D (2019) Indications for treatment of sarcoidosis. Curr Opin Pulm Med 25:505–518

Stoevesandt J, Morbach H, Martin TM, Zierhut M, Girschick H, Hamm H (2010) Sporadic Blau syndrome with onset of widespread granulomatous dermatitis in the newborn period. Pediatr Dermatol 27(1):69–73. ► https://doi.org/10.1111/j.1525-1470.2009.01060.x

Valeyre D, Prasse A, Nunes H, Uzunhan Y, Brillet PY, Muller-Quernheim J (2014) Sarcoidosis. Lancet 383:1155–1167

Wang C, Liu H, Zhang T, Su H, Shen J, Feng J, Sun L (2019) Acute kidney injury as a rare manifestation of pediatric sarcoidosis: a case report and systematic literature review. Clin Chim Acta 489:68–74

28

Recurring Fever Spikes, But not Always an Infection

Henner Morbach

Contents

29.1 Medical History

A 4-year-old girl has been experiencing recurring **fever episodes** since about the 4th month of life, which occur every 2 months and last about 5 days. These fever episodes also occur during the summer months, and a strict periodicity of the episodes cannot be determined from the medical history. During the episodes, there is usually a fine-spotted **maculopapular rash**, cervical lymphadenopathy, diarrhea, and leg pain. Additional infection symptoms such as cough or runny nose are usually not present during the fever episodes. Compared to her 2-year-old sister, however, fever occurs more frequently and intensely during respiratory infections and also after the administered vaccinations. Between the fever episodes, the girl is not impaired. Her psychomotor development so far has been unaffected.

29.2 Examination Findings

Upon presentation in the outpatient clinic, the 4-year-old girl is fever-free and unaffected. Apart from mild cervical Lymphadenopathy (maximum diameter of the lymph nodes 2 cm), the lymphatic system appears unremarkable. The skin and joint findings, as well as the abdominal findings, are also unremarkable. There are also no abnormalities in the oral cavity.

29.3 Laboratory Values and Imaging

29.3.1 Laboratory Values

The blood count showed a borderline high leukocyte count (16,740 leukocytes/μl) with a neutrophil emphasis (**70% neutrophils**, 22% lymphocytes, 2% monocytes). A moderate hypochromic-microcytic ane-

mia was also noted (**Hb 9.6 g/dl; MCH 23.7 pg; MCV 30.9 fl**). The **inflammatory parameters** were **elevated (CRP 4.0 mg/dl; ESR 36 mm/h)**. The overview values of clinical chemistry (electrolytes, renal retention parameters, transaminases, cell decay parameters) were unremarkable. In the examination of the **serum immunoglobulins**, age-appropriate values for IgG and IgM were found with slightly elevated **IgA (155 mg/dl, reference range 25–147)** and **IgD (19.7 mg/dl, reference range <15)**.

29.3.2 Imaging

The sonographic examination of the abdomen showed an unremarkable finding, in particular no hepatosplenomegaly, no conspicuous or enlarged intra-abdominal lymph nodes, no intestinal wall thickening or free abdominal fluid. The cervical lymph nodes appeared somewhat enlarged with a maximum diameter of 2.5 cm, but otherwise of unremarkable morphology. The echocardiographic examination showed normal cardiac anatomy without indications of inflammatory changes.

29.4 Educational Questions

1. How would you classify the fever episodes and the raised laboratory parameters in terms of differential diagnosis?
2. What further diagnostics would you initiate?
3. What therapeutic options are available?

29.5 Differential Diagnostic Considerations

Recurring fever episodes in early childhood initially suggest an infectious cause such as frequent respiratory infections. These could occur as part of a physiological susceptibility to infection in toddlers. If there are further warning signs and indications of a pathological susceptibility to infection, the presence of a **primary immune deficiency** should also be included in the differential diagnostic considerations. Noteworthy in the child were - apart from the diarrhea - the absence of infection-typical symptoms, such as rhinitis, bronchitis. The fever episodes did not occur more frequently seasonally and also during the summer months, which argues against typical viral respiratory infections as the cause. The symptomatology of the fever episodes also appeared **very stereotypical** and was always accompanied by a **rash**. This constellation could indicate a periodic fever syndrome/ an autoinflammatory disease. Even though the long course over several years makes a malignant disease as the cause of the fever episodes unlikely, this should always be included in the differential diagnosis for unclear fever episodes.

29.6 Further Course

In the further course, the length of the respective fever episodes decreased slightly, but they continued to occur approximately every 4-6 weeks and lasted 2-3 days. When these fever episodes occurred, the parents applied symptomatic therapy with ibuprofen. Due to the recurring fever episodes, a human genetic examination for autoinflammatory diseases/periodic fever syndromes was initiated. This revealed a compound heterozygous mutation in the **MVK gene** (L234P/V377I). Each of the parents had one of these mutations in the heterozygous state. The diagnosis of **Hyper-IgD Syndrome/Mevalonate Kinase Deficiency** was made.

At the age of 7, there was a one-time unilateral parotitis, which was treated with anti-inflammatory therapy with ibuprofen and additionally with antibiotics. At the age of 8, following a fever episode, petechiae and palpable purpura occurred, predominantly on the legs, which was interpreted as Schönlein-Henoch purpura. There were no indications of abdominal or renal involvement. In this context, there was also monoarthritis of the left knee joint. The Borrelia serology and autoimmune serology (ANA) were negative. Currently - at the age of 10 - the fever episodes only occur 3 to 4 times a year and can be well treated with symptomatic therapy with ibuprofen. Regular examinations of the laboratory parameters in the fever-free interval showed no elevated inflammation parameters (CRP, **S100A8/9, Serum Amyloid A [SAA]**).

29.7 Educative Answers

- **1. How would you classify the fever episodes and the laboratory parameters obtained in terms of differential diagnosis?**

Noteworthy in the patient are the frequently occurring fever episodes with fine-spotted maculopapular exanthema and often diarrhea as stereotypical accompanying symptoms. The absence of other infection-typical symptoms and the occurrence of episodes in the summer months make respiratory viruses - as the most common cause of physiological infection susceptibility in toddlers - unlikely. Even though the long course over several years in the patient argues against a malignant disease as the cause of the fever episodes, a differential diagnostic clarification should be carried out in this regard. A manual differential blood count, cell decay parameters, and an ultrasound of the abdomen with the question of leukemia/lymphoma, and the determination of catecholamine metabolites in the urine with the question of neuroblastoma would be suitable for this. However, the previous course and the diagnostics carried out in the patient have not provided any indication of a malignancy.

The most likely differential diagnosis for the child is a disease from the group of autoinflammatory diseases, which are characterized by chronic recurrent systemic inflammations (Sangiorgi and Rigante 2022). Even though the term periodic fever syndromes is often used synonymously, it rather characterizes a subgroup of **autoinflammatory diseases**, in which recurrent fever is the leading symptom. The "classic" periodic fever syndromes with known genetic etiology include familial Mediterranean fever (FMF), cryopyrin-associated periodic syndrome (CAPS), tumor necrosis factor-associated periodic syndrome (TRAPS), and mevalonate kinase deficiency/hyper-IgD syndrome (HIDS) (Gattorno et al. 2019). The most common periodic fever syndrome is certainly the **PFAPA syndrome** (periodic fever, aphthous stomatitis, pharyngitis, adenitis), which, unlike the other diseases mentioned, is not due to a monogenetic change. The individual periodic fever syndromes are characterized by typical symptom constellations (◘ Table 29.1), which are used for classification and are helpful for diagnosis (Gattorno et al. 2019). However, the symptoms of a patient often cannot be exactly assigned to a specific phenotype, so that the clinical picture of the respective patient often appears undifferentiated and not classifiable. The latter patients are increasingly summarized under the term **SURF (Syndrome of Undifferentiated Fever)** (Sutera et al. 2022).

The symptoms of the fever episodes in the described patient fit well with the characteristic symptoms of HIDS, although a CAPS can also present with similar symptoms. The recurring exanthema is not compatible with a PFAPA syndrome. In TRAPS, longer episodes typically occur (but not always) (Gattorno et al. 2019).

- **2. What further diagnostics would you initiate?**

The differential diagnosis of recurrent fever episodes in childhood is broad and includes infectious, malignant, and immunological diseases. After excluding infectious and malignant causes, the collection of laboratory findings during a fever episode and in the fever-free interval is suitable for the question of periodic fever syndrome. The latter serve in particular to investigate a subclinically existing chronic inflammation.

◘ Table 29.1 Clinical symptoms of various periodic fever syndromes

	Duration of attacks (days)	Possible accompanying symptoms	Affected gene	Possible therapy
FMF	1–3	Serositis (peritonitis, pleuritis, arthritis), erythema	MEFV	Colchicine IL-1 blockade
CAPS	A few days to continuous	Exanthema (partly urticarial), conjunctivitis, progressive sensorineural deafness, arthralgia, arthritis	CIAS1	IL-1 blockade
TRAPS	Days/weeks	Myalgia, arthralgia, erythema, serositis, conjunctivitis	TNFRSF1a	IL-1 blockade
HIDS	3–7	Cervical lymphadenopathy, oral aphthae, exanthema, abdominal pain, diarrhea	MVK	IL-1 blockade
PFAPA	4–7	Oral aphthae, pharyngotonsillitis, cervical lymphadenopathy	–	Corticosteroids Colchicine Tonsillectomy

In addition to CRP, **SAA** is particularly suitable for this. The examination of the inflammation values during the fever episode aims to recognize possible characteristic patterns. For example, CRP is usually significantly increased during a PFAPA episode and can thus be used for orientation to differentiate from viral infections. In FMF, very high levels of S100A8/9 (calprotectin) can often be detected in the serum during episodes. Serum IgD levels are elevated in many patients with HIDS, but an increase in IgD neither confirms the diagnosis nor does normal IgD levels exclude the diagnosis (van der Hilst et al. 2008).

Genetic diagnostics are useful for the precise diagnosis and classification of autoinflammatory diseases. If a clear suspicion of a disease can be worked out from the anamnesis and clinical symptoms (e.g. FMF), targeted diagnostics can be carried out with Sanger sequencing. Otherwise, diagnostics are carried out using panel sequencing or mostly exome/genome-based sequencing with subsequent bioinformatic panel on known genes. Genetic examinations often yield gene variants of unclear significance, the direct meaning of which for the clinical symptoms is unclear. Close consultation with human genetics is therefore important for the evaluation of the genetic examination results. The offered genetic diagnostics usually do not cover somatic gene variants. However, these can be disease-causing in various autoinflammatory diseases. If the genetic findings are inconspicuous and there is a clear clinical suspicion, specialized diagnostics should be carried out on this. In the described patient, the diagnosis of mevalonate kinase deficiency/HIDS could be made due to the presence of two mutations classified as pathogenic in the **compound heterozygous state**.

Mevalonate kinase deficiency/HIDS is an autosomal recessive disease in the metabolism of **isoprenoid biosynthesis** (van der Hilst et al. 2008). While severe courses of the disease additionally manifest with neurological symptoms and psychomotor retardation (**mevalonic aciduria**), HIDS is characterized by fever episodes accompanied by cervical lymphadenopathy, exanthema, oral aphthae, and gastrointestinal symptoms. The changes in isoprenoid synthesis result in an activation of pyrin (which is altered in FMF) and an inflammasome/caspase-1-mediated release of IL-1β.

■ **3. What therapeutic options are available?**

The therapy of HIDS is based on the severity of the disease and takes into account the frequency of fever episodes and the presence of a subclinically occurring chronic inflammation (Jeyaratnam and Frenkel 2020). In mild courses with rarely occurring episodes and normal inflammation values in the interval, a demand therapy with ibuprofen and/or paracetamol during the episode is usually sufficient (Hansmann et al. 2020). If the episodes cannot be fully controlled by this, corticosteroids can be added if necessary. In case of a high frequency of episodes or signs of a persistent inflammatory reaction, continuous therapy is aimed for (Hansmann et al. 2020). This is particularly aimed at preventing late effects (**amyloidosis**) due to chronic inflammation. For this purpose, targeted IL-1 blockade is particularly suitable. Under therapy with canakinumab, depending on the dosage, complete remission was achieved in about 30-50% of patients (De Benedetti et al. 2018).

29.8 Summary

29.8.1 Etiology

HIDS follows an autosomal recessive inheritance pattern and is caused by mutations in the MVK gene.

29.8.2 Pathogenesis/Clinic

Changes in the metabolism of isoprenoid biosynthesis lead to increased IL-1β secretion, which explains the inflammatory episodes of the disease. These manifest as fever episodes accompanied by cervical lymphadenopathy, a fine-spotted maculopapular exanthema, enoral aphthae, and/or gastrointestinal manifestations. In addition to arthralgia or arthritis, purpura-like skin efflorescences are also described.

29.8.3 Therapy

In mild to moderate disease activity, demand therapy of fever episodes with ibuprofen/paracetamol can be carried out, possibly supplemented by corticosteroids.

29.8.4 Diagnosis

The diagnosis is confirmed by genetic examination of the MVK gene.

> **Conclusion**
> Recurrent fever episodes with accompanying exanthema may indicate the presence of an autoinflammatory disease.

References

De Benedetti F, Gattorno M, Anton J, Ben-Chetrit E, Frenkel J, Hoffman HM, Kone-Paut I, Lachmann HJ, Ozen S, Simon A, Zeft A, Calvo Penades I, Moutschen M, Quartier P, Kasapcopur O, Shcherbina A, Hofer M, Hashkes PJ, Van der Hilst J, Hara R, Bujan-Rivas S, Constantin T, Gul A, Livneh A, Brogan P, Cattalini M, Obici L, Lheritier K, Speziale A, Junge G (2018) Canakinumab for the treatment of autoinflammatory recurrent fever syndromes. N Engl J Med 378(20):1908–1919. ▶ https://doi.org/10.1056/NEJMoa1706314

Gattorno M, Hofer M, Federici S, Vanoni F, Bovis F, Aksentijevich I, Anton J, Arostegui JI, Barron K, Ben-Cherit E, Brogan PA, Cantarini L, Ceccherini I, De Benedetti F, Dedeoglu F, Demirkaya E, Frenkel J, Goldbach-Mansky R, Gul A, Hentgen V, Hoffman H, Kallinich T, Kone-Paut I, Kuemmerle-Deschner J, Lachmann HJ, Laxer RM, Livneh A, Obici L, Ozen S, Rowczenio D, Russo R, Shinar Y, Simon A, Toplak N, Touitou I, Uziel Y, van Gijn M, Foell D, Garassino C, Kastner D, Martini A, Sormani MP, Ruperto N, Eurofever R, the Paediatric Rheumatology International Trials O (2019) Classification criteria for autoinflammatory recurrent fevers. Ann Rheum Dis 78(8):1025–1032. ▶ https://doi.org/10.1136/annrheumdis-2019-215048

Hansmann S, Lainka E, Horneff G, Holzinger D, Rieber N, Jansson AF, Rosen-Wolff A, Erbis G, Prelog M, Brunner J, Benseler SM, Kuemmerle-Deschner JB (2020) Consensus protocols for the diagnosis and management of the hereditary autoinflammatory syndromes CAPS, TRAPS and MKD/HIDS: a German PRO-KIND initiative. Pediatr Rheumatol Online J 18(1):17. ▶ https://doi.org/10.1186/s12969-020-0409-3

van der Hilst JCH, Bodar EJ, Barron KS, Frenkel J, JPH D, van der JWM M, Simon A, International HSG (2008) Long-term follow-up, clinical features, and quality of life in a series of 103 patients with hyperimmunoglobulinemia D syndrome. Medicine (Baltimore) 87(6):301–310. ▶ https://doi.org/10.1097/MD.0b013e318190cfb7

Jeyaratnam J, Frenkel J (2020) Management of mevalonate kinase deficiency: a pediatric perspective. Front Immunol 11:1150. ▶ https://doi.org/10.3389/fimmu.2020.01150

Sangiorgi E, Rigante D (2022) The clinical chameleon of autoinflammatory diseases in children. Cell 11(14). ▶ https://doi.org/10.3390/cells11142231

Sutera D, Bustaffa M, Papa R, Matucci-Cerinic C, Matarese S, D'Orsi C, Penco F, Prigione I, Palmeri S, Bovis F, Volpi S, Caorsi R, Gattorno M (2022) Clinical characterization, long-term follow-up, and response to treatment of patients with syndrome of undifferentiated recurrent fever (SURF). Semin Arthritis Rheum 55:152024. ▶ https://doi.org/10.1016/j.semarthrit.2022.152024

When Sweating and Drafts Repeatedly Cause Fever

Hermann Girschick

Contents

© The Author(s), under exclusive license to Springer-Verlag GmbH, DE, part of Springer Nature 2024
C. Huemer and H. Girschick (eds.), *Clinical Examples in Pediatric Rheumatology*,
https://doi.org/10.1007/978-3-662-68732-1_30

30.1 Medical History

An 11-year-old girl developed a variably pronounced urticaria in December of one year, ultimately with a "for years" existing tendency to "hectic" erythematous "spots", which were mainly shown on the face and thigh area. The hives occurred primarily after physical activity and ultimately led to the impossibility of any sports activity (◘ Fig. 30.1a, b). In April of the following year, a fever episode occurred over a period of 3 weeks, daily up to 40 °C, increasing in the afternoon/evening (◘ Fig. 30.2). An initially possible fever reduction by ibuprofen changed to a continua.

30.2 Examination Findings

The inpatient admission in an external clinic showed a trunk-accentuated, erythematous-flat rash with significant itching,

which partly appeared as **urticaria**. The suspected diagnosis of systemic juvenile idiopathic arthritis (sJIA) was made and in the differential diagnostic clarification of a bacterial infection, a probatory calculated multimodal antibiotic therapy with meropenem and vancomycin intravenously was carried out. Supportively, the patient received ibuprofen three times a day. Under this, the itching and temperature could be moderately slowed down at best.

On the 4th day, additional glucocorticoid medication with prednisone 100 mg daily, corresponding to about 2 mg per kg body weight/day, was started. Under this, there was a very rapid clinical improvement. During the high fever phase, there was polyarthralgia mainly of the hands, fingers, feet, knees, and toes, so that a clear **polyarthritis** could be described. It was noticeable that the itching and rash increased after sweating activity and then also had a urticarial character (◘ Fig. 30.1 and 30.2).

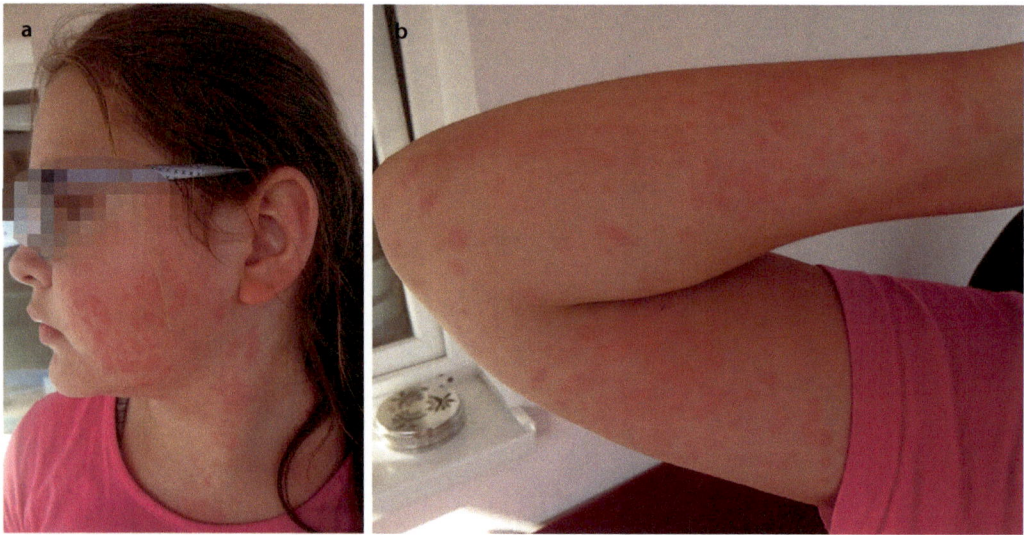

◘ **Fig. 30.1   a, b** Urticarial rash after sports in APLAID syndrome. The images show the urticarial rash that occurred after sports and stress and led to the diagnosis

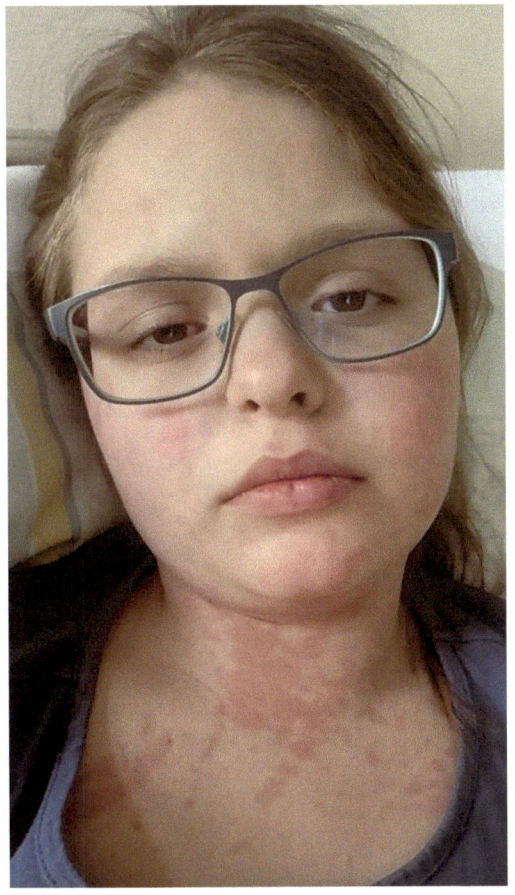

◙ Fig. 30.2 APLAID syndrome with fever-malaise. Urticarial rash in the context of a fever episode with significant impairment of general well-being

30.3 Laboratory Values and Imaging

30.3.1 Laboratory Values

The high inflammation parameters with leukocytosis 12000/μl (84% granulocytes), **CRP 126 mg/l**, **Ferritin 1214 ng/ml** and a moderate increase of the soluble **Interleukin-2 receptors to 805 U/ml** were ultimately interpreted as systemic juvenile idiopathic arthritis (pathological values in bold) - especially be-cause the antibiotic therapy showed no significant effect. Supportively, the girl received cetirizine and vitamin D.

There were no indications of an immune defect. There was a normal immunoglobulin distribution IgG, IgA, IgM, furthermore IgE. Serologically, there were no indications of the presence of Lyme disease or a **Mycoplasma infection**, furthermore herpes virus infections (CMV, VZV, EBV). HIV status and parvovirus B19 serology were inconspicuous. Influenza was ruled out by PCR nasal swab. Blood cultures and stool diagnostics remained inconspicuous, Calprotectin was not increased in the stool. There were no indications of tuberculosis either in the skin test or in the γ-interferon release test. Autoantibodies against nuclear structures were not detectable (ANA). A rheumatoid factor-IgG was moderately increased, while IgM and IgA were inconspicuous.

30.3.2 Imaging

Imaging examinations with chest X-ray, echocardiography several times in the course and an MRI examination of the left knee were inconspicuous except for a slight accumulation of fluid in the dorsal knee joint space. An ultrasound of the abdomen showed a slightly enlarged spleen, echocardiographically a mild pericardial effusion was visible, without restriction of heart function. An ECG was inconspicuous, as was an ophthalmological examination of the fundus, no evidence of uveitis.

30.4 Educational Questions

1. What suspected diagnosis should be considered due to the 3-week fever, urticarial rash, polyarthralgia, and high inflammation parameters?

2. Can a prioritization of possible differential diagnoses be carried out at this point in time?
3. Would further diagnostic strategies be considered under the assessment "fever of unknown origin"?
4. What therapeutic steps could be considered in addition to NSAID, antiallergics, glucocorticoids, and vitamin D?

30.5 Differential Diagnostic Considerations

In the differential diagnosis, due to the prolonged fever reaction with urticarial rash and polyarthralgia with high inflammation parameters, ultimately, primarily **autoinflammatory-rheumatic diseases should be considered**. Generally, an oncological underlying disease, especially a leukemia from the myeloid series, should be considered in the differential diagnosis. Inflammatory components are also possible in the skin area with fever reactions. However, the peripheral blood picture analysis was normal, so the bone marrow puncture to be considered under the view of a fever of unknown origin was deliberately postponed in the patient.

Infectious diseases are to be considered as the third major differential diagnosis, especially **Parvovirus B19** and various herpes viruses. There were no serological indications for this. Formally, tuberculosis and even HIV infection are possible. However, it seemed unlikely due to the clinical symptoms. The absence of significant infection events in the past made a primary immune defect seem unlikely. A solid humoral immunity with a normal blood picture and normal vaccination antibodies confirmed this assessment. The lack of response of the inflammation parameters under antibiotic therapy reinforced the differential diagnostic impression of an autoinflammatory disease or immune dysregulation, as did the rapid response to systemic oral glucocorticoid therapy.

The girl was then assigned to us for further differential diagnostic assessment of systemic juvenile idiopathic arthritis/Still's disease. At this point, we could suspect a **sweating**/physical cooling associated **urticaria** as a fever syndrome disease. The family history then provided further clues at this point: The mother herself suffered from a chronic urticarial rash in the area of the inner thigh, and also from a non-specific chronic inflammatory bowel disease. The girl did not develop a classic polyarthritis, as typical for Still's disease. Also, the immediate triggering of the skin rash after physical activity and sweating argued against a sJIA. Thus, a monogenetic urticarial basic disease with fever syndrome character was considered as the main suspected diagnosis.

30.6 Further Course

To better assess possible triggering by cold/evaporative cold, we conducted an **ice cube test**. Pure exposure to cold by applying an ice cube did not lead to erythema. Only when the ice cube was removed and drying of the skin was induced by a cool breeze/also cold hairdryer air, urticaria could be triggered. Over a period of about 6 months, fever episodes occurring every 6 weeks, which lasted for 3-6 days, occurred under ibuprofen and low-dose glucocorticoid therapy (prednisone 5 mg/day), cetirizine medication, and calcium/vitamin D substitution. The particularly triggering power of sweating episodes remained.

In month 5 after taking over care, an autoinflammatory-genetic diagnosis was made based on Next generation sequencing, a **panel diagnosis for fever syndrome diseases** with special inclusion of the NLRP3 inflammasome, familial Mediterranean fever, but also various urticaria variants (the panel included MEFV, TNFRSF1A, MVK, NLRP3, NLRP12, PLCG2, NLRC4, IL1RN, NOD2). This genetic diagnosis was informative: It revealed a heterozygous mutation in the **Phospholipase-CG2 gene** (c.1014C>T;p.=). This mutation was also detectable in the patient's mother, the father did not show such a mutation. Thus, an autosomal dominant inheritance could be assumed. The diagnosis of "**familial cold urticaria with variable immune defect syndrome**, Type 3" was made (OMIM reference 614468). In "Autoinflammation with PLCG2-associated antibody deficiency and immune dysregulation" (APLAID; OMIM reference 614878), mutations in the PLCG2 gene were described. The mutation described in the patient leads to altered splicing in the digital prediction and was therefore seen as causative for the clinically seen urticaria of the patient.

Due to the symptoms, the patient's previous athletic activity was no longer possible. After detailed explanation, an individual attempt at healing was made using Interleukin-1 blockade/Anakinra. This required a 6-month application process with the cost carriers, so that ultimately a first therapy was possible 14 months after taking over care. The dose was 2 mg/kg body weight s.c., applied daily. An immediate effect was evident. Since then, urticaria has only sporadically occurred in minimal form on the face and inner thigh. The provoking ice cube test was no longer triggerable. The patient was in clinical remission. Therefore, it was possible to switch to an antibody-based interleukin-1 blockade after approval of this individual attempt at healing after 3 months of use. The dose of 150 mg subcutaneously every 8 weeks was chosen, corresponding to 2.4 mg/kg body weight. The complete remission of the patient could be maintained and the girl has gradually been able to resume her previous physical activity with high-performance sports. The multimodal anti-inflammatory and anti-allergic therapy used within the first 12 months was able to be stopped immediately after the start of the interleukin-1 blockade.

30.7 Educational Answers

- **1. What suspected diagnosis should be considered due to the 3-week fever, urticarial rash, polyarthralgia, and high inflammation parameters?**

Formally, in the case of a continuous fever reaction, especially in the afternoon and evening hours, rising to 40 °C, which also shows a fine-spotted rash, further serositis of the pericardium and splenomegaly, sJIA should be considered, especially when high inflammation parameters are present. However, the detailed clinical examination findings were strictly speaking untypical for **sJIA**. A triggering of the rash or fever reaction by physical activity/sweating or cold exposure would be untypical for Morbus Still. Ultimately, the development of polyarthritis was also lacking, so this differential diagnosis could finally be discarded. Classic autoimmune diseases, such as **systemic lupus erythematosus**, would be differential diagnoses to consider. However, the clinical picture of the skin rash was untypical for this. The antinuclear antibody, a classic entry criterion for lupus diagnostics, was also missing. Various viral or bacterial infectious diseases, e.g. mycoplasmas, were not confirmed by the diagnostics, and seemed unlikely due to the prolonged course. Since the haemato-oncological assessment of the peripheral blood count gave no indications of leukaemia, a bone marrow puncture and lumbar puncture could be calculatedly postponed in the patient. However, in the situation of unclear fever, these two diagnostic steps would conceptually be considered.

- **2. Can a prioritization of possible differential diagnoses be carried out at this point in time?**

Main suspected diagnosis: a monogenetic urticarial primary disease with fever syndrome character.

- **3. Would further diagnostic strategies be considered under the assessment of fever of unknown origin?**

Bone marrow puncture especially in case of suspicion of leukemia and lumbar puncture in case of suspicion of infection or sJIA.

- **4. What therapeutic steps could be considered in addition to antibiotics, NSAID, antiallergics, glucocorticoids, and vitamin D?**

If the response is insufficient, an interleukin-1 blockade should be considered due to clinical proximity to NLRP3-dependent cold urticaria.

30.8 Summary

30.8.1 Etiology

A rare variant of familial atypical cold urticaria triggered by sweating and skin cooling was identified. This was first described by Gandhi in 2009 (Gandhi et al. 2009). The genetic resolution of the disease occurred in 2012 by Zhou et al. (Zhou et al. 2012). The causative mutation in the PLCG2 gene results in a clinically highly variable underlying disease with cold urticaria, triggered by minor temperature fluctuations or sweating (Schade et al. 2016). Autoimmunity phenomena and signs of immunodeficiency are described (Gandhi et al. 2009; Zhou et al. 2012).

30.8.2 Pathogenesis/Clinic

Our patient typically showed urticaria and arthralgia. Autoantibodies were not detectable except for rheumatoid factor-IgG. The patient's mother, but not the patient herself, had an undefined enterocolitis. There were no indications of an immunodeficiency in the family. The mutation of the PLCG2 associated with functional enhancement was already described in the mouse model in 2005. It was shown that particularly in B cells, an increased calcium influx was detectable and furthermore, cells of the innate immune system experienced a significant expansion (Yu et al. 2005). The PLCG2 was assigned a key role in triggering autoimmunity/autoinflammation. Especially in B cells, it was shown that the PLCG2, in co-action with Bruton's tyrosine kinase, activates signal activation via the nuclear factor-κB (NF-κB). The B cell receptor can ultimately not transfer any signal into the B cell in case of complete mutation failure of the PLCG2. Corresponding mouse models show a severe humoral immunodeficiency (Petro and Khan 2001).

In general, it has been shown that phospholipases of group C can control a wide range of immunoregulatory interactions up to oncogene activations (Bunney and Katan 2011). In 2015, activation of the NLRP3 inflammasome, among other things triggered by increased intracellular calcium concentrations, was demonstrated in the context of mutations in the PLCG2 gene (Chae et al. 2015). This also shows the clinical proximity of the APLAID disease to the classic NLRP3-dependent cold urticaria, although cold exposure does not lead to an increase in rash and fever reaction in our patient.

30.8.3 Diagnosis

Our patient ultimately did not show signs of an immune defect. An immune phenotyping, especially of the humoral B cell compartment, revealed a reduced total number of B cells and within that a reduction of memory B cells. However, CD21-negative,

CD38-negative anergic autoreactive B cells were somewhat increased. The measurement of peripheral immunoglobulin levels was unremarkable. The patient's mother had a normal number of B cells, but within these, a reduction of memory B cells was found. Mother and daughter otherwise showed an unremarkable distribution of B cell populations. Compared to further descriptions of this very rare variant of an autoinflammatory syndrome in the literature (Novice et al. 2020; Martín-Nalda et al. 2020), our patient has clear signs of NLRP3 inflammasome activation with urticaria and high inflammation parameters, but shows a relatively moderate restriction of peripheral B cell numbers without significant influence on immunoglobulins.

Diagnostically, an autoinflammation panel with a focus on **urticaria and fever syndromal diseases** was clearly indicative. This made the diagnosis of APLAID syndrome possible (Novice et al. 2020).

30.8.4 Therapy

Therapeutically, an excellent positive effect with interleukin-1 blockade was achieved with permanent remission.

30.8.5 Diagnosis

"Autoinflammation with PLCG2-associated antibody deficiency and immune dysregulation" (APLAID; OMIM reference 614878). Mutations were found in the PLCG2 gene.

30.8.6 Prophylaxis

If realistic in everyday life, patients should avoid sweating.

Conclusion

Next-generation sequencing concepts including so-called autoinflammation panels enable a targeted diagnosis of monogenetic autoinflammatory diseases and support a pathogenesis-based, targeted immunological basic therapy, specifically in our patient an interleukin-1 blockade.

References

Bunney TD, Katan M (2011) PLC regulation: emerging pictures for molecular mechanisms. Trends Biochem Sci 36:88–96. ▶ https://doi.org/10.1016/j.tibs.2010.08.003

Chae JJ, Park YH, Park C, Hwang IY, Hoffmann P, Kehrl JH, Aksentijevich I, Kastner DL (2015) Connecting two pathways through Ca 2+ signaling: NLRP3 inflammasome activation induced by a hypermorphic PLCG2 mutation. Arthritis Rheumatol 67:563–567. ▶ https://doi.org/10.1002/art.38961

Gandhi C, Healy C, Wanderer AA, Hoffman HM (2009) Familial atypical cold urticaria: description of a new hereditary disease. J Allergy Clin Immunol 124:1245–1250. ▶ https://doi.org/10.1016/j.jaci.2009.09.035

Martín-Nalda A, Fortuny C, Rey L, Bunney TD, Alsina L, Esteve-Solé A, Bull D, Anton MC, Basagaña M, Casals F, Deyá A, García-Prat M, Gimeno R, Juan M, Martinez-Banaclocha H, Martinez-Garcia JJ, Mensa-Vilaró A, Rabionet R, Martin-Begue N, Rudilla F, Yagüe J, Estivill X, García-Patos V, Pujol RM, Soler-Palacín P, Katan M, Pelegrín P, Colobran R, Vicente A, Arostegui JI (2020) Severe autoinflammatory manifestations and antibody deficiency due to novel hypermorphic PLCG2 mutations. J Clin Immunol 40:987–1000. ▶ https://doi.org/10.1007/s10875-020-00794-7

Novice T, Kariminia A, Del Bel KL, Lu H, Sharma M, Lim CJ, Read J, Lugt MV, Hannibal MC, O'Dwyer D, Hosler M, Scharnitz T, Rizzo JM, Zacur J, Priatel J, Abdossamadi S, Bohm A, Junker A, Turvey SE, Schultz KR, Rozmus J (2020) A germline mutation in the C2 domain of PLCγ2 associated with gain-of-function expands the phenotype for PLCG2-related diseases. J Clin Immunol 40:267–276. ▶ https://doi.org/10.1007/s10875-019-00731-3

Petro JB, Khan WN (2001) Phospholipase C-gamma 2 couples Bruton's tyrosine kinase to the NF-kappaB signaling pathway in B lymphocytes. J Biol Chem 276:1715–1719. ▶ https://doi.org/10.1074/jbc. M009137200

Schade A, Walliser C, Wist M, Haas J, Vatter P, Kraus JM, Filingeri D, Havenith G, Kestler HA, Milner JD, Gierschik P (2016) Cool-temperature-mediated activation of phospholipase C-γ2 in the human hereditary disease PLAID. Cell Signal 28:1237–1251. ▶ https://doi.org/10.1016/j.cellsig.2016.05.010

Yu P, Constien R, Dear N, Katan M, Hanke P, Bunney TD, Kunder S, Quintanilla-Martinez L, Huffstadt U, Schröder A, Jones NP, Peters T, Fuchs H, de Angelis MH, Nehls M, Grosse J, Wabnitz P, Meyer TP, Yasuda K, Schiemann M, Schneider-Fresenius C, Jagla W, Russ A, Popp A, Josephs M, Marquardt A, Laufs J, Schmittwolf C,

Wagner H, Pfeffer K, Mudde GC (2005) Autoimmunity and inflammation due to a gain-of-function mutation in phospholipase C gamma 2 that specifically increases external Ca2+ entry. Immunity 22:451–465. ▶ https://doi.org/10.1016/j.immuni.2005.01.018

Zhou Q, Lee GS, Brady J, Datta S, Katan M, Sheikh A, Martins MS, Bunney TD, Santich BH, Moir S, Kuhns DB, Long Priel DA, Ombrello A, Stone D, Ombrello MJ, Khan J, Milner JD, Kastner DL, Aksentijevich I (2012) A hypermorphic missense mutation in PLCG2, encoding phospholipase Cγ2, causes a dominantly inherited autoinflammatory disease with immunodeficiency. Am J Hum Genet 91:713–720. ▶ https://doi.org/10.1016/j.ajhg.2012.08.006

30

Back Pain in School Children—Overuse or More?

Annette Holl-Wieden

Contents

31.1 Medical History

Mia, aged 8 9/12 years, was presented for the investigation of recurring **bone pain**. Eight weeks ago, she had severe pain in the lumbar spine area for a week, these pains now only occur with certain twisting movements of the spine. For the past 6 weeks, she has been complaining about pain in the right hip joint. When running, a reduced load on the right leg is noticeable. The pains are becoming more frequent and increasing in intensity. Questions about fatigue, lethargy, night sweats, weight loss, fever, abdominal pain, and diarrhea were denied. A trauma or infection did not precede the complaints.

31.2 Examination Findings

31

The clinical examination showed no passive movement restriction in the area of the right hip joint, but the movement was painful in all directions. When running, a reduced load on the right leg was noticeable. The rest of the examination findings were unremarkable.

31.3 Laboratory Values and Imaging

31.3.1 Laboratory Values

The blood count with differential blood count was unremarkable. The ESR was at most slightly elevated (ESR 20 mm/h), the CRP was negative. The other overview laboratory values showed no abnormalities.

31.3.2 Imaging

The sonography of the hip joints was unremarkable. An MRI of the pelvis showed

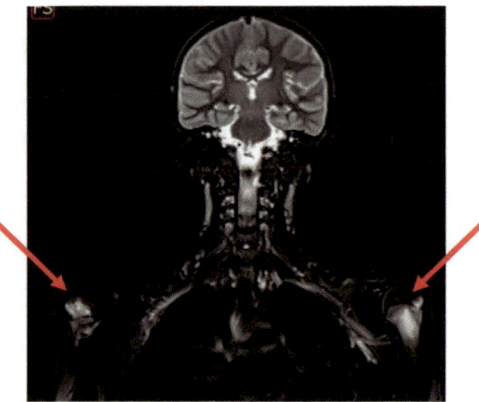

◻ Fig. 31.1 Whole-body MRI (TIRM sequence) at initial diagnosis: Flat T2w signal elevations in the humeral head on both sides. (With kind permission from Dr. Clemens Benoit, Institute for Diagnostic and Interventional Radiology, University Hospital Würzburg)

a flat **bone edema** with corresponding contrast enhancement of the apophysis of the right trochanter major and the adjacent femur metaphysis.

A subsequent **whole-body MRI** showed, in addition to the bone edema of the right proximal femur, **bone edemas with corresponding contrast uptake** in the left proximal tibia, in the humeral head on both sides, in T9 and L4 (◻ Fig. 31.1, 31.2, 31.3, and 31.4). This was followed by an MRI of the spine in 2 planes. In addition to the known bone edemas in T9 and L4, slight irregularities of the endplate of T9 and the base and endplate of L4 were found. However, there were no major structural abnormalities of the vertebral bodies.

31.4 Educational Questions

1. What differential diagnoses should be considered based on Mia's history, examination, laboratory findings, and imaging?
2. What therapy should be administered?

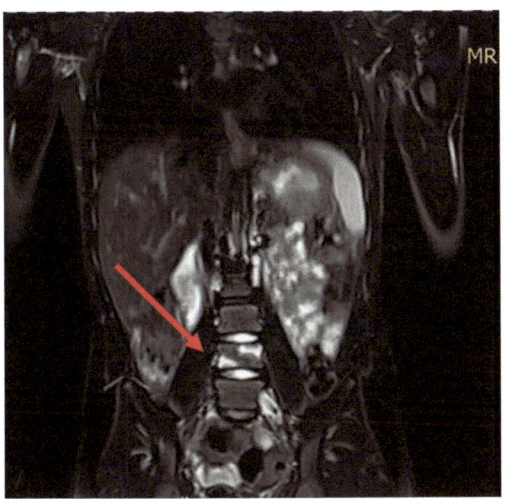

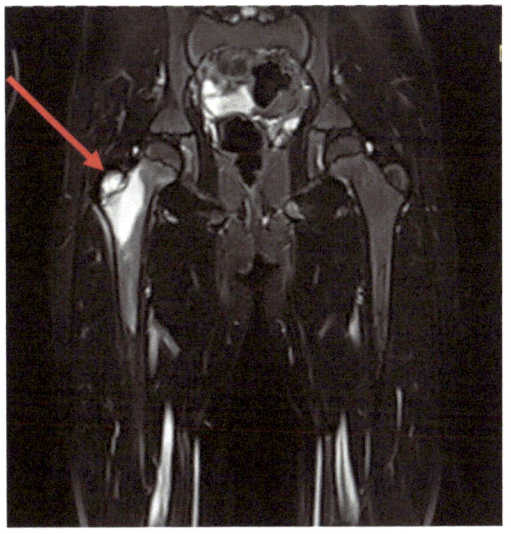

○ Fig. 31.2 Whole-body MRI (TIRM sequence) at initial diagnosis: Flat T2w signal elevations in L4. (With kind permission from Dr. Clemens Benoit, Institute for Diagnostic and Interventional Radiology, University Hospital Würzburg)

○ Fig. 31.4 Whole-body MRI (TIRM sequence) at initial diagnosis: Flat T2w signal elevation of the apophysis of the trochanter major and the adjacent femur metaphysis with periosteal reaction and corresponding contrast enhancement in T1 weighting (not shown). (With kind permission from Dr. Clemens Benoit, Institute for Diagnostic and Interventional Radiology, University Hospital Würzburg)

31.5 Differential Diagnostic Considerations

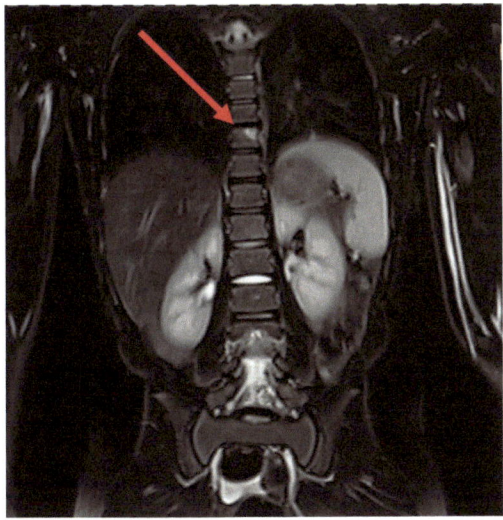

○ Fig. 31.3 Whole-body MRI (TIRM sequence) at initial diagnosis: Flat T2w signal elevations in T9. (With kind permission from Dr. Clemens Benoit, Institute for Diagnostic and Interventional Radiology, University Hospital Würzburg)

A variety of diseases must be considered in the case of bone pain. Even if the clinical examination is inconspicuous, comprehensive diagnostics should be carried out. Important differential diagnoses are **injuries**, bacterial infections such as **bacterial osteomyelitis** or **arthritis**, and especially **malignant or benign bone tumors**, but also other malignant diseases such as **leukemias, lymphomas** or **Langerhans cell histiocytosis**. Mia had no fever, the inflammation parameters were only slightly elevated, so bacterial osteomyelitis was rather unlikely.

The blood count with manual differential blood count showed no abnormalities, the cell decay parameters were not elevated, so there was no indication of leukemia. The key in bone pain is imaging, and here an MRI is best. Based on the MRI of the pelvis showing a bone edema of the apophysis of the right trochanter major and the adjacent femur metaphysis, a malignant oncological finding was considered, but chronic non-bacterial osteomyelitis (CNO) was already suspected. In CNO, one usually finds other osteomyelitis lesions in other places, which are typically possible symmetrically (◻ Fig. 31.1), but can be asymptomatic for the patient. The whole-body MRI then showed further bone edemas. The location of the bone edemas and the distribution were consistent with a CNO. It was decided not to perform a bone biopsy. In the case of unifocal findings or bone edemas atypical for CNO or also atypical locations of the bone edemas, however, a biopsy should be performed, especially to exclude a malignant disease (Hedrich et al. 2020).

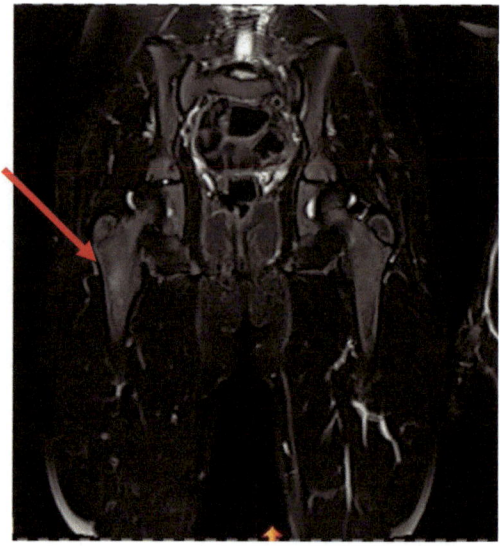

◻ **Fig. 31.5** Whole-body MRI (TIRM sequence), 3 months after the start of therapy: Extensive T2w signal increase of the apophysis of the right trochanter major and the adjacent femur metaphysis clearly regressing. (With kind permission from Dr. Clemens Benoit, Institute for Diagnostic and Interventional Radiology, University Hospital Würzburg)

31.6 Further Course

After the diagnosis of CNO, the parents were informed about the various therapy options. Due to the involvement of the vertebral bodies, we recommended therapy with Adalimumab, a TNF-α blocker. A therapy with a conventional synthetic DMARD was, in our estimation, too weak for Mia's disease. Since there were no structural abnormalities of the vertebral bodies, we initially decided against therapy with bisphosphonates (see summary, ► Sect. 31.8). Therapy with Adalimumab 20 mg s.c. (24 mg/m² BSA) every 2 weeks was initiated. Mia was symptom-free after just 4 weeks. The next whole-body MRI 3 months after the start of therapy showed the multiple signal increases known from the preliminary examination clearly regressing with discrete residual findings (◻ Fig. 31.5). The

therapy was continued, the next MRI is planned in 3 months.

31.7 Educational Answers

- **1. What differential diagnoses should be considered based on Mia's history, examination, laboratory findings, and imaging?**

A variety of diseases must be considered. Important differential diagnoses of chronic non-bacterial osteomyelitis are injuries, malignant or benign bone tumors, leukemias, lymphomas, Langerhans cell histiocytosis, and bacterial osteomyelitis.

- **2. What therapy should be administered?**

After the diagnosis of CNO with vertebral body involvement, therapy with csDMARDs, Bisphosphonates or TNF blockers should be initiated. Close clinical follow-up and MRI follow-up are necessary.

31.8 Summary

Chronic nonbacterial osteomyelitis (CNO) is an **autoinflammatory disease of the bone**. There are different courses, from mild, self-limiting monofocal to chronically active or recurrent multifocal courses. The latter course is also referred to as chronic recurrent multifocal osteomyelitis (CRMO). Adult rheumatologists often also refer to CNO as **SAPHO syndrome** (Synovitis, Acne, Pustulosis, Hyperostosis, Osteomyelitis). However, the term SAPHO syndrome should only be used for patients who also have skin involvement such as **acne or pustulosis** (Zhao et al. 2021).

31.8.1 Pathogenesis

The pathogenesis is still not fully understood. There is an **imbalance** between the production of proinflammatory and anti-inflammatory cytokines. Proinflammatory cytokines such as interleukin (IL)-1 and IL-6 as well as TNF-α are released in increased amounts and anti-inflammatory cytokines such as IL-10 or IL-19 are released in reduced amounts. This leads to chronic inflammation, activation of osteoclasts, destruction of bone and in some cases to hyperostosis and sclerosis of bone (Hedrich et al. 2020).

31.8.2 Clinic

The disease mainly occurs in children and adolescents and only rarely in adults. Children between 7 and 9 years of age are most commonly affected. Girls are more frequently affected than boys. Most children present with bone pain. Some children have local swelling and movement restrictions (Hedrich et al. 2020). Other organ systems can also be affected. Up to 20% of CNO patients develop skin manifestations such as a **palmoplantar pustulosis**, severe acne (possibly **acne conglobata**) and **psoriasis**. A **chronic inflammatory bowel disease (IBD)** occurs in about 10% of patients (Girschick et al. 2018; Hedrich et al. 2020).

31.8.3 Diagnosis

The diagnosis of CNO is made after **excluding differential diagnoses** and includes clinical examination, laboratory tests, imaging and possibly a biopsy (Schwarz et al. 2018). The clinical examination is often unremarkable. Sometimes there is local tenderness, warmth or swelling of the bone and overlying soft tissues. The inflammation parameters (ESR, CRP) are usually slightly elevated. X-rays show lytic lesions, sclerosis, hyperostosis, but can also be unremarkable. The most important examination is the MRI. Here, bone edema is shown as a sign of inflammation. It is then important to perform a **whole-body MRI** to search for further bone lesions, especially clinically **"silent"** lesions. The whole-body MRI is now considered the diagnostic gold standard, if established locally. The metaphyses of the long tubular bones are often affected, especially in the area of the lower extremity near the knee joints and ankle joints. In 20% of patients, symmetrical lesions are found. The pelvis, vertebral bodies, clavicle and lower jaw are considered "classic" locations of CNO. In unclear cases, a **biopsy** is performed to exclude malignant diseases, infections or other systemic diseases (Zhao et al. 2021). Proposed diagnostic criteria for CNO are available, which are not validated, but can be helpful for diagnosis (Jansson et al. 2007; Roderick et al. 2016).

31.8.4 Therapy

There is no major prospective therapy study and thus little controlled evidence for treatment. National and international Treat-to-Target protocols, such as the **CARRA recommendations** (Childhood Arthritis and Rheumatology Research Alliance) of North American and the **PRO-KIND recommendations** (Protocols for classification, monitoring, and therapy in pediatric rheumatology) of German pediatric rheumatologists, are based on experience and data from small case series, but also large international cohorts (Zhao et al. 2018; Schwarz et al. 2018; Girschick et al. 2018). Initial treatment is usually with nonsteroidal anti-rheumatic drugs (NSAIDs). If there is no response to NSAIDs or involvement of the vertebral bodies, treatment with conventional synthetic DMARDs such as methotrexate or sulfasalazine or biological DMARDs, especially TNF-α blockers like adalimumab or etanercept, or with bisphosphonates should be carried out. If there is vertebral body involvement **with structural changes**, many authors recommend treatment with bisphosphonates. Vertebral body involvement with structural changes already implies a fracture and the risk of further vertebral body collapses. This may result in spinal deformities and neurological deficits. Through therapy with bisphosphonates, one hopes to improve inflammation, but also structural changes in the sense of stabilization and reconstruction. In cases of vertebral body involvement without structural changes, TNF-α blockers are usually used. Short-term use of glucocorticoids can also be helpful (Hedrich et al. 2020; Schwarz et al. 2018; Zhao et al. 2018).

31.8.5 Prognosis

Earlier reports suggested that CNO may be a self-limiting disease that usually comes to a standstill after 12–18 months. Recent data show that many patients achieve clinical remission under medication after 12 months, but 50% on average experience a relapse after a total of 29 months (Schnabel et al. 2017). The most common complications are **vertebral compression fractures, leg length differences, bone thickening or deformities** (Schnabel et al. 2017; Zhao et al. 2021).

Conclusion

In case of bone pain in childhood, even if the examination is inconspicuous, CNO must also be considered and further diagnostics must be carried out.

References

Girschick H, Finetti M, Orlando F, Schalm S, Insalaco A, Ganser G, Nielsen S, Herlin T, Kone-Paut I, Martino S, Cattalini M, Anton J, Mohammed Al-Mayouf S, Hofer M, Quartier P, Boros C, Kuemmerle-Deschner J, Pires Marafon D, Alessio M, Schwarz T, Ruperto N, Martini A, Jansson A, Gattorno M, Paediatric Rheumatology International Trials O, the Eurofever r (2018) The multifaceted presentation of chronic recurrent multifocal osteomyelitis: a series of 486 cases from the Eurofever international registry. Rheumatology (Oxford) 57(7):1203–1211. ▶ https://doi.org/10.1093/rheumatology/key058

Hedrich CM, Morbach H, Reiser C, Girschick HJ (2020) New insights into adult and paediatric chronic non-bacterial osteomyelitis CNO. Curr Rheumatol Rep 22(9):52. ▶ https://doi.org/10.1007/s11926-020-00928-1

Jansson A, Renner ED, Ramser J, Mayer A, Haban M, Meindl A, Grote V, Diebold J, Jansson V, Schneider K, Belohradsky BH (2007) Classification of non-bacterial osteitis: retrospective study of clinical, immunological and genetic aspects in 89 patients. Rheumatology (Oxford) 46(1):154–160. ▶ https://doi.org/10.1093/rheumatology/kel190

Roderick MR, Shah R, Rogers V, Finn A, Ramanan AV (2016) Chronic recurrent multifocal osteomyelitis (CRMO) – advancing the diagnosis. Pediatr Rheumatol Online J 14(1):47. ▶ https://doi.org/10.1186/s12969-016-0109-1

Schnabel A, Range U, Hahn G, Berner R, Hedrich CM (2017) Treatment response and longterm outcomes in children with chronic nonbacterial osteomyelitis. J Rheumatol 44(7):1058–1065. ► https://doi.org/10.3899/jrheum.161255

Schwarz T, Oommen PT, Windschall D, Weissbarth-Riedel E, Trauzeddel R, Grote V, von Bismarck P, Morbach H, Hofmann C, Holl-Wieden A, Hügle B, Schnabel A, Dedeoglu F, Ferguson PJ, Zhao Y, Borte M, Haas JP, Hufnagel M, Hedrich V, Girschick HJ, Jansson AF (2018) Protokolle zur Klassifikation, Überwachung und Therapie in der Kinderrheumatologie (Pro-Kind): Chronisch nicht-bakterielle Osteomyelitis (CNO). Arthritis Rheumatol 38:282–288

Zhao DY, McCann L, Hahn G, Hedrich CM (2021) Chronic nonbacterial osteomyelitis (CNO) and chronic recurrent multifocal osteomyelitis (CRMO). J Transl Autoimmun 4:100095. ► https://doi.org/10.1016/j.jtauto.2021.100095

Zhao Y, Wu EY, Oliver MS, Cooper AM, Basiaga ML, Vora SS, Lee TC, Fox E, Amarilyo G, Stern SM, Dvergsten JA, Haines KA, Rouster-Stevens KA, Onel KB, Cherian J, Hausmann JS, Miettunen P, Cellucci T, Nuruzzaman F, Taneja A, Barron KS, Hollander MC, Lapidus SK, Li SC, Ozen S, Girschick H, Laxer RM, Dedeoglu F, Hedrich CM, Ferguson PJ, Chronic Nonbacterial Osteomyelitis/Chronic Recurrent Multifocal Osteomyelitis Study G, the Childhood A, Rheumatology Research Alliance Scleroderma VA, Rare Diseases S (2018) Consensus treatment plans for chronic nonbacterial osteomyelitis refractory to nonsteroidal antiinflammatory drugs and/or with active spinal lesions. Arthritis Care Res (Hoboken) 70(8):1228–1237. ► https://doi.org/10.1002/acr.23462

When a Child's Hip Hurts and It's not Rheumatism

Hermann Girschick and Moritz Klaas

Contents

32.1 Medical History

The 6 ½ year old Iko was presented acutely in the emergency department because he had been experiencing discomfort in the area of both hips with pain and protective posture for a week. Clinically, there was a limitation of hip joint mobility on the right in flexion/extension of 120°/0°/0° and reduction of internal to external rotation to 45° each. The left hip was clinically unremarkable in terms of mobility. Generally, there was an over-mobility/hypermobility of the joints. Other joints were not affected by arthritis. The pediatric-internal whole body examination was also unremarkable. The body length was on the 75th percentile, as was the body weight. His own medical history and family history were unremarkable in terms of musculoskeletal diseases.

32.2 Examination Findings

At the initial presentation, there was a significant limitation of hip joint mobility on the right with general hypermobility, no other signs of a chronic disease, age-appropriate examination findings.

32.3 Laboratory Values and Imaging

32.3.1 Laboratory Values

There was an unremarkable blood count with normal leukocytes and their differentiation. The CRP was negative. Serum overview values including creatine kinase and alkaline phosphatase were unremarkable. LDH and uric acid were normal, no pathological laboratory values were found. This was followed by an ANA antibody determination. It was assessed as "borderline" with a titer of 1:200. The fluorescence pattern

was reported as homogeneous in the cell nucleus. Other inflammation parameters such as ferritin or serum-IgG, -IgA, -IgM were unremarkable.

32.3.2 Imaging

The sonographic examination of both hips revealed a thickening and detachment of the capsule, and also a slight effusion, so the diagnosis of **Coxitis** on both sides with emphasis on the right was made (◘ Fig. 32.1a).

32.4 Educational Questions

1. What suspected diagnosis should be considered based on the one-week painful history and clinical oligoarthritis of both hips as well as the absence of inflammation parameters?
2. What laboratory diagnostics are to be considered sufficient/reasonable at this point?
3. Should osseous differential diagnoses be considered given the above symptoms?
4. What therapeutic steps appear sensible?

32.5 Differential Diagnostic Considerations

In the case of "arthritic" complaints that have been present for just a few days or a few weeks, with pain, limited mobility, and protective posture, the differential diagnosis of a **reactive arthritis** is at the forefront. If the hip is affected, this is also referred to as "hip cold" in layman's terms. Even if an infection event in the respiratory tract or gastrointestinal tract or a viral childhood disease, e.g., erythema infectiosum, was not reported, reactive arthritis remains the most likely differential diagnosis. The first manifestation of juvenile idiopathic arthritis (JIA) cannot

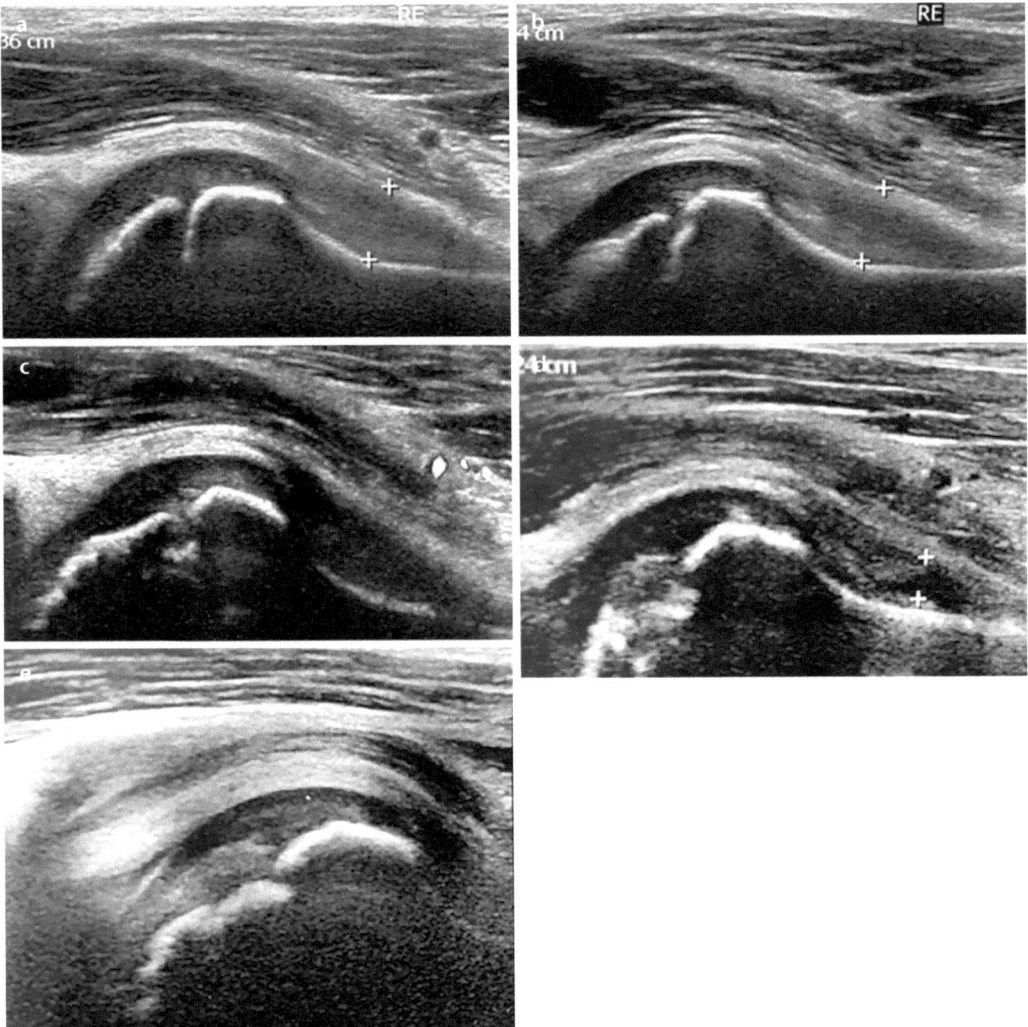

◻ Fig. 32.1 **a–e** Sonography of 6-year-old Iko with arthritis and subsequent Morbus Perthes of the right femoral head. **a–e** show the situation starting from **a** recording, **b** after one, **c** after 6, **d** after 13 and **e** after 21 months. Initially there was inflammation/Coxitis, then increasing structural unrest of the epiphyseal bone core, then cartilaginous expansion laterally and forward, with reduction of the bony and cartilaginous superstructure. (Containment reduced)

naturally be ruled out. According to the currently used ILAR criteria, the diagnosis of chronic arthritis (JIA) can be made after 6 weeks of documentation in the course. Additional indicative aspects in the clinical examination picture as well as in the family, e.g., psoriasis, were not detectable. "Limited" arthritides and musculoskeletal complaints should also be considered in systemic diseases in the broadest sense, especially hematological-oncological diagnoses such as **leukemia**, Langerhans cell histiocytosis, or osseous/musculoskeletal-tumorous space-occupying lesions. The latter can represent benign lesions, such as cartilaginous exostoses, osteomas, enchondromas, or juvenile bone cysts/fibrous bone dysplasia. Malignant osseous lesions should always be considered in the differential diagnosis - especially if it is a monofocal problem. Rare skeletal dysplasias and joint malpositions/ dislocations round off the differential diagnosis. Chronic osseous inflammation, which can occur uni- or multifocally, should be considered, as well as the consequences of trauma/injury. As in the differential diagnosis of childhood rheumatism, bleeding disorders and rare metabolic diseases (gout, hypophosphatasia) may play a role.

32.6 Further Course

After the blood count showed no indications of a hematological-oncological underlying disease, an anti-inflammatory therapy with ibuprofen at a dosage of 30 mg/ kg body weight/day was initiated. Under this, the clinical symptom picture improved quickly. Already after 4 weeks, the patient was symptom-free in everyday life and signaled that he wanted to participate unrestrictedly in recreational sports again. A moderate sports restriction had been recommended. However, above all, the **external and internal rotation restriction of the hip** persisted, so that follow-up checks every 2 weeks were aimed for.

32.7 Educative Answers

- **1. What suspected diagnosis should be considered based on the one-week painful history and clinical oligoarthritis of both hips as well as the simultaneous absence of inflammation parameters?**

In the differential diagnosis, in addition to post-infectious-reactive arthritides or the onset of JIA, oncological underlying diseases should also be considered, starting with **leukemia** and **Langerhans cell histiocytosis** up to benign or malignant bone tu-

mors. Also, osseous dysplasias, bone metabolic diseases should be considered in the differential diagnosis.

- **2. What laboratory diagnostics are to be considered sufficient/sensible at this point in time?**

At the initial presentation, a blood count with differential blood count, laboratory overview values including creatine kinase, alkaline phosphatase, LDH and uric acid, furthermore CRP and ESR are usually sufficient to achieve a good orientation in the differential diagnosis. If the symptom picture persists for 4-6 weeks, then "rheumatological parameters" such as an antinuclear antibody titer should be considered in the differential diagnosis. The determination of a rheumatoid factor IgM, of CCP antibodies (antibodies against cyclic citrullinated antigens) appears necessary only in the presence of polyarthritis/an extended oligoarthritis. The determination of creatine kinase helps to capture muscular differential diagnoses, such as regional myositides. The **alkaline phosphatase** helps, on the one hand, to exclude a vitamin D metabolic disorder/**rickets** in case of an increase and, on the other hand, a genetic hypophosphatasia in case of a decrease. Infection serologies to search for possibly triggering infectious agents are not absolutely necessary in clinical practice. However, in the case of persistent mono- or oligoarthritis, a **Lyme borreliosis** should be ruled out, as in our patient. Thus, the diagnostics in clinical practice only expand after about 4-6 weeks, should there be no other alarm signs for a systemic disease, such as hepatosplenomegaly or lymph node pathology, a conspicuous accompanying anemia or thrombocytopenia.

- **3. Should osseous differential diagnoses be considered in the above symptomatology?**

The sonographic examination does not rule out a primary osseous pathology. The early form of bone circulatory disorders/ osteonecrosis also appears structurally externally inconspicuous in the initial stage (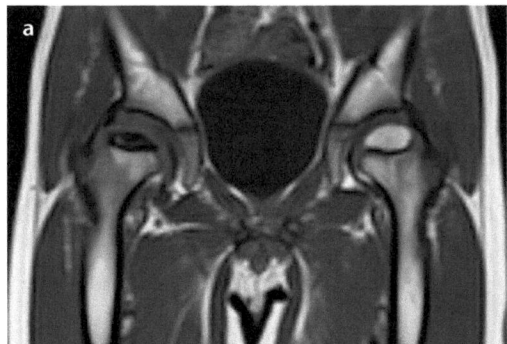 Fig. 32.1a). The differential diagnosis **osteonecrosis** and in our case aseptic hip necrosis remains therefore still existent, as well as a unifocal chronic non-bacterial osteomyelitis (CNO). A septic osteomyelitis seems essentially excluded in the absence of clinical parameters, fever or previous infection events, and also in the case of inconspicuous inflammation parameters. However, it should be noted that individual bacterial infection pathogens, such as *Borrelia burgdorferi, Kingella kingae*, can be associated with low or absent inflammation parameters.

■ **4. What therapeutic steps seem sensible?**
Initially, a symptomatically anti-inflammatory therapy with non-steroidal drugs, e.g. Ibuprofen or Naproxen, seems sensible and sufficient. If no significant improvement can be achieved within a maximum of 2 weeks, then the sonographic imaging diagnostics should be repeated and expanded

to include other imaging, e.g. conventional X-rays or an MRI examination.

Iko remained conspicuous in the clinical examination over several weeks, although he no longer reported any complaints in everyday life. Specifically, the internal and external rotation of the right hip under Ibuprofen therapy, which was reduced to 15 mg/ kg body weight/day over time, remained restricted. The subsequent sonography after 4 weeks showed a structural unrest in the **right hip head** epiphysis, with persistent capsular thickening and arthritis (■ Fig. 32.1b). Therefore, the suspicion of aseptic hip head necrosis (**Morbus Perthes**) was raised. An MRI examination including contrast agent confirmed this suspected diagnosis after 2 months (■ Fig. 32.2a, b). An interdisciplinary orthopedic evaluation also confirmed this suspected diagnosis. A conservative approach involving physiotherapy and continuation of the anti-inflammatory therapy was recommended. A sporting rest in everyday life was also recommended, but not implemented by the boy. A conventional X-ray at the time of 6 (■ Fig. 32.3a, b) and 9 months

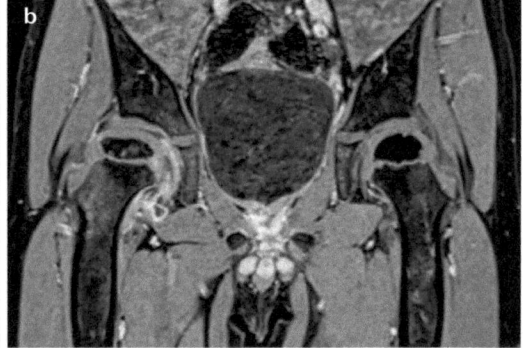

■ **Fig. 32.2   a, b** MRI of Iko's pelvis with arthritis and subsequent Morbus Perthes of the right hip head. The images show the situation 2 months after the first presentation already with the beginning of the osteodestructive disturbance of the epiphysis, condensation and coxitis (here contrast agent uptake), furthermore diffuse contrast medium uptake in the femoral neck, near the epiphyseal plate and missing perfusion in the epiphysis (**a** T1, with Gadolinium contrast agent). In the T2 weighting, there is also an edema in the middle of the femoral neck and in the epiphyseal core, furthermore a synovitis especially medial from the femoral neck(**b**). (With kind permission of Prof. Dr. J. Wagner, Institute for Radiology and Interventional Therapy, Vivantes Klinikum im Friedrichshain, Berlin)

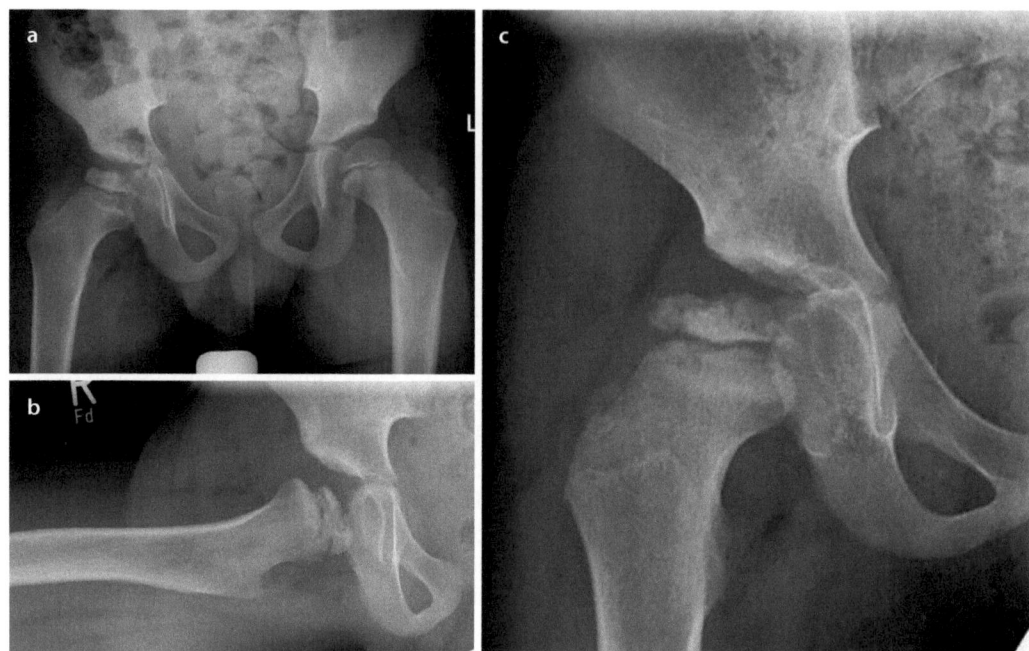

◘ Fig. 32.3 **a–c** Conventional X-ray of Iko's right hip with Perthes disease. **a, b** Situation 6 and **c** 9 months after the onset of symptoms. There is a severe, still increasing trophic disorder of the epiphysis (Caterall stage 4; stage B/C according to Herring). (With kind permission from Prof. Dr. J. Wagner, Institute for Radiology and Interventional Therapy, Vivantes Klinikum im Friedrichshain, Berlin)

32

(◘ Fig. 32.3c) after the onset of symptoms documented the trophic disturbance of the right hip head/epiphysis, and also the **widening of the femoral neck**. According to the various classification divisions, a stage IV according to **Caterall**, a stage B/C according to Herring with approximately 50% preservation of the lateral pillar was classified (◘ Fig. 32.3a–c) (Hefti 2015). The morphological description of the course stages of a Morbus Perthes with **condensation/fragmentation** and subsequent signs of **repair** could be traced in the boy. There was a moderate widening of the femoral neck and a reduced **containment**/hip socket overbuilding in the context of the cartilaginous-bony expansion of the hip head laterally (◘ Fig. 32.1c–e). The accompanying anti-inflammatory therapy was ended after 8 months. 13 months after diagnosis, the boy was symptom-free in everyday life. The clinically definable hip

joint mobility was inconspicuous. To document the physical performance, we also used a mechanograph, which impressively showed Iko's sparing of the affected right leg side, which was no longer detectable in the course! The overall performance was also pleasingly not restricted (◘ Fig. 32.4).

32.8 Summary

32.8.1 Etiology

The cause of a child's aseptic hip necrosis is ultimately still unclear. Genetic factors are discussed, especially in the construction of collagen type II (Hefti 2015) or the disease is generally seen in relation to systemic basic problems such as increased body size/obesity and hypothyroidism (Hailer and

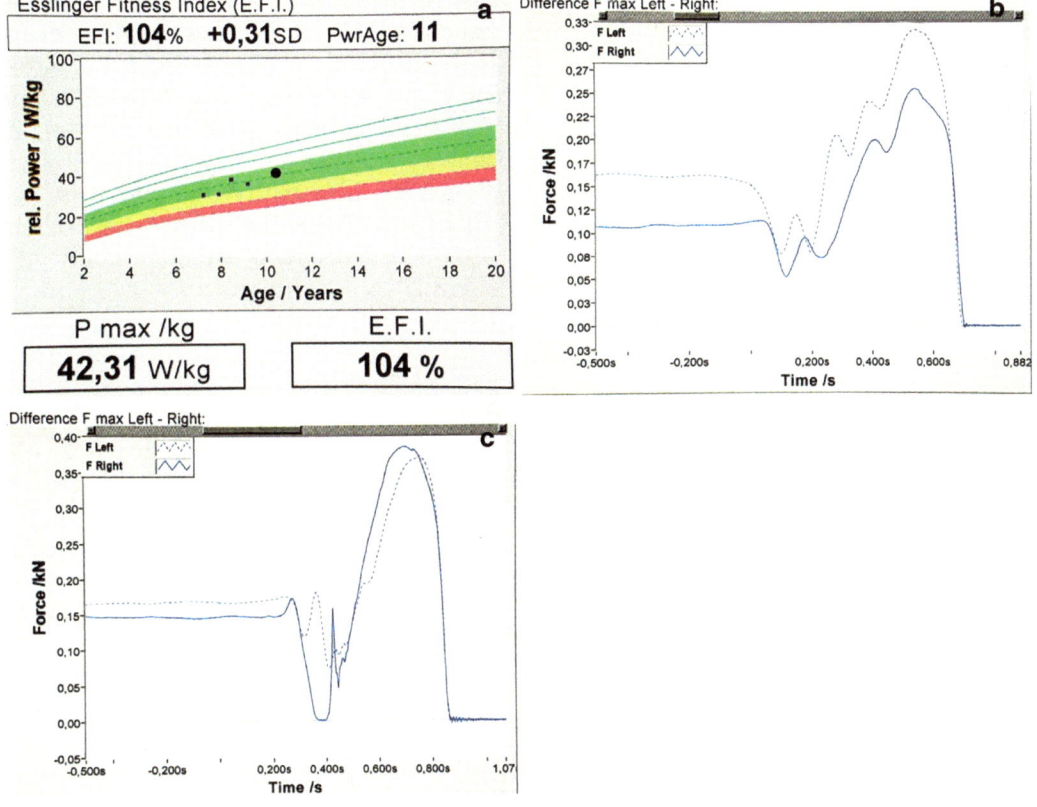

□ Fig. 32.4 **a–c** Biodynamic mechanograph analysis with two-legged jump initially and after 8 months. **a** shows the pleasing development of Iko's jumping power over 4 years after the onset of symptoms in the 6th year of life. **b** Initially, there was a clear side difference with weakness/protection on the right (temporal power development in the jump, force plate analysis), **c** which had normalized 8 months later and remained the same on both sides in the course. (Measurement analysis with Leonardo force plate, Stratec, Pforzheim; normalization by a same-age control cohort from Baden-Württemberg)

Hailer 2018). Ultimately, however, a unifactorial cause, e.g. an isolated gene defect, cannot be specified. Mechanistic considerations, which particularly take into account the blood supply to the head of the hip, have been discussed again and again. From a rheumatological point of view, the question arises to what extent a unifocal arthritis/coxitis could not lead to a circulatory disorder in the **ligamentum capitis femoris** and the **arteria capitis femoris** located there. Almost as a rule, patients with Perthes disease show very early or at the beginning of the disease a thickening of the joint cap-

sule, effusion formation and increased synovial blood flow, all signs of arthritis (□ Fig. 32.1a–e and 32.2a, b). A resulting **malnutrition of the head of the hip** is therefore not to be excluded from the authors' point of view, even if this question does not receive sufficient evaluation in the orthopedic literature. Hefti summarizes a multifactorial genetic etiology with aspects of skeletal maturation disorder and growth delay at the age of 3-5 years as possible causes (Hefti 2015). There is a preference for boys. Here, physical-sporting aspects/load aspects may play a role? The hypermobility seen in our patient is not documented in the literature as a possible risk factor.

32.8.2 Pathogenesis/Clinic

From a rheumatological point of view, the possibly initial inflammatory component should not be neglected. We generally have the impression in patients with Perthes disease treated by us that a **consistent anti-inflammatory therapy** can have positive effects on the long-term course, not only in terms of purely symptomatic pain reduction, but also with regard to structural destruction.

32.8.3 Diagnosis

As a rule, in orthopedic literature, reliance is placed on the conventional X-ray in the course of time. For the assessment of various structural disorders within the framework of morphological classification, follow-up examinations are necessary. Initially, in addition to the a.p. image, an axial image (◘ Fig. 32.3c) (Lauenstein image) is recommended, especially to document the **subchondral fracture** (Hefti 2015). From a rheumatological point of view, sonographic diagnostics using a linear transducer and also power Doppler examination are of significant relevance when performed by an experienced examiner. **An MRI examination can support early diagnosis** (◘ Fig. 32.2a, b). Here, the recommendations of the orthopedic and rheumatological professions differ, with the latter recommending this. For the assessment of the differential diagnosis, a blood count, differential blood count, inflammation parameters, a limited bone metabolism diagnosis, possibly a coagulation analysis are useful. In this context, hematological primary diseases such as hemoglobinopathies should be assessed, which are also associated with an increased risk of femoral head necrosis. Bone metabolic diseases such as achondroplasia or epiphyseal dysplasias should be distinguishable within the framework of the clinic and conventional radiological imaging. In this context, a general clinical whole-body examination, also with regard to liver and spleen size (storage diseases?) as well as neurological disorders should be considered (Hefti 2015).

32.8.4 Therapy

Hefti formulates as central goals for the therapy of Morbus Perthes on the one hand the improvement of mobility, on the other hand the relief and depending on the progression of the disease a **centering treatment** to improve the **joint congruence/containment** (Hefti 2015). From a rheumatological point of view, the already described anti-inflammatory therapy and regular physiotherapy to improve mobility/its restriction are considered. From an orthopedic point of view, the injection of botulinum toxin into adductors is described as pain-reducing and indirectly an adductor spasm is seen as possibly causing the patient's pain sensation. Various mobilization measures, partly under anesthesia, including the use of an extension table, should certainly be placed in the hands of a very experienced orthopedic expert team (Hefti 2015). Arthroscopic measures to reduce the consequences of Morbus Perthes and in particular an **impingement** problem on the femoral head, on the acetabulum and on the labrum (Goyal et al. 2021), appear to be very helpful in experienced hands. Surgical measures to reduce the size of the femoral head, which is destroyed in the course of the disease, but also decentered, and measures for recentering should also be placed in the hands of experienced teams, as possible complications with femoral head necrosis (quasi on top) postoperatively need to be considered (Randelli et al. 2021). A centering treatment was mainly historically performed with abduction splints. They significantly restrict children in their everyday activities, so the pros and cons of a surgical approach versus the conservative abduction splint must be carefully weighed (Maleki et al. 2021). Patients who are more than 8 years old at manifestation seem to benefit from a better, more forced containment setting and thus surgical intervention. Patients who are younger than 6 years old generally have a good prognosis and seem to be amenable to conservative therapy. For patients between 6 and 8 years old, it is recommended to identify factors that consider the femoral head as "at risk". **Risk factors for the femoral head** include the extent of the **necrosis**, the **degree of subluxation** and the remaining **percentage of coverage** as well as the condition of the lateral pillar (Hefti 2015).

32.8.5 Diagnosis

Morbus Legg-Calvé-Perthes, Morbus Perthes, childhood aseptic femoral head necrosis

32.8.6 Prophylaxis

There is no prophylaxis to fundamentally prevent femoral head necrosis.

Conclusion

Children with Morbus Perthes are still primarily cared for by pediatric orthopedics today. From a pediatric rheumatological point of view, anti-inflammatory therapy is quite opportune and sensible - not only to treat symptomatically anti-inflammatory and pain-reducing, but also to reduce assumed pathophysiological inflammatory processes that can contribute negatively to the outcome. Interdisciplinary joint care, as in our patient, appears medically sensible.

References

Goyal T, Barik S, Gupta T (2021) Hip arthroscopy for sequelae of Legg-Calve-Perthes disease: a systematic review. Hip Pelvis 33:3–10. ▶ https://doi.org/10.5371/hp.2021.33.1.3

Hailer YD, Hailer NP (2018) Is Legg-Calvé-Perthes disease a local manifestation of a systemic condition? Clin Orthop Relat Res 476:1055–1064. ▶ https://doi.org/10.1007/s11999.0000000000000214

Hefti F (2015) Morbus Perthes. In: Hefti F (Hrsg) Kinderorthopädie in der Praxis, Bd 3. Springer, Berlin, S 241–255

Maleki A, Qoreishy SM, Bahrami MN (2021) surgical treatments for Legg-Calvé-Perthes disease: comprehensive review. Interact J Med Res 10:e27075. ▶ https://doi.org/10.2196/27075

Randelli F, Papavasiliou A, Mazzoleni MG, Fioruzzi A, Basile G, Ganz R (2021) Femoral head necrosis and progressive osteoarthritis of a healed intracapital osteotomy in a severe sequelae of Legg-Calvé-Perthes disease with aplasia of tensor fasciae latae. J Hip Preserv Surg 8:i16–i24. ▶ https://doi.org/10.1093/jhps/hnab019

Immediate Hip Pain After Sports and Jumping

Hermann Girschick

Contents

© The Author(s), under exclusive license to Springer-Verlag GmbH, DE, part of Springer Nature 2024
C. Huemer and H. Girschick (eds.), *Clinical Examples in Pediatric Rheumatology*,
https://doi.org/10.1007/978-3-662-68732-1_33

33.1 Medical History

To illustrate the **Epiphyseolysis capitis femoris**, two adolescent patients are presented, a 14-year-old girl Ella and a nearly 18-year-old patient Otto at the time of first presentation.

▪▪ Ella

The girl had fallen off a skateboard a week before presentation. Immediately afterwards, she experienced pain in her right hip and was unable to stand up. This pain was of a changing character. Even before the fall, she had been experiencing recurring pain in her right hip over a period of 2 weeks, unrelated to the fall.

▪▪ Otto

At the beginning of his 17th year, the boy fell during a stair jump and immediately felt pain in his left hip. Prior to this, the boy had no complaints. No bone or joint problems were reported. Since the complaints persisted, a CT scan was carried out externally in the outpatient department 7 months later. Here, suspicion of a **slipped capital femoral epiphysis** (SCFE) on the left side was raised. In addition, cystic changes on the femoral head, a **cartilage defect** anterior to the femoral neck, and osseous structural disturbances in the area of the acetabulum were already described (◘ Fig. 33.1a–d). A CT-guided biopsy of the femoral neck was performed, which did not yield any clear findings. Therefore, an open exploration of the left hip was decided upon. Since a significant **osteolysis** of the acetabulum with structural weakness was seen intraoperatively, there was suspicion that it was a **bacterial osteomyelitis.** Therefore, an initial 2-fold oral antibiotic therapy with cefuroxime (14 days) and clindamycin for a total of 6 weeks was carried out. Four months later, no improvement of the still painful hip condition could be achieved. An MRI examination revealed a significant bone edema

in the area of the femoral neck and in the femoral head (◘ Fig. 33.2a, b). Furthermore, a significant **synovitis** was described and a rheumatic event was suspected. Suspicion of a **villonodular synovitis** was raised. No therapy concept resulted from this. For a deeper osteological and rheumatological assessment, the boy was finally included in a rheumatological evaluation 16 months after the trauma. Here, the previous imaging was completely analyzed again. The MRI examination from the time 10 months after trauma (◘ Fig. 33.2a, b) was evaluated as significant synovitis, but also as osseous inflammation in the area of the acetabulum, the femoral head, and the femoral neck. Another 7 months later, the structural disturbance in the MRI increased, the bone edema extended into the upper diaphysis of the femoral neck. Significant structural deficits were identified in the T1 weighting both in the area of the acetabulum and in the area of the femoral neck and femoral head (◘ Fig. 33.2c, d). Thus, the inflammatory process had progressed further, so that at the time of presentation, chronic inflammation and significant structural deficits on the femoral head could already be described. Formally, the diagnosis of a **chronic non-bacterial osteomyelitis (CNO)** with subsequent structural disturbances, or **osteoarthritis,** most likely on the basis of an untreated SCFE could be made.

33.2 Examination Findings

▪▪ Ella

The slightly obese patient (body weight 70 kg, 92nd percentile; BMI 24.5 kg/m^2 BSA) presented with painful leg mobility, external rotation position in the hip due to pain (**Drehmann's sign**), the mobility in the hip was therefore not testable. There was groin pressure pain on the right leg without local swelling, redness or overheating. The remaining joint status, tendon status and

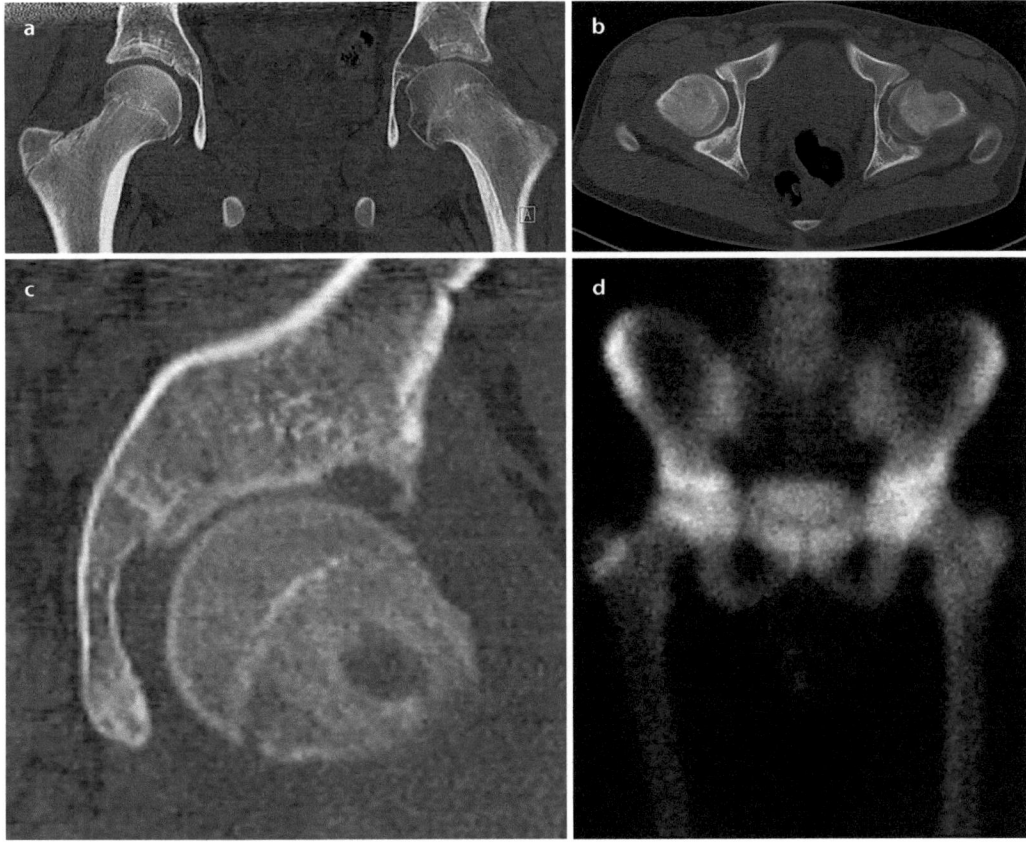

◪ **Fig. 33.1** **a–d** Computed tomography of the 16-year-old patient Otto with chronic epiphyseal detachment and osteolysis. **a–c** Situation upon admission to the external clinic 7 months after stair fall and subsequent chronic pain. The CT scan described an osteolytic disturbance of the femoral neck, and the hip socket and a chronic SCFE. **d** Late phase of a 3-phase 99m-Technetium bone scintigraphy with slight over-occupancy of the nuclide in the femoral head and socket

assessment of the connective tissue status revealed no abnormalities.

■■ **Otto**

17 months after trauma, the normal weight patient (body weight 69 kg, 75th percentile; body length 1.86 m, 90th percentile) showed an almost stiff, end-stage significantly painful hip mobility on the left with still slight flexion ability of 45°, with missing rotation. The left leg was about 2 cm shorter. The remaining joint status, tendon status and assessment of the connective tissue status revealed no abnormalities except for moderate hypermobility.

33.3 **Laboratory Values and Imaging**

33.3.1 **Laboratory Values**

■■ **Ella**

Due to the urgent clinical suspicion of epiphysiolysis, the collection of laboratory values was omitted.

■■ **Otto**

Inflammatory laboratory parameters could not be identified, the ESR was not accelerated at 16 mm/h. A CRP was negative. The

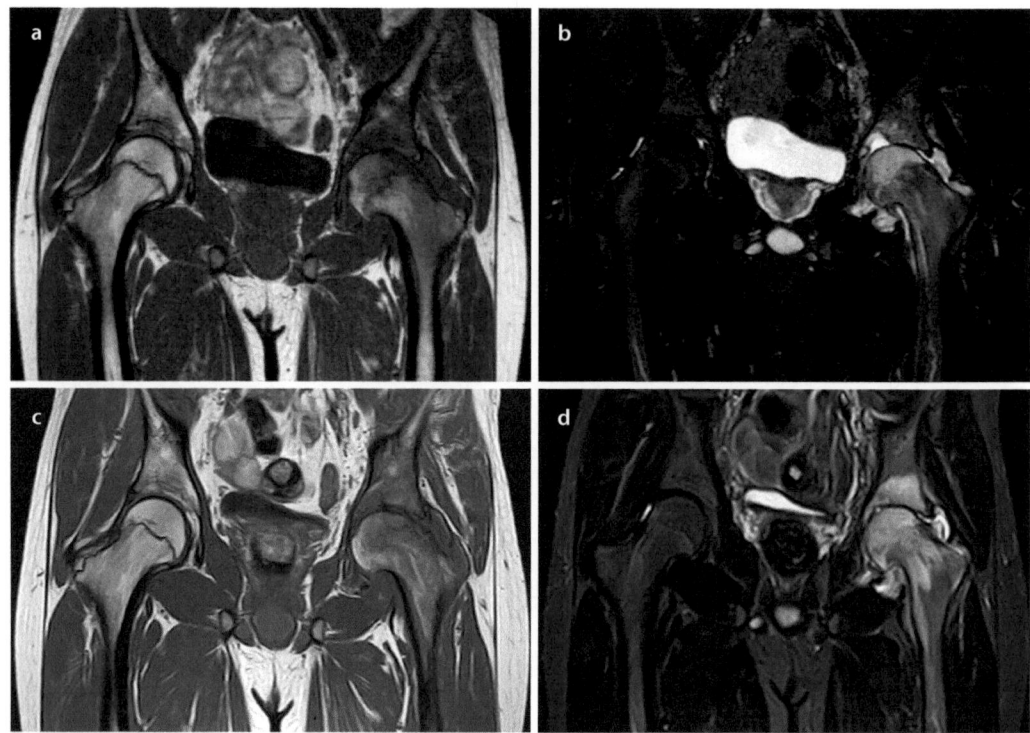

◘ Fig. 33.2   a–d MRI of Otto's pelvis with chronic epiphyseal detachment of the left femoral head and osteoar-thritis/arthritis. **a, b** Situation 10 months after stair fall: osteodestructive disturbance of the femoral neck and the hip socket on the basis of the unaddressed chronic SCFE (T1, TIRM weighting, resp.). **c, d** Further increasing destruction of the femoral head and the spread of inflammation into the ilium and the femoral neck (T1, TIRM weighting, resp.) 17 months after trauma

33

rheumatological diagnostics revealed no antinuclear antibodies. The complement system was unremarkable, there was no vitamin D deficiency, Lyme arthritis could be ruled out. The alkaline phosphatase showed age-appropriate normal values, so a general osteopathy of metabolic origin was rather unlikely.

33.3.2 Imaging

■■ **Ella**

A conventional X-ray pelvic overview with additional axial representation of the right hip confirmed the suspected diagnosis of

"acute-on-chronic" existing epiphysiolysis with "tilting of the epiphysis medially and dorsally in relation to the femoral neck". There were already trophic changes on the femoral neck with remodeling processes and signs of shortening, so a longer existing process was to be assumed.

■■ **Otto**

The conventional X-rays taken for the first time in domo (17 months after trauma) showed severe **osteodestruction and osteoarthritis** of both the hip head in "detached", displaced position and a significant **joint space narrowing** The initial diagnosis of ECF was confirmed (◘ Fig. 33.3a, b).

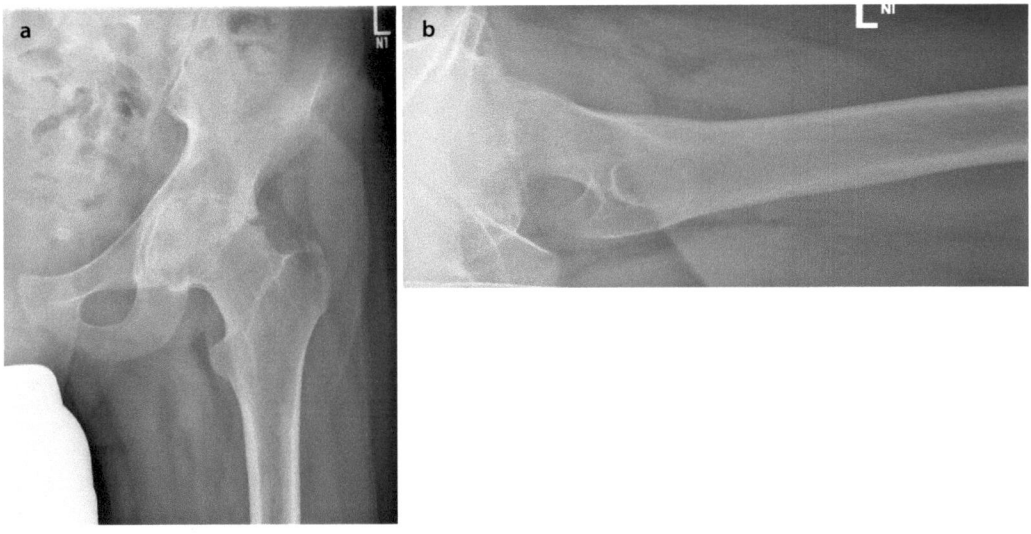

■ Fig. 33.3 **a, b** Conventional X-ray of Otto's left hip with chronic ECF and osteoarthritis/-osis 17 months after trauma. **a** Situation with fall history 17 months ago. There is a severe trophic disorder of the epiphysis and the femoral neck, hence the diagnosis of severe chronic ECF with osteoarthritis. **b** Tilting of the epiphysis in Lauenstein position. (With kind permission of Prof. Dr. J. Wagner, Institute for Radiology and Interventional Therapy, Vivantes Klinikum im Friedrichshain, Berlin)

33.4 Educational Questions

1. What suspected diagnoses arise in the adolescent patient due to a 1 ½-year course with pain and protection in a joint region, specifically the hip?
2. Can a prioritization of possible differential diagnoses already be carried out at this point in time?
3. What therapeutic steps can currently be considered in addition to general analgesia?

33.5 Differential Diagnostic Considerations

■ ■ Ella

Since no significant additional differential diagnostic considerations were necessary, a consecutive surgical fixation of the epiphysis was performed using three Kirschner wires (■ Fig. 33.4a–c).

■ ■ Otto

The differential diagnosis of a destructive monoarthritis is firstly the genuine rheumatic disease of the adolescent (enthesitis-associated arthritis or psoriasis arthritis). Since various family members had psoriasis, the patient himself showed pitting nails as a manifestation of nail psoriasis and accompanying bone diseases, e.g. in the paternal grandfather, even led to a knee joint replacement, a familial predisposition to bone lesions in the context of psoriasis could be suspected. An infectious genesis seemed unlikely, the differential diagnosis was most likely to be rheumatic. Since no signs of an infectious event were reported beforehand, and inflammation parameters were also negative, bacterial osteomyelitis and septic arthritis as possible structural disorders in our patient could be ruled out. Lyme disease could also be ruled out. Differentially, a CNO with lesions in the area of the femur and the acetabulum could be considered. However,

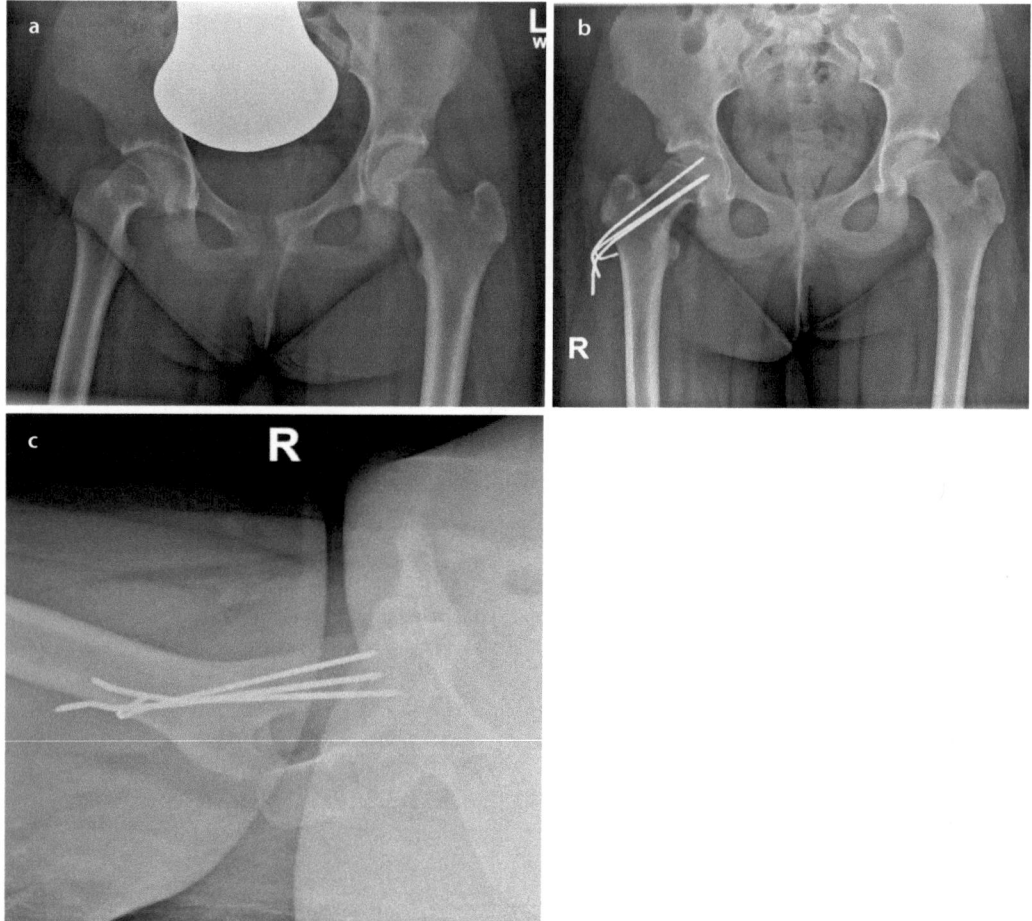

■ **Fig. 33.4   a–c** Conventional X-ray of the 14-year-old patient Ella with acute on chronic ECF of the right femoral head. **a** Situation upon admission. With a history of falling 2 weeks ago, there is already a trophic disorder of the right femoral neck, hence the diagnosis of acute on chronic ECF. **b** Surgical care/fixation of the epiphysis with three Kirschner wires in p.a. and **c** in Lauenstein position. (With kind permission from Prof. Dr. J. Wagner, Institute for Radiology and Interventional Therapy, Vivantes Klinikum im Friedrichshain, Berlin)

33

the significant osseous structural disorder already present 4 months after the onset of symptomatology argues against the diagnosis of CNO. In this case, there is usually an osteoplastic component/**hyperostosis** on the peripheral skeleton, which is triggered by chronic inflammation. General osteoporosis or a vitamin D metabolic disorder/rickets could be ruled out in the boy, and also seemed unlikely based on the im-

aging. A possibly already existing unilateral **hip dysplasia** seemed ultimately unlikely due to the tilting of the femoral head relative to the femoral neck. The focus of the differential diagnosis was therefore an untreated ECF. The deformity of the femoral head-neck transition (CAM deformity) with particularly pronounced osteolysis of both the acetabulum and lesions on the femoral neck/femoral head were seen as secondary to the epiphysiolysis (Weinmann et al. 2020; Slongo et al. 2010). However, a familial tendency towards joint inflammation was assumed.

33.6 Further Course

▪▪ Ella

During the operative fixation, the epiphysis of the femoral head on the right side was fixed with 3 Kirschner wires, inserted through the major trochanter (◘ Fig. 33.4c). The postoperative representation showed a satisfactory fixation. The family has declined fixation of the opposite side at this time. The immediate postoperative course was without complications. This rapid approach has likely created a good starting position for Ella, so that in the long term the possible complications of an ECF, such as hip head necrosis, the development of osteoarthritis and further tilting of the hip head with subsequent femoroacetabular hip head disorder/deformity (CAM deformity) can be avoided. The patient Otto illustrates this danger.

▪▪ Otto

A symptomatic anti-inflammatory therapy with ibuprofen and Wobenzyme® was started, with only minor therapeutic efficiency/improvement. To better assess the inflammatory nature of the synovitis, a minimally invasive biopsy was performed through **mini-arthrotomy**. The histology revealed a significant **lymphocytic infiltrate**. A 14-day long-term culture for the search of bacteria remained aerobic and anaerobic sterile. Based on the histological picture in conjunction with the imaging, a symptomatic basic therapy with methotrexate orally once a week (20 mg as a single dose) was initiated. This resulted in moderate improvement and slight pain reduction, with

good general condition. However, the mobility of the hip (extension/flexion 0–0–45°, lack of rotation ability) had not improved as expected. In general, however, the boy had gained 5 kg in weight (74 kg at a body length of 186 cm). From an orthopedic point of view, a hip joint replacement was advised and explained. In the case of **CAM impingement** and severe advanced structural destruction, a **realignment osteotomy** in the femoral neck as a therapy strategy for better adjustment of the hip head into the socket no longer seemed timely. The destructive finding was too far advanced for this. Due to reaching the age limit, the boy was no longer under our care. A year later, the operative replacement of the socket and femoral neck of the left hip was performed with excellent improvement of hip function. After intensive rehabilitation, the young man feels no restrictions in everyday life.

33.7 Educative Answers

▪ **1. What suspected diagnoses are made for the adolescent patient Otto due to a 1 ½-year course with pain and protection in a joint region, specifically the hip?**

Chronic pain and protection of a joint region may primarily correspond to chronic arthritis on a rheumatic basis. As a differential diagnosis, an immunological osteomyelitis/CNO must be included. A bacterial genesis with septic arthritis/osteomyelitis seemed unlikely based on history, findings, and laboratory parameters. A bone structural disorder as a possible starting point, e.g., a **hip dysplasia**, or an epiphyseolysis capitis femoris, furthermore a **Morbus Perthes** can be discussed. Since the hip head initially appeared structurally normal, Morbus Perthes was ruled out. The tilting of the epiphysis relative to the femoral neck made chronic ECF highly likely.

■ **2. Can a prioritization of possible differential diagnoses be carried out at this point?**

The prioritization of the diagnostic assessment thus results in a chronic, surgically untreated ECF with secondary CAM impingement, accompanying osteolysis of the acetabulum and femoral neck, and severe osteoarthritic coxitis (Weinmann et al. 2020; Hellmich and Krieg 2019).

■ **3. What therapeutic steps can currently be considered in addition to general analgesia?**

In this late phase of an ECF, a **Dunn realignment osteotomy** no longer seems possible (Bittersohl et al. 2015). From our point of view, the operative hip replacement with simultaneous installation of a neo-socket was the main focus for the boy.

33.8 Summary

33.8.1 Etiology

ECF mainly affects adolescents before the closure of the growth plate, with a gender ratio of 1.5:1 in favor of male adolescents. Increased body weight or general **connective tissue weakness** can be considered as additional risk factors. However, the exact cause of ECF is unknown. Structural disorders of the growth plates and loosening, possibly based on mechanical stress or trauma, are possible (Hellmich and Krieg 2019).

33.8.2 Pathogenesis/Clinic

Hormonal influences during the puberty growth spurt may lead to a **loosening of the growth plates**. Additional risk factors include, for example, growth hormone therapy in the context of short stature. The

hypothyroidism and **hypogonadism** are also seen as possible accompanying causes (Hellmich and Krieg 2019). Patients often report pain after a sports trauma, which significantly increases over time. The pain can radiate into the groin and thigh region and even throughout the entire leg. This sometimes uncharacteristic symptom constellation often leads to a delayed diagnosis, as happened with Otto. Here, the particular difficulty was that MRI-based imaging already showed significant remodeling processes in the cartilage and bone of the femoral head as well as the acetabulum, so that an inflammatory differential diagnosis **osteoarthritis** up to bacterial osteomyelitis was foregrounded (Hedrich et al. 2020). In retrospect, however, these infectious differential diagnoses had to be discarded. The chronic ECF can be seen as the cause of this complex disease pattern.

33.8.3 Diagnosis

A good orientation is provided by the sonographic representation of the hip using a linear transducer. The deviation of the femoral neck axis in cross-section is as indicative as the tilting of the epiphysis dorsally. Conventional X-rays in **Imhäuser projection** or **Lauenstein position** provide excellent radiological clues for this tilting of the hip (Hesper et al. 2017). MRI-based examinations can additionally document inflammatory components. However, in our patient, this led to an **overemphasis of the inflammatory differential diagnosis**. A bone scintigraphy at the time 4 months after the onset of symptoms showed at most a slight increase in signal intensity in the area of the left hip. Strictly speaking, this examination would rule out bacterial osteomyelitis with several months of progression. A CT scan of the hip can be helpful in the differential diagnosis of tumorous diseases/osteoid osteoma (Hesper et al. 2017). The structural representation of the femoral neck-femoral head anatomy is also helpful. However, attention must be paid to radiation exposure in the intimate area! Ella's story shows that conventional radiology alone can be sufficient for the diagnosis of ECF.

33.8.4 Therapy

The focus is on the planned rapid fixation of the epiphysis by **Kirschner wire** management/alternatively by a **dynamic hip screw**, as happened with Ella (Hellmich and Krieg 2019). This is intended to prevent further slippage of the epiphysis and ideally also enable partial repositioning/repositioning. Severe subsequent damage such as avascular necrosis of the femoral head, chondrolysis, CAM deformity/CAM impingement and long-term loss of the hip should be avoided. These goals are generally not achievable with purely conservative measures, as Otto's story shows. Therefore, surgical treatment is paramount. From an orthopedic point of view, preoperative extension treatment is often considered helpful (Bittersohl et al. 2015). If an intracapsular hematoma is suspected in the case of acute slippage, then after relief of the bloody joint effusion, a subsequent closed repositioning with the insertion of several Kirschner wires or a dynamic hip glide screw should be aimed for (Weinmann et al. 2020). These fixing metal implants remain in the body until the completion of the **epiphyseal growth** and until the completion of the **epiphyseal plate closure** and can then be removed. If the femoral head slips by more than 30° in relation to the respective anatomical axis of the femoral neck and epiphysis, then an **intertrochanteric osteotomy** should be performed. The aim of this procedure is to reposition the epiph-

ysis ventrally and in particular to improve the internal rotation movement. The osteotomy is then fixed with angle plates. Possible complications of these procedures are avascular necrosis of the femoral head and also cartilage damage (Samelis et al. 2020). According to current data, the operative intertrochanteric correction osteotomy with modified Dunn technique is currently the recommended procedure for a slip angle of more than 50° (Slongo et al. 2010).

33.8.5 Diagnosis

The diagnosis of ECF is usually possible in the conventional overview image in combination with the Lauenstein projection (the patient shown is Ella). Sonography is helpful for the anatomical **assessment of the axial reference from epiphysis to femoral neck**, inflammatory processes can also be well assessed. Further imaging examinations such as computed tomography, MR tomography or skeletal scintigraphy carry the risk that the primary morphological finding of the ECF, for example, the description of inflammatory or osteolytic diagnoses, is given less importance in terms of prioritization (see Otto's story).

- Patient Ella: Epiphyseolysis capitis femoris, acute on chronic course
- Patient Otto: Epiphyseolysis capitis femoris, chronic course, secondary cartilage, bone and structural deformity with accompanying osteoarthritic destruction, CAM impingement

33.8.6 Prophylaxis

A basic prophylaxis of an epiphyseolysis capitis femoris is naturally not possible. Chronic-destructive osteoarthritic courses can be avoided through a consistent operative fixation strategy of the femoral head.

Conclusion

The use of supposedly higher-quality imaging diagnostics compared to conventional X-ray imaging may cloud the diagnostic view of the ECF and even prevent timely surgical care.

References

Bittersohl B, Hosalkar HS, Zilkens C, Krauspe R (2015) Current concepts in management of slipped capital femoral epiphysis. Hip Int 25:104–114. ▶ https://doi.org/10.5301/hipint.5000189

Hedrich CM, Morbach H, Reiser C, Girschick HJ (2020) New insights into adult and paediatric chronic non-bacterial osteomyelitis CNO. Curr Rheumatol Rep 22:52. ▶ https://doi.org/10.1007/s11926-020-00928-1

Hellmich HJ, Krieg AH (2019) Slipped capital femoral epiphysis – etiology and pathogenesis. Orthopade 48:644–650. ▶ https://doi.org/10.1007/s00132-019-03743-4

Hesper T, Zilkens C, Bittersohl B, Krauspe R (2017) Imaging modalities in patients with slipped capital femoral epiphysis. J Child Orthop 11:99–106. ▶ https://doi.org/10.1302/1863-2548-11-160276

Samelis PV, Papagrigorakis E, Konstantinou AL, Lalos H, Koulouvaris P (2020) Factors affecting outcomes of slipped capital femoral epiphysis. Cureus 12:e6883. ▶ https://doi.org/10.7759/cureus.6883

Slongo T, Kakaty D, Krause F, Ziebarth K (2010) Treatment of slipped capital femoral epiphysis with a modified Dunn procedure. J Bone Joint Surg Am 92:2898–2908. ▶ https://doi.org/10.2106/jbjs.i.01385

Weinmann D, Adolf S, Meurer A (2020) Slipped capital femoral epiphysis. Z Orthop Unfall 158:417–431. ▶ https://doi.org/10.1055/a-0917-7940

A 15-Year-Old Boy with Episodically Occurring Severe Back Pain

Christian Huemer

Contents

34.1 Medical History

A 15-year-old boy is presented in the rheumatology clinic, referred by the orthopedist with a history of episodic **back pain** that has been present for a year. He describes the peak of the back pain in the area of the thoracic/lumbar spine transition. At no time was there evidence of preceding trauma or inflammatory diseases. The patient is very athletic, plays football, and cannot rule out a minor injury. So far, he has been seen by a specialist in orthopedics and for outpatient physiotherapy, but no specific diagnosis has been defined and there has been no significant improvement with physiotherapy. He takes ibuprofen as needed, which does provide some relief for individual episodes, which occur about once a month. General medical history is completely unremarkable. Family history is unremarkable.

34.2 Examination Findings

15-year-old adolescent in excellent general and nutritional condition. No abnormalities in the internal status. In the musculoskeletal status, no evidence of palpable synovitis or enthesopathy in peripheral joints. On examination of the back, there is slight tenderness to pressure at the transition of the thoracic/lumbar spine, also palpable slight muscular hardening here. Slight pain in the lumbar spine area at the end range of lateral flexion. Modified Schober test 18 cm (thus slightly restricted).

34.3 Laboratory Values and Imaging

34.3.1 Laboratory Values

Blood count, CRP unremarkable, ESR unremarkable, rheumatoid factor and antinuclear antibodies negative; Anti-CCP negative; HLA-B27 negative.

34.3.2 Imaging

Plain X-ray of the entire spine a.p. and lateral: shows typical X-ray changes with marginal hernias, disc narrowing and wedge vertebrae formations (from Hefti 2006).

34.4 Educational Questions

1. What differential diagnoses would you discuss for this pain symptomatology of the adolescent patient?
2. What further diagnostic steps would be sensible?

34.5 Differential Diagnostic Considerations and Educational Answers

Back pain in childhood and especially in adolescence is a common symptom, which can have many causes. In the case of pronounced pain symptoms, a basic distinction must be made between inflammatory and non-inflammatory causes. In our patient, there was no evidence of inflammation, no fever, no preceding inflammatory diseases, no existing additional focal findings, so a non-inflammatory process is assumed. In the case of signs of inflammation such as fever, high CRP and changes in the blood count, a local inflammatory disease should always be considered, e.g. a **spondylodiscitis**, so that imaging diagnostics are always indicated in the case of symptoms and increased inflammation parameters. In the case of negative inflammation signs, a plain X-ray would initially be sufficient to differentiate non-inflammatory degenerative changes, especially from the spectrum of osteodystrophies.

34

34.6 Further Course

In the adolescent, a plain X-ray of the spine a.p. and lateral was subsequently performed at the first presentation, which showed a clear finding: In the area of the 11th and 12th thoracic vertebrae, there was clear evidence of wedge vertebrae formation as well as a narrowing of the intervertebral discs, as a typical finding in the sense of the confirmed diagnosis of Scheuermann's disease, typical Schmorl's nodules were also shown in the plain X-ray. The patient was presented to a pediatric orthopedist with the confirmed diagnosis of Scheuermann's disease. Intensive physiotherapy and a slight reduction in stress from leisure and school sports led to almost complete freedom from symptoms within a few months. The patient was completely symptom-free and fully resilient again 6 months after the first presentation.

34.7 Summary

Scheuermann's disease is defined as a growth disorder of the spine with narrowing of the intervertebral discs, formation of wedge vertebrae, endplate fractures, and kyphosis in the affected area. Scheuermann's disease is a typical pediatric orthopedic diagnosis in adolescents, a multifactorial event is discussed, where mechanical factors (tall adolescents, competitive sports as well as endogenous factors), familial predisposition (postural abnormalities) and also psychological factors are discussed (Hefti et al 2006; Aufdermauer 1981).

Pathogenetically, Scheuermann's disease leads to a weakening of the cartilaginous ring apophyses of the base and endplates of the vertebral bodies, these ring apophyses are the actual growth zones of the vertebral bodies. During the pubertal growth spurt, there can be a reduction in the mechanical strength of this cartilage, this favors the development of **degenerative changes** and the formation of **Schmorl's nodes** or endplate fractures, which reflect the pathophysiological events at the ventral edge of the vertebral body (❏ Fig. 34.1) (Lowe 1999).

The clinical symptoms of Scheuermann's disease in adolescence strongly depend on the location, with the main complaints being load-dependent pain of relatively high intensity without signs of inflammation.

The therapy for Scheuermann's disease mainly consists of intensive physiotherapy, only in selected cases, with a very pronounced thoracic kyphosis of more than

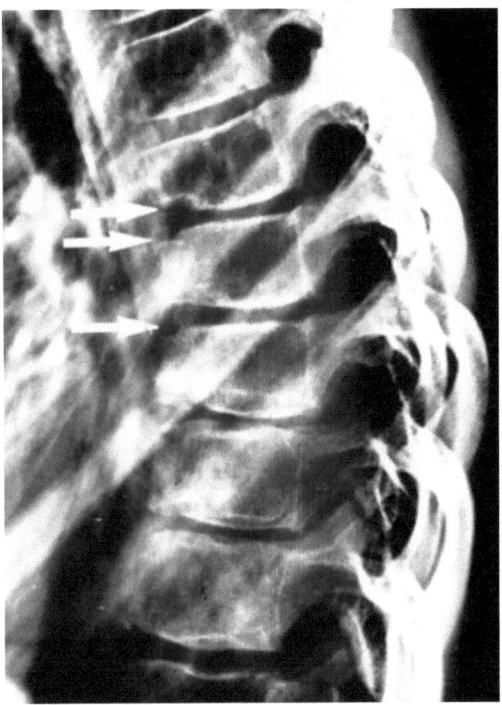

❏ **Fig. 34.1** X-ray changes in the area of the thoracic spine in a boy with Scheuermann's disease. One can see marginal hernias, disc narrowing and wedge vertebrae formations. (From Hefti 2006)

50°, would a corset treatment be discussed (Sachs et al. 1987; Poolman et al. 2002).

The prognosis for Scheuermann's disease is therefore favorable, with long-term impairments extremely rare.

Conclusion

Chronic back pain in adolescents can be differentiated well by clinical assessment and possibly imaging diagnostics, the spectrum of osteodystrophies and Scheuermann's disease as part of this spectrum is always to be considered for pediatric rheumatology in the initial assessment of childhood pain conditions.

References

Aufdermauer M (1981) Juvenile kyphosis (Scheuermann's disese: radiography, histology and pathogenesis). Clin Othop 154:166.74

Hefti F (2006) Morbus Scheuermann. In: Hefti F, Brunner R, Freuler F, Hasler C, Jundt G (Hrsg) Kinderorthopädie in der Praxis. Springer, Berlin/Heidelberg, S 94–101

Lowe T (1999) Scheuermanns's disease. Orthop Clin North Am 30:475–487

Poolman R, Been H, Ubags L (2002) Clinical outcome and radiographic results after operative treatment of Scheuermann's disease. Eur Spine J 11:561–569

Sachs B, Bradford D, Winr R, Lonstein J, Moe J, Wilson S (1987) Scheuermann kyphosis. Follow-up of Milwaukee-brace treatment. J Bone Joint Surg Am 69:50–57

A Toddler with an Unusually Early Tibia Fracture—What's Behind It?

Christian Huemer

Contents

© The Author(s), under exclusive license to Springer-Verlag GmbH, DE, part of Springer Nature 2024
C. Huemer and H. Girschick (eds.), *Clinical Examples in Pediatric Rheumatology*,
https://doi.org/10.1007/978-3-662-68732-1_35

35.1 Medical History

The 12-month-old girl was presented via the emergency department due to an unusual medical history and left tibia fracture: the child had stumbled at home on the carpet and twisted her leg slightly, followed by presentation in the trauma surgery department and diagnosis of a tibia shaft fracture. From the perspective of the trauma surgery department and the family doctor, the accident history was "suspicious", therefore, she was referred to the children's clinic to rule out child abuse or a basic disease in the area of bone metabolism.

Social history unremarkable, birth without problems, the child was fully breast-fed until the 8th month, and developed excellently. Nutrition normal, vitamin D prophylaxis was also carried out regularly since birth. Milestones also unremarkable. The child had started to take her first free steps a few weeks before the initial presentation, the parents again deny having found any further obstacles or hard objects at the reported fall of the child.

Family history not precisely ascertainable due to both parents' limited German skills, however, there is the impression that the child's father has also had frequent fractures since childhood.

35

35.2 Examination Findings

1-year-old girl in good general and nutritional condition, slight microcephaly, suggested triangular shape of the facial skull, otherwise no further signs of dysmorphia. Internal status completely unremarkable without focal signs of inflammation.

Musculoskeletal status shows slight muscular atrophy in the area of the left lower leg after plaster treatment, suggested leg length difference of 5 mm left < right. Callus palpable on the left tibia.

Skin unremarkable. ENT findings without focal signs of inflammation. Eyes show bluish livid discoloration of the sclera on both sides.

35.3 Laboratory Values and Imaging

35.3.1 Laboratory Values

Blood count, CRP, sedimentation rate unremarkable. Liver function parameters, calcium, phosphate, **alkaline phosphatase, vitamin D status**, celiac disease screening unremarkable. Urine findings unremarkable

35.3.2 Imaging

The native X-ray at the time of diagnosis showed a spiral fracture of the distal tibia shaft, no further abnormalities, no evidence of osteopenia, no evidence of pathological fracture. The ◘ Fig. 35.1 shows a later fracture after already performed bisphosphonate therapy with typical densification lines in the metaphyses (◘ Fig. 35.1).

35.4 Educational Questions

1. What differential diagnoses would you consider in this constellation of findings and history?
2. What further diagnosis can verify the primary suspicion?
3. What treatment concepts are currently available?

35.5 Differential Diagnostic Considerations and Educative Responses

In the case of unusually early fractures in the infant period or in early childhood, a very rapid differentiation is necessary. In pediatrics, this scenario primarily requires a rapid, often very complex assessment of whether there is suspicion of child abuse ("**battered child syndrome**"). Prior to this

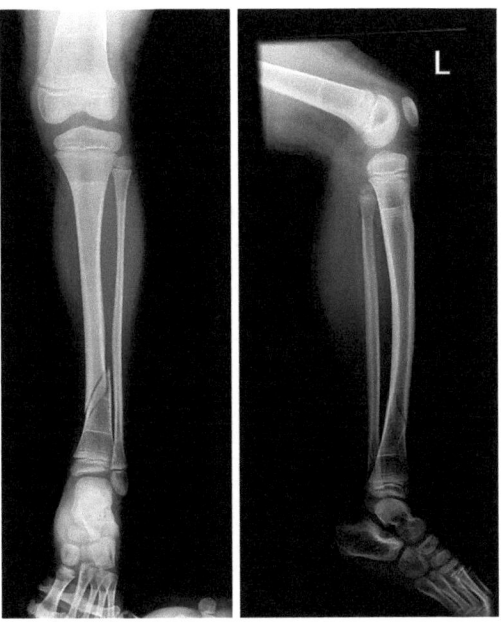

☐ Fig. 35.1 Spiral fracture of the tibia in osteogenesis imperfecta: In native radiology, in addition to the multi-fragment fracture in the tibial plateau/transition to the metaphysis, typical horizontal ossification densification lines are seen, as an expression of bisphosphonate therapy, also in the distal tibial metaphysis and in the femur

suspicion, it is quickly necessary to assess whether possible underlying diseases predispose to fractures. Secondary, endocrinological or metabolically induced forms of **osteoporosis/osteomalacia** are not so rare, but usually need to be differentiated in the clinical context. The involvement of clinical genetics and - based on often existing additional clinical stigmata - a targeted molecular genetic examination are routine today (Steinmann et al. 2020). A thorough family history with documentation of other family members with notably frequent fractures or other stigmata (blue sclerae, dental abnormalities, hearing loss, etc.?) support this joint diagnosis with clinical genetics. Ultimately, in these case scenarios, a suspicion of physical abuse often remains initially; the rapid involvement of the responsible

child protection group and interdisciplinary assessment together with the responsible authority for child and youth protection are necessary to by no means expose the child to a conceivable further risk. In the case described, the more detailed extended family history provided the decisive clue: the child's father had also had multiple (a total of 12!) fractures, especially of the long tubular bones, since childhood, and he also had blue sclerae and unclear hearing loss. This history quickly allowed the suspicion of a genetically determined **osteogenesis imperfecta** to be assumed for the child presented. A molecular genetic examination of the **Col1A1 gene** subsequently confirmed the presence of **osteogenesis imperfecta type I**. This enabled the rapid initiation of established therapy options with **bisphosphonatetherapy**.

35.6 Further Course

The fracture healing in the toddler proceeded quite normally. The detailed clinical examination showed no further evidence of previous fractures. The metabolic evaluation initially did not provide a conclusive finding. In view of the clinical picture (blue sclerae) and the family history (comparable symptoms in the child's father), molecular genetics were carried out on this child immediately after the initial presentation: the sequence analysis of both then-strands of the Col1A1 gene showed that a nonsense mutation (stop mutation) was present in exon 31(31*). This stop mutation had already been described in the literature in connection with **osteogenesis imperfecta (OI)** - the diagnosis of OI type I, autosomal dominantly inherited, was thus confirmed (Körkkö et al. 1998). The child was presented to Pediatric Endocrinology and subsequently underwent therapy with bisphosphonate for a total of 3 years: in the first 2 years pamidronate at 3-month intervals (a total of 9 mg/year), in the 3rd year switch to zoledronic acid at 6-month intervals (0.05 mg/kg body weight). This therapy was well tolerated. In a follow-up period of 3 years, there was no further fracture.

35.7 Summary

Osteogenesis imperfecta is a clinically and genetically heterogeneous group of diseases, characterized not only by abnormal formation and homeostasis of the bone matrix, but also by generally abnormal soft connective tissue, it is primarily characterized by increased bone fragility and is therefore also known as so-called brittle bone disease. The incidence of all types of osteogenesis imperfecta is likely to be 1-2 per 10,000.

35.7.1 Pathogenesis

Crucial for most variants of OI is the disruption of collagen type 1 biosynthesis. This collagen consists of two α-1 and one α-2 chain, which are twisted together in the endoplasmic reticulum. This results in procollagen 1 with the structure of a triple helix. Several proteins modify this triple helix post-translationally. Proteins involved include cyclophilin B, osterix, and a variety of other enzymes (Van Dijk and Sillence 2014). Procollagen 1 is then further processed in the Golgi apparatus: After removal of the propeptides by bone morphogenetic protein 1 (BMP1), collagen type 1 is formed, which is then exported into the extracellular matrix and subjected to a linking of the various fibrils with each other. Many of these collagen type 1 fibrils then form the collagen fiber, which represents the decisive, non-mineral basic substance of the bone.

35.7.2 Classification

Osteogenesis imperfecta is divided into a number of subgroups:
- Type I—non-deforming OI with blue sclerae
- Type II—perinatally lethal OI
- Type III—progressively deforming type
- Type IV—variable OI type with normal sclerae
- Type V—OI with calcifying interosseous membranes

In type I, fractures rarely occur in the newborn period, but there is a significant long-term impairment of growth. Blue sclerae are typically found as a secondary finding, and tooth development in this form of osteogenesis imperfecta is usually inconspicuous. Patients also show very thin skin with low skin turgor, moderately hyperextensible joints, and premature hearing loss. The molecular genetic confirmation of the diagnosis of this disease, which is autosomal dominant, is possible by detecting the COL1A1 and COL1A2 genes.

In type II, the perinatally lethal form of osteogenesis imperfecta, there are often breech and transverse positions, underweight premature babies with short and curved limbs.

Other forms include type III as a progressively deforming form, type IV as a moderately severe form, and type V as osteogenesis imperfecta with hyperplastic callus formation (Fauch and Glorieux 2004).

35.7.3 Clinic

Even in the milder OI variants I and IV, the clinical symptom of bone fracture is predominant. Newer bone density examinations, up to peripheral quantitative computed tomography, ultimately describe a reduced bone density in all patients. The fragility of the bone is due to both the defective connective tissue framework and a secondary brittleness caused by osteoporosis.

35.7.4 Diagnosis

Standard, serum, and overview values such as calcium phosphate, parathyroid hormone, and also vitamin D are usually not changed. Only the alkaline phosphatase is increased as part of the increased bone formation. A vitamin D deficiency can usually be distinguished by determining the monohydroxylated form (25-hydroxyvitamin D_3) and the borderline low calcium and the significant increase in parathyroid hormone. The various variants of phosphate diabetes are characterized by the reduced phosphate concentration in the serum with simultaneous increase in alkaline phosphatase.

For the diagnosis, often important secondary findings are blue, pale-gray, but also white sclerae, a conductive and mixed hearing loss due to fractures of the ossicles, and a dentinogenesis imperfecta with gray-blue or amber-colored translucent teeth. The diagnosis is suspected clinically and radiologically and should always be proven molecular genetically, also with regard to other affected family members and prenatal diagnostics. The course depends very much on the impact of the individual biochemical defect, severely affected patients die shortly after birth from respiratory insufficiency, other forms already have numerous fractures at birth and also suffer many fractures afterwards. In all types, the tendency to fracture decreases spontaneously around puberty, but increases somewhat again in old age.

35.7.5 Therapy

Therapeutic goals are to improve the patient's well-being and to reduce the frequency of fractures. Therefore, the focus is on strengthening muscle power and increasing general physical activity. This can be achieved by reducing bone pain in the context of microfractures. Therefore, bisphosphonates are at the forefront of OI therapy.

Causal therapy is (still) not possible, conservative and surgical-orthopedic measures are applied. The currently common therapy with bisphosphonates leads to a reduction in the tendency to fracture (Dwan et al. 2014), still experimental therapeutic approaches include antibodies against Rankl and antibodies against sclerostin (Sagar et al. 2019; Cardinal et al. 2019)

It is important to provide **genetic counseling** for this disease, osteogenesis imperfecta, as in about 80% of cases there is autosomal dominant inheritance. The **fracture healing is generally normal**, occasionally with excessive callus formation. Life expectancy is limited by pulmonary insufficiency, cor pulmonale, and brainstem compression due to basilar impression.

> **Conclusion**
>
> Early occurrence of fractures: A highly challenging differential diagnosis; especially due to the necessity to quickly rule out any form of child abuse, an immediate interdisciplinary approach in cooperation with child protection is extremely valuable. Recently available molecular genetic possibilities support a clear diagnosis, therefore, involving clinical geneticists is very sensible.

References

Cardinal M, Tys J, Roels T et al (2019) Sclerostin antibody reduces long bone fractures in the oim/oim model of osteogenesis imperfecta. Bone 124:137–147

Dwan K, Pillipi CA, Steiner RD, Basel D (2014) Bisphosphonate therapy for osteogenesis imperfecta. Cochrane Database Syst Rev 7:CD005088

Fauch F, Glorieux FH (2004) Osteogenesis imperfecta. Lancet 363:1377–1385

Körkkö J, Ala-Kokko L, De Paepe A, Nuytinck L, Earley J, Prockop DJ (1998) Analysis of the

COL1A1 and COL1A2 genes by PCR amplification and scanning by conformation-sensitive gel electrophoresis identifies only COL1A1 mutations in 15 patients with osteogenesis imperfecta type I: identification of common sequences of null-allele mutations. Am J Hum Genet 62(1):98–110. ► https://doi.org/10.1086/301689

Sagar R, Gotherstrom C, David AL, Westgren M (2019) Fetal stem cell transplantation and gene therapy. Best Pract Res Clin Obstet Gynaecol 58:142–153

Steinmann B, Rohrbach M, Matyas G (2020) Hereditäre Bindegewebserkrankungen. In: Hoffmann GF (Hrsg) Pädiatrie. Springer, Berlin/Heidelberg, S 2835–2840

Van Dijk FS, Sillence DO (2014) Osteogenesis imperfecta: clinical diagnosis, nomenclature and severity assessment. Am J Med Genet A 164A(6):1470–1481

A Walk Like Charlie Chaplin

Hermann Girschick

Contents

© The Author(s), under exclusive license to Springer-Verlag GmbH, DE, part of Springer Nature 2024
C. Huemer and H. Girschick (eds.), *Clinical Examples in Pediatric Rheumatology*,
https://doi.org/10.1007/978-3-662-68732-1_36

36.1 Medical History

As a 4-week-old infant, the now 26-year-old Karl was found to have an unusually elongated head shape, and a diagnosis of premature sagittal suture ossification/**sagittal synostosis** was made. Since the child was cared for in a center for bone metabolism disorders, the differential diagnosis included a genetic disorder of the **alkaline phosphatase (AP)** (Mornet et al. 2014): Biochemically, the AP was significantly reduced for his age, with values around 50 IU/l. Over time, a compound heterozygous mutation constellation was identified, with evidence of a paternal and a maternal mutation in the TNSALP gene. Due to the very early age of manifestation, a diagnosis of an early childhood/infantile form of **hypophosphatasia (HPP)** could have been made. However, the long-term course was somewhat mild, and an assignment to the somewhat milder "child subtype" would also have been possible. At that time, there was suspicion of increased intracranial pressure, so a craniectomy of the bony calvaria was performed, although rapid reossification occurred. It should be noted that desmal ossification in hypophosphatasia is not necessarily disturbed, and may even be pathologically enhanced in the sense of premature suture synostoses. As signs of increased intracranial pressure persisted, a frontoorbital advancement and calvarial remodeling were performed neurosurgically at just under 2 years of age. In early childhood and school age, **musculoskeletal problems** existed, including delayed walking, **muscle weakness** in the legs, **general leg pain**, as well as feeding disorders with swallowing difficulties, loss of appetite, and general **failure to thrive**. Conceptually, Naproxen and Meloxicam were used as a pain and anti-inflammatory treatment concept. It showed very good clinical efficacy (Girschick et al.

2006; Girschick et al. 1999b). In later school age, a quite passable athletic activity, fitness exercises, and musculoskeletal stabilization were possible. Possibly also in the context of athletic activities, fractures of the talus, metatarsal V, and most recently also in the tibia shaft were recorded. In this context, the patient received an **enzyme replacement therapy** with a recombinant preparation for alkaline phosphatase (Strensiq [R]) for a duration of 6 months in his 25th year of life (Hofmann et al. 2015). For the current case report, musculoskeletal complaints in the 16th year of life are to be particularly considered: Diffuse leg pain and myalgia continued to occur, especially after physical exertion, and there were no clear clinical signs of arthritis.

36.2 Examination Findings

Musculoskeletally, Karl's general lower leg muscle tenderness and the hypophosphatasia-typical "stilt-like" gait were prominent. Accompanying the underlying bone disease, Karl also had **hypermobility**/connective tissue weakness, specifically flat spread feet on both sides (◘ Fig. 36.1b) (Beck et al. 2009b). An X-leg position seen in early childhood was no longer present (◘ Fig. 36.1a in the 2nd year of life). There were no signs of rickets or bone fractures and no impressive arthritis. A 3/6 systolic heart murmur was audible over Erb, the pulmonary auscultation was unremarkable, arterial hypertension with 170/84 mmHg was diagnosed. A Gower's sign as in early childhood was no longer present. There were still moderate signs of the previous craniosynostosis and the postoperative condition of the skull cap. Muscle-strengthening exercises, physiotherapy, and a phosphate-binding calcium carbonate therapy were recommended (Beck et al. 2009b).

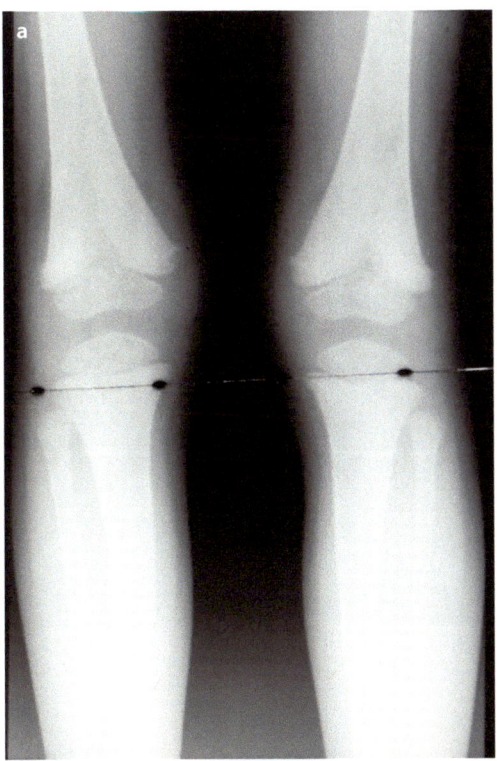

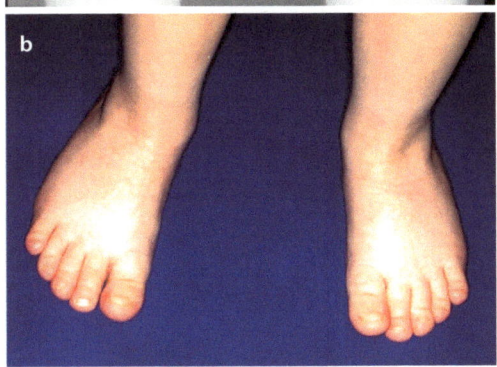

Fig. 36.1 a,b Karl's clinic at 2 years - flat spread feet on both sides, moderate X-leg position, radiological representation of the knees. **a** Conventional radiology of Karl's legs with moderate X-leg position and meta- and epiphyseal structural disorders. **b** Clinically, there was a bilateral flat foot and a connective tissue weakness/hypermobility

36.3 Laboratory Values and Imaging

36.3.1 Laboratory Values

Inflammatory parameters (blood sedimentation, ferritin, CRP) were normal, as were the blood count and overview values for "liver and muscle". The **AP was at 11 IU/l** significantly below the age-appropriate normal range (for men, postpubertal status >60 IU/l) (Beck et al. 2009b). Autoimmune diagnostics: Autoantibodies ANA were negative.

36.3.2 Imaging and Functional Examinations

A whole-body MRI examination was performed using TIRM technology. This is a screening examination that provides a very quick overview of possible multifocal inflammatory processes (❏ Fig. 36.2) (Beck et al. 2011). The oncological tumor search is also successful with this. There were signal abnormalities in the sense of a multifocal bone edema, especially in the distal metaphyses of both femurs, in the cranial metaphyses of both upper arms, further at the lateral ends of the clavicles and also at a thoracic vertebral body. In addition, there were moderate fluid accumulations in the area of the knee joint space, which was interpreted as mild arthritis. A conventional X-ray was not repeated at this time. However, it would be expected that the hypophosphatasia typical "brightening zones" (Looser zone) in the central metaphysis of the femur near the knee joint

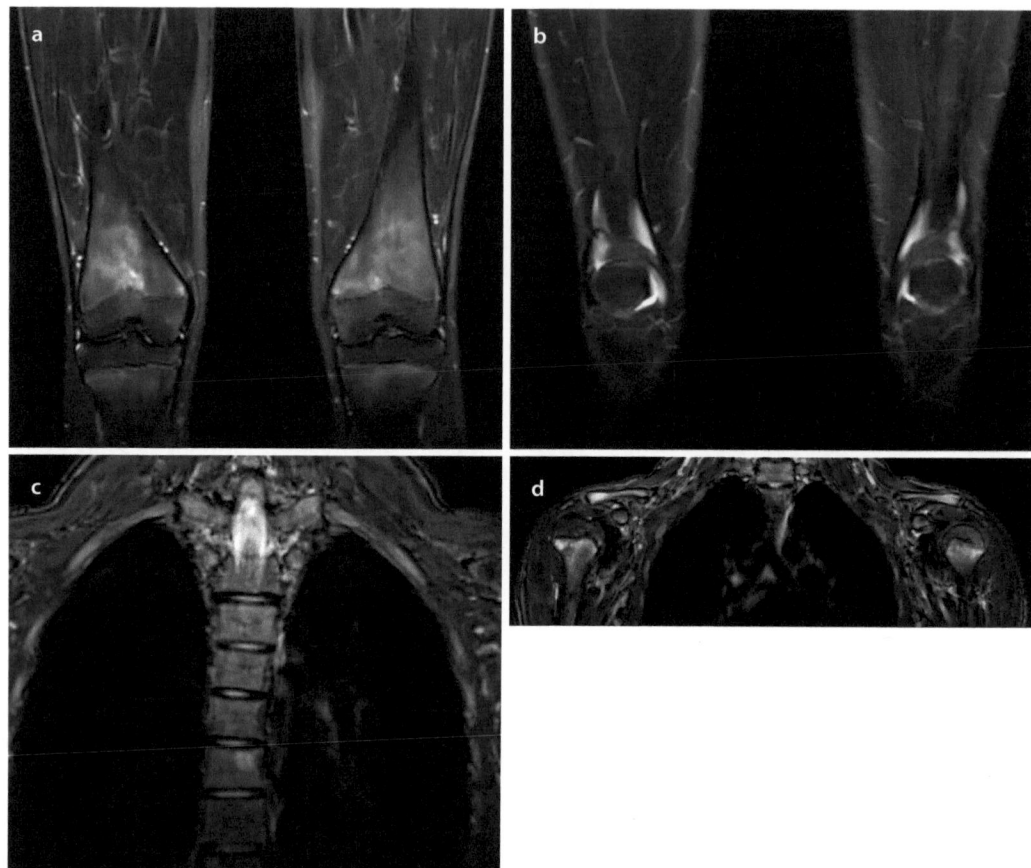

Fig. 36.2 **a–d** Karl's MRI at 16 years – whole-body MRI in TIRM technology. **a** Signal increases in the distal metaphyses in the knee on both sides (**a**), in BWK 6 (**c**), in the cranial humerus metaphyses and in the area of the lateral clavicle (**d**). The knees show mild signs of arthritis with moderate effusion formation on both sides (**b**)

36

would continue at least on the right side (see **Fig. 36.1**). An ultrasound of the abdomen showed a moderate increase in echogenicity in the area of the kidneys, echocardiographically the patient was inconspicuous.

36.4 Educational Questions

1. What differential diagnosis do you consider for the symptoms of gait disturbance, leg pain, bow legs?
2. What significance does imaging have here?

3. What role does genetics and inflammation play in the laboratory diagnosis of hypophosphatasia?
4. What therapeutic considerations should be taken into account, especially with the therapy goal of pain reduction?

36.5 Differential Diagnostic Considerations

From an osteological perspective, in cases of chronic recurrent pain in the musculoskeletal system, particularly in the lower extremities and spine, which persist over years, vitamin D deficiency, "idiopathic" osteoporosis, osteogenesis imperfecta, various bone dysplasias, and benign bone tumors, e.g., osteoid osteoma, should be considered (Beck et al. 2011). Very rarely, syndromal primary diseases based on genetic factors, e.g., Camuratti-Engelmann syndrome (CES), can also be considered. The latter is associated with hyperostosis of the long tubular bones and recurrent leg pain. The gait is similar to stiltlike, and muscle weakness is present. In hypophosphatasia, paradoxically increased bone density values have been measured (Girschick et al. 1999). The latter are attributed to an excess of non-mineralized osteoid. In our own studies, we have seen a clearly irregular mineralization with osteolysis on the one hand (◘ Fig. 36.1a, Looser zone in the center of the distal femur metaphyses) and osseous condensations, especially in the area of the main stress lines of the long tubular bones, on the other hand, the compacta of the tubular bone may even appear densified (Hyperostosis) (Girschick et al. 1999). However, the periosteal increased calcification and/or the compacta hyperostosis, as seen in CES, is atypical for HPP in this form.

From a rheumatological perspective, chronic nonbacterial osteomyelitis (CNO), which can also take a recurrent, undulating course (CRMO), cannot be clinically distinguished in individual cases (Girschick et al. 2007). The multifocal distribution pattern of bone edema seen in MRI would be quite compatible with CRMO, as would the occurrence of mild bilateral gonarthritis (◘ Fig. 36.2). Although the bone edema signal in its coarseness and regional distribution pattern at the single lesion is not 100% typical compared to CRMO, "in everyday life" the finding as in ◘ Fig. 36.2 could also be subsumed under CRMO (Girschick et al. 2007; Beck et al. 2009).

Crucial for making the differential diagnosis of HPP, which is very similar to that of CNO, is the laboratory determination of alkaline phosphatase. The performance of conventional radiographic diagnostics in combination with generously applied MRI diagnostics (whole-body MRI) is relevant. Cranial and spinal MRI imaging with a view to possible craniosynostosis/abnormality in the cranio-cervical transition, possible formation of hydrocephalus or spinal cord split formation (syringomyelia) should be mentioned as a co-indication for the MRI. Sonographically, nephrocalcinosis should be assessed at regular intervals (Beck et al. 2009).

36.6 Further Progress

The patient benefited significantly from the use of NSAIDs for his musculoskeletal complaints, and a remarkably intensive fitness program could be completed. Injuries that occurred as a result of minor traumas were counterproductive, including a talus fracture at 21 years, a metatarsal fracture of the 5th ray at 24, and a tibia fracture at 26 years. Since the metatarsal fracture had a poor, insufficient healing tendency and recurrent complaints, an **enzyme substitution therapy** was temporarily carried out for 6 months with success. It should be noted that the indication for enzyme substitution requires a so-called bone phenotype with hypophosphatasia manifested in childhood and adolescence (Hofmann et al. 2015). This condition is given in the young man on the one hand by the clinic on the musculoskeletal system and radiological diagnostics in early childhood. The manifestation on the neurocranium does not strictly count as this indication, as a positive effect of enzyme substitution on the pathology of desmal ossification of the neurocranium has not been clearly demonstrated. Under ACE inhibition, the blood pressure was adequately adjustable. Dietary measures helped to control the patient's hyperphosphatemia and thus prevent further renal calcification.

36.7 Educative Responses

- **1. What differential diagnosis do you consider for the symptoms of gait disturbance, leg pain, bow legs?**

In addition to the osteological and rheumatological differential diagnoses already described above, neurological disorders in the area of the posterior columns and the extrapyramidal motor system should also be considered in relation to the stilt-like gait pattern (Beck et al. 2009b, 2011a). However, these should be quickly ruled out by clinical examination. Diseases related to metabolic disorders with effects on various organ systems, which are associated with **hyperprostaglandinism**, such as **hypertrophic osteoarthropathy/pachydermoperiostosis**, should be added. Our own studies have shown a significant increase in systemic prostaglandins in hypophosphatasia patients (Girschick et al. 2006). Activation of inflammatory cascades triggered by pyrophosphates and involvement of the **NLRP3 inflammasome** are suspected (Beck et al. 2009a). These diphosphates are not sufficiently degraded in HPP and lead to inflammatory changes, such as **crystal-induced synovitis** or possibly the described multifocal bone inflammation (❏ Fig. 36.2).

- **2. What is the significance of imaging in this context?**

Conventional radiological diagnosis of HPP is now supplemented and expanded by whole-body MRI diagnostics due to reduced radiation exposure (Beck et al. 2011b). The main focus here is on **bone dysplasia** in the broadest sense and **inflammatory changes**, but also neurological manifestations in the CNS and craniocervical junction. Abdominal sonography is of great importance for nephrological follow-up diagnostics. Bone density examination in the hands of an experienced examiner may be helpful, but there are various uncertainties which make the interpretation of findings very difficult, e.g. paradoxically high density values (Girschick et al. 1999a).

- **3. What role do genetics and inflammation play in the laboratory diagnosis of hypophosphatasia?**

For diagnosis, a biochemical determination of alkaline phosphatase in serum or plasma is a basic prerequisite. Since AP uses zinc in its catalytic center, a significant **zinc deficiency** also simulates HPP in laboratory chemistry. Therefore, it should be ruled out. Severe consuming diseases, including anorexia, can lead to "reactively" low AP values during growth stop. Substrates of AP (phosphoethanolamine, pyridoxal phosphate, possibly also pyrophosphate) can be measured increased in the blood (Beck et al. 2009). The final proof can be provided by a genomic sequencing of the TNSALP gene with its exons and the respective flanking intron regions (Mornet et al. 2014). The medical assessment of findings is complicated by the possibility of a so-called **dominant negative mutation detection**. If the single mutation affects the binding area of the AP enzyme, which usually acts as a duet or in a quartet, then the enzyme action can also be disturbed by just one mutation alone. The inheritance of this form of inheritance, which exists in about up to 15% of patients, then follows a dominant characteristic (Mornet et al. 2014). In the vast majority of clinically much more severely affected patients, however, there is a **double heterozygosity** with paternal and maternal mutations. In special stress situations of life such as long immobility, postpartum lactation phase, even in heterozygous carriers (one mutation) a mild "bone phenotype" with osteoporosis, fractures or joint inflammations can occur. Standard laboratory parameters for detecting inflammation (CRP, ESR, ferritin, blood count) are usually inconspicuous. Special diagnostics regarding the inflammasome or the **prostaglandin**metabolism are currently reserved for purely scientific questions (Beck et al. 2009a).

36

■ **4. What therapeutic considerations should be taken into account, especially with the therapy goal of pain reduction?**

A symptomatic anti-inflammatory therapy with NSAID has been proven effective in HPP. A negative effect on ossification was not seen with prostaglandin synthesis blockade. Single reports from adulthood about interleukin-1 blockade are circulating, but have not yet been found in the scientific literature. **Enzyme replacement therapy** can significantly improve the musculoskeletal status in the long term, especially the walking distance and bone mineralization increases (Hofmann et al. 2015). Due to a very rapid onset of therapy effect, it is assumed that a **crystal synovitis** and **myositis** induced by pyrophosphates represents a decisive factor for the symptom picture and that the clinical improvement is essentially due to the blockade of this pathophysiological component. Data that possibly the chronic bone inflammation also experiences a positive effect through enzyme substitution is not yet available in international experience.

36.8 Summary

36.8.1 Etiology

HPP is predominantly an autosomal recessive genetic disease with a subsequent defect in the enzymatic activity of AP. Biochemical metabolic substrates can induce additional secondary effects in the metabolism of the affected person.

36.8.2 Pathogenesis/Clinic

The complex inflammatory disorder of bones, muscles, and joints can lead to systemic effects in the kidney or in the central or peripheral nervous system. The enzyme AP is also directly present in many organ systems outside of the bone.

36.8.3 Diagnosis

In addition to a detailed medical history (including family) and clinical examination, the determination of the age- and gender-related AP value is paramount (Beck et al. 2009b). The smaller the AP value, the more clinically pronounced is the phenotype. Subsequently, genetic testing can describe the mode of inheritance and also provide an additional assessment of the severity (Mornet et al. 2014).

36.8.4 Therapy

In addition to the use of NSAIDs, indicated enzyme replacement therapy can be helpful for complaints in the musculoskeletal system, especially for immediate pain reduction. Positive effects on bone formation are possible through this (Hofmann et al. 2015).

36.8.5 Diagnosis

The diagnosis is primarily based on the clinical picture of the disease, the determination of the age- and gender-related AP value, conventional and MRI imaging, and also genetic testing.

36.8.6 Prophylaxis

There is no prophylaxis to prevent the disease. Close connection to a specialized interdisciplinary center for pediatric osteology and also rheumatology is desirable (Vogt et al. 2020).

Conclusion

Patients with rare diseases of the musculoskeletal system, here using the example of HPP, require an interdisciplinary diagnostic and therapeutic approach. In HPP, in addition to osteology, rheumatology/immunology, nephrology, neurosurgery, and dentistry are important. This is flanked by intensive physiotherapy, a promotion of musculoskeletal fitness, and thus also of bone formation.

References

Beck C, Morbach H, Richl P, Stenzel M, Girschick HJ (2009a) How can calcium pyrophosphate crystals induce inflammation in hypophosphatasia or chronic inflammatory joint diseases? Rheumatol Int 29:229–238. ▸ https://doi.org/10.1007/s00296-008-0710-9

Beck C, Morbach H, Stenzel M, Schneider P, Collmann H, Girschick G, Girschick HJ (2009b) [Hypophosphatasia]. Klin Padiatr 221:219-226. ▸ https://doi.org/10.1055/s-0029-1220718

Beck C, Beer M, Morbach H, Raab P, Girschick HJ (2011a) Differentialdiagnosen von Knochenschmerzen im Kindes- und Jugendalter. Chir Praxis 74:471–486. ▸ https://doi.org/10.1186/1471-2431-7-3

Beck C, Morbach H, Wirth C, Beer M, Girschick HJ (2011b) Whole-body MRI in the childhood form of hypophosphatasia. Rheumatol Int 31:1315–1320. ▸ https://doi.org/10.1007/s00296-010-1493-3

Girschick HJ, Schneider P, Kruse K, Huppertz HI (1999a) Bone metabolism and bone mineral density in childhood hypophosphatasia. Bone 25:361–367. ▸ https://doi.org/10.1016/s8756-3282(99)00164-7

Girschick HJ, Seyberth HW, Huppertz HI (1999b) Treatment of childhood hypophosphatasia with nonsteroidal antiinflammatory drugs. Bone 25:603–607. ▸ https://doi.org/10.1016/s8756-3282(99)00203-3

Girschick HJ, Schneider P, Haubitz I, Hiort O, Collmann H, Beer M, Shin YS, Seyberth HW (2006) Effective NSAID treatment indicates that hyperprostaglandinism is affecting the clinical severity of childhood hypophosphatasia. Orphanet J Rare Dis 1:24. ▸ https://doi.org/10.1186/1750-1172-1-24

Girschick HJ, Mornet E, Beer M, Warmuth-Metz M, Schneider P (2007) Chronic multifocal non-bacterial osteomyelitis in hypophosphatasia mimicking malignancy. BMC Pediatr 7:3. ▸ https://doi.org/10.1186/1471-2431-7-3

Hofmann C, Jakob F, Seefried L, Mentrup B, Graser S, Plotkin H, Girschick HJ, Liese J (2015) Recombinant enzyme replacement therapy in hypophosphatasia. Subcell Biochem 76:323–341. ▸ https://doi.org/10.1007/978-94-017-7197-9_15

Mornet E, Hofmann C, Bloch-Zupan A, Girschick H, Le Merrer M (2014) Clinical utility gene card for: hypophosphatasia – update 2013. Eur J Hum Genet 22. ▸ https://doi.org/10.1038/ejhg.2013.177

Vogt M, Girschick H, Schweitzer T, Benoit C, Holl-Wieden A, Seefried L, Jakob F, Hofmann C (2020) Pediatric hypophosphatasia: lessons learned from a retrospective single-center chart review of 50 children. Orphanet J Rare Dis 15:212. ▸ https://doi.org/10.1186/s13023-020-01500-x

36

When the Skin and Neck Stretch

Hermann Girschick

Contents

© The Author(s), under exclusive license to Springer-Verlag GmbH, DE, part of Springer Nature 2024
C. Huemer and H. Girschick (eds.), *Clinical Examples in Pediatric Rheumatology*,
https://doi.org/10.1007/978-3-662-68732-1_37

37.1 **Medical History**

Due to the broad spectrum of connective tissue diseases associated with "**hyperextensibility**" in childhood and adolescence, the following presents two patients with their histories.

■■ Neo

Neo was born prematurely at 34 weeks of gestation, and "**club feet**" were noticed on both sides at birth. He underwent orthopedic treatment according to Ponsetti. An umbilical hernia was reported. General developmental abnormalities were observed in the first year of life, and a general connective tissue weakness/**hypermobility** was diag-

nosed at 1.5 years (■ Fig. 37.1d). An echocardiogram revealed **valve insufficiencies** of the tricuspid, mitral, and pulmonary valves. Neo learned to walk at 17 months. General skin vulnerability as a toddler led to the suspected diagnosis of **Ehlers-Danlos Syndrome** (EDS). Between the ages of 4 and 7, the boy repeatedly sustained extensive injuries from trivial falls, and there was scar and keloid formation (■ Fig. 37.2). Due to an increasing pes cavus position with a reasonably well-developed foot arch, an operation was performed on the midfoot bone with cuboid wedge osteotomy, bone transfer into the medial cuneiform bone, and a relocation of the tendon of the anterior tibialis muscle, on both sides (■ Fig. 37.1 and 37.2).

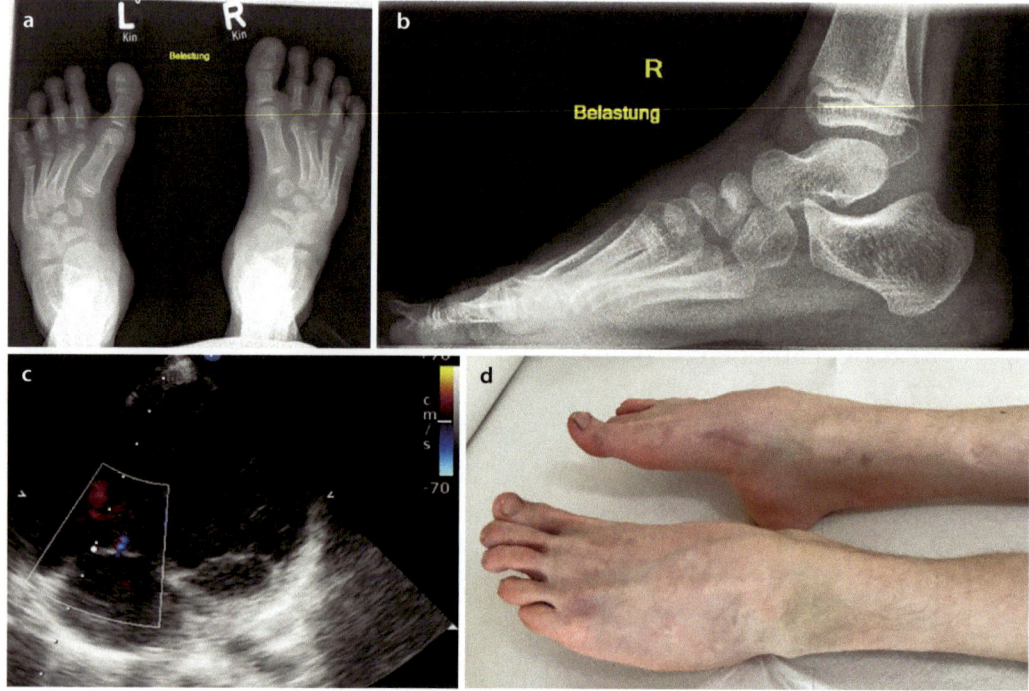

■ **Fig. 37.1   a–d** Neo at 7 years old – pes cavus on both sides, radiologically before surgery and clinical impression 5 years postoperatively. **a, b** Conventional radiology of Neo's feet with the clear pes cavus position with a reasonably well-developed foot arch (status after Ponsetti care in infancy; 7th year of life). **c** Echocardiography showing mild mitral insufficiency. **d** Clinical impression after another 5 years with scar formation, hyperextensibility

37

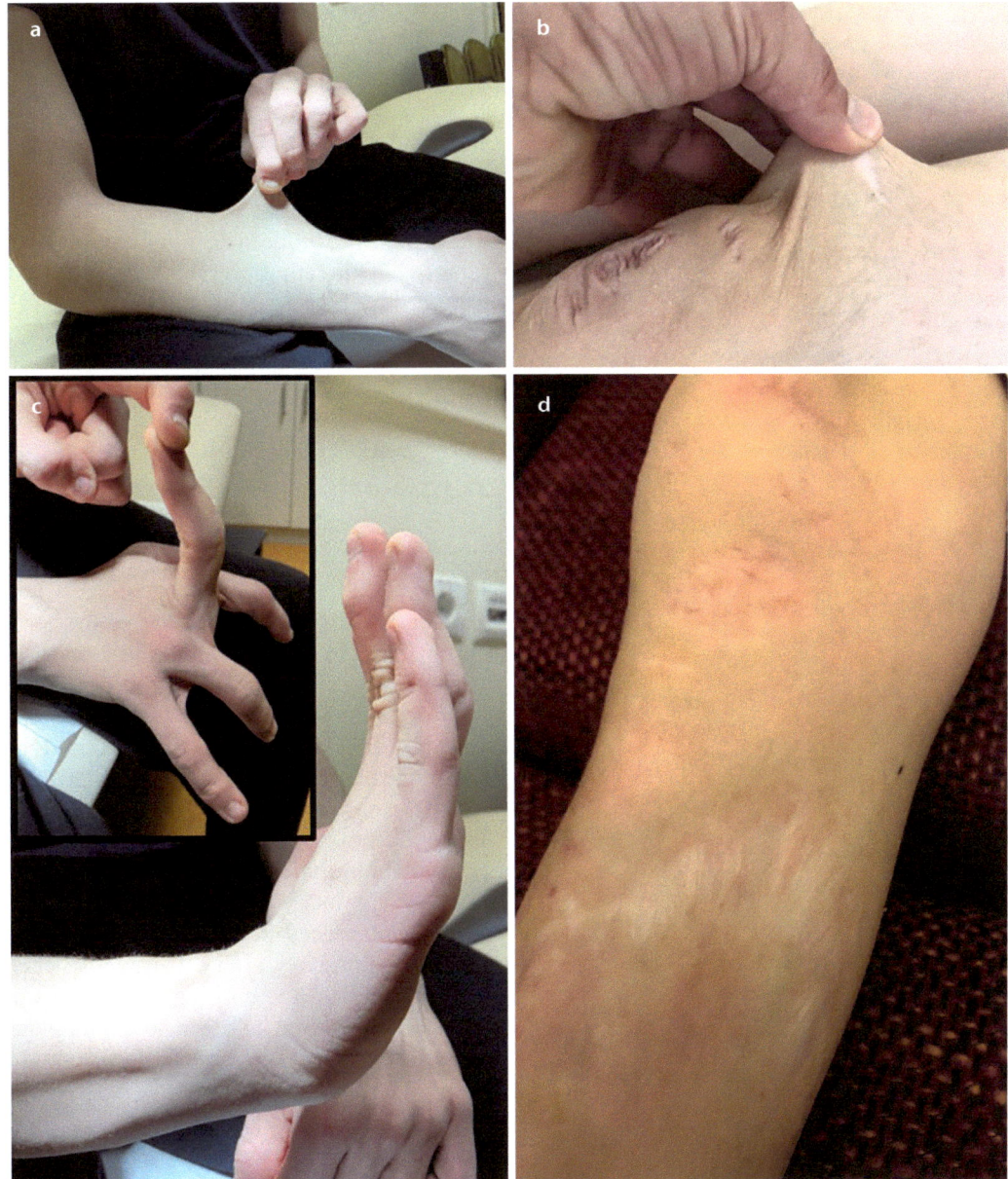

Fig. 37.2 a–d Neo's clinic at 14 years old – significant hypermobility and dermal vulnerability, tendency to dehiscence. The images show the connective tissue pathology with vulnerability, keloid formation during healing, loss of pigmentation

▪▪ Toni

At the age of 5, the parents noticed a varying neck swelling at the transition to the chest, especially during excitement, crying, or straining. This swelling was not painful, the voice had not changed, there were no indications of gastroesophageal reflux, swallowing disorders, or tendency to aspiration. Toni's mother had general hypermobility, otherwise musculoskeletal diseases in the family were denied. No other problems are reported.

37.2 Examination Findings

▪▪ Neo

The body length progressed along the 3rd percentile until the age of 11, as did the body weight, the body structure was overall delicate. Nighttime leg orthoses were used in early childhood for about 2 years, but were then no longer tolerated. At the age of 10, a bone age of 8 years was diagnosed. From the age of 12, there was a decrease in skin vulnerability. This period coincides with the start of muscular vibration training/physiotherapy on the device. At the transition to the 13th year of life, a significant growth spurt occurred, reaching the 50th percentile for body length and weight. The connective tissue pathology with vulnerability, **keloid** formation during healing, loss of pigmentation with scarring and hyperextensibility continued to exist (◻ Fig. 37.2b, d).

▪▪ Toni

There were soft skin and connective tissue structures as an expression of generalized **hypermobility**, accompanied by significant postural weakness with hollow and round back and a non-fixed scoliosis. There were no indications of a **Cutis laxa**. When a Valsalva maneuver was triggered, a significant balloon-like protrusion of the entire lower neck region with emphasis on the right side occurred. No pulsatility of this space-occupying lesion. After the end of the pressure maneuver, there was a complete regression of the protrusion (◻ Fig. 37.3a–c).

37.3 Laboratory Values and Imaging

37.3.1 Laboratory Values for Neo and Toni

There were no noticeable inflammation parameters (sedimentation rate, ferritin, CRP), likewise the blood count and overview values for "liver, kidney, muscle, bone" were normal. Autoimmune diagnostics were not performed.

37.3.2 Imaging and Functional Examinations

▪▪ Neo

The diagnostics focused on the sonography of the heart, the joints, and occasionally orthopedically intended, conventional X-ray examinations of the feet. Here, the pronounced sickle foot position could be documented at the age of 7 with a sufficiently good foot arch (◻ Fig. 37.1a, b). The midfoot operation was performed. Echocardiographically, over about 14 years without significant changes, there was a valve insufficiency in the area of the atria and the pulmonary artery. It was also classified as mild in the course. Further examinations, including large devices, were not necessary.

▪▪ Toni

Echocardiographically, a significant aneurysmatic protrusion of the internal jugular vein was found. After the end of the Valsalva maneuver, the circular protrusion completely regressed (◻ Fig. 37.3d, e). The aneurysm partially displaced the thyroid to the right (◻ Fig. 37.3e). The maximum diameter was 1.5 cm. There was no intraluminal thrombus. On the right side, an inconspicuous internal jugular vein was shown. Intracardiac structures and also heart-related vessels, furthermore the heart valves were inconspicuous (■ Fig. 37.3d). Evidence of the involvement of other "internal" organs, vessels was not found.

37.4 Educational Questions

1. What differential diagnosis do you consider for hypermobility, soft skin structures, poorly healing skin lesions after trauma?

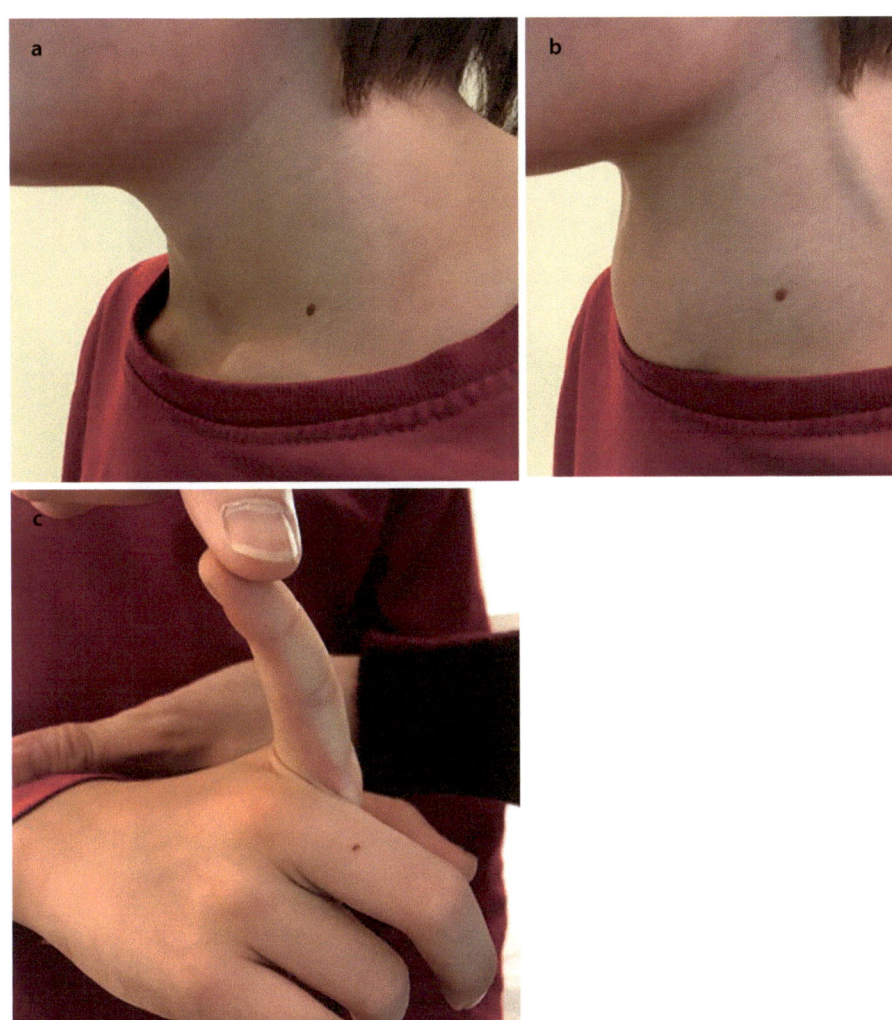

■ **Fig. 37.3** **a–c** Toni's clinical aspect: frog neck and hypermobility and the echocardiographic diagnosis. **a, b** Toni during straining/breath holding, a "frog neck" develops. **c** Significant hypermobility. **d, e** Echocardiographically, a significant aneurysmatic saccular protrusion of the internal jugular vein was found. (**d, e** with kind permission of Dr. P. Barikbin, Vivantes Klinikum im Friedrichshain, Berlin)

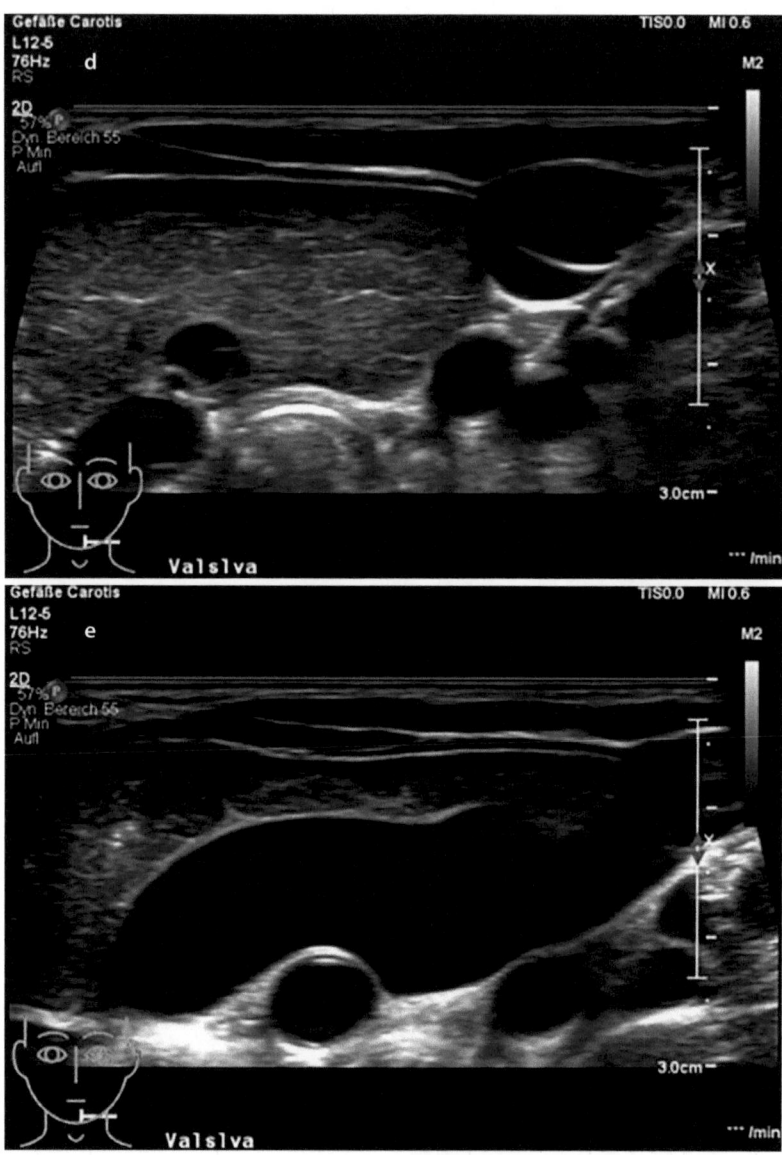

◘ Fig. 37.3 (continued)

2. Can the symptoms of the two teenagers be assigned to classification systems?
3. How do you design the diagnostics?
4. What therapeutic considerations should be taken into account, especially in the absence of controlled therapy studies in childhood and adolescence?

37.5 Classification

Connective tissue weakness in childhood is physiological to a certain extent, especially in early childhood (Cattalini et al. 2015) (Gedalia and Brewer 1993). In the case of clear structural diseases of the skin, tendons or joints such as Osteogenesis imperfecta or Hypophosphatasia, in addition to the actual bone problem, the connective tissue structure may also appear "weak" (Sillence and Rimoin 1978; Girschick et al. 2006). The **benign hypermobility** of the toddler often goes hand in hand with joint pain in the evening or at night. A dependence on physical, athletic stress is seen. The frequency is given as up to 20% of toddlers (Gedalia and Brewer 1993). Additional phenomena, such as a cracking of the joints, lead to uncertainty. A restriction of sports activities may even intensify the connective tissue weakness subsequently, so that therapeutically muscle strengthening, physiotherapy and possibly also supportive measures such as shoe inserts or tape bandages can play a role. Anti-inflammatory drugs for pain reduction seem sensible. Measurement systems, which allow to estimate the extent of hypermobility, are used in special clinics, e.g. the **Beighton-Score** (Beighton et al. 1998). Here, the hypermobility in the area of the wrist, the elbow, the thumb, also in the area of the knee is mainly checked. This summation score grades the degree of hypermobility. If this is significant, a genetic basis of the hypermobility should also be considered, cardiac and ophthalmological diagnostics are then additionally required.

The Ehlers-Danlos syndrome comprises a group of monogenic diseases with multisystemic expression (De Paepe and Malfait 2012). Principally affected is usually the structure of the **collagen**, it represents the main component of the extracellular matrix proteins (collagen 1, 2, 3, 5, 11). Collagens form fibrillar structures, which are additionally molecularly cross-linked and thus stabilized among each other. Intracellularly, precursors are synthesized, which are intensively modified intra- and extra-cellularly, e.g. by hydroxylation or glycosylation, furthermore by the removal of propeptides. According to the **Villefranche classification**, 6 subgroups are described in this classification, supplemented by 3 further subgroups with molecular definition: Ehlers-Danlos syndrome classic type (EDS I and II), hypermobile type (EDS III), vascular type (EDS IV), kyphoscoliotic type (EDS VI), arthrochalasis type (EDS VIIA and EDS VIIB), Dermatosparaxis (EDS VIIC), unspecified forms (Beighton et al. 1998; Mayer et al. 2013).

37.6 Further Course

▪▪ Neo
Through years of intensive physiotherapeutic accompaniment, also using oscillation devices, it was possible to accompany the musculoskeletal development of the boy and even stabilize a good general physical fitness and athletic activity in later adolescence. Thus, the boy's quality of life was considered high. The body length percentile then pleasingly rose to the 70% range.

▪▪ Toni
Once it became clear that the diagnosed aneurysm was an expression of the general connective tissue weakness in the context of the predisposition, the family restricted themselves in everyday life to avoiding Valsalva maneuvers. Within a 4-year follow-up control, no complications have arisen. Spontaneous ruptures are not documented in the literature. If the patient shows swallowing disorders, thrombosis of this venous ectasia or also the development of a Horner's syndrome due to pressure on neural structures, then surgical intervention may be indicated.

37.7 Educational Answers

- **1. What differential diagnosis do you consider for hypermobility, soft skin structures, poorly healing skin lesions after trauma?**

Depending on the severity of the connective tissue weakness and possible healing disorders, genetically caused structural connective tissue diseases such as Ehlers-Danlos or **Marfan** syndrome must be considered (Beighton 1972; Beighton et al. 1998). A variety of bone metabolism disorders, e.g. osteogenesis imperfecta or hypophosphatasia, regularly also go hand in hand with a weakness of the connective tissue (Girschick et al. 2007). Since the bone also has a non-mineral matrix, the disturbance of the formation of collagen fibrils is of great importance for the entire musculoskeletal system. If there is only moderate hypermobility without signs of skin injury, without scarring and without cutis laxa, then the clinical assessment appears sufficient. Otherwise, genetic diagnostics would be possible after informing the family.

- **2. Can the symptoms of the adolescents be classified into classification systems?**

Classification systems exist for Ehlers-Danlos syndrome from a clinical point of view, but also on the basis of molecular foundations (Beighton et al. 1998).

- **3. How do you design the diagnostics?**

The diagnostics are crucially dependent on the severity of the clinic. The clinical examination can diagnose hypermobility as part of the Beighton score. In addition, ultrasound examinations of the musculoskeletal system, and also of vessels, seem sensible. General fitness tests including the use of mechanical force analyses can provide an incentive for physical fitness/sporting activity for the person affected. In case of suspected genetically caused connective tissue weakness, a **skin biopsy** for the presentation of **collagen fibrils** may be sensible. Molecular diagnostics can help to capture the molecular basis in a panel analysis based on next generation sequencing today (Sobey 2015).

- **4. What therapeutic considerations should be taken into account, especially in the absence of controlled therapy studies in children and adolescents?**

Therapeutic strategies essentially aim to strengthen the musculoskeletal unit and support muscle building. Painful sensations can be limited by appropriate medication, e.g. NSAID (Sobey 2014). Physiotherapeutic exercise treatment serves to strengthen the muscular balance of the joint structures as well as bandages and possibly splints. In case of injuries, careful **layer-by-layer suturing technique** should be observed. Overall, multidisciplinary care is at the forefront or is desirable.

37.8 Summary

37.8.1 Etiology

The etiology of Neos and Tonis' connective tissue weakness is ultimately still unclear. A genetic analysis was not desired in either patient. A molecular genetic analysis could certainly define a collagen formation disorder.

37.8.2 Pathogenesis/Clinic

A complex disorder of the connective tissue structure of skin, subcutis, tendons, joint capsule and also muscles ultimately leads to many stresses, painful sensations. Medium and long term, stresses/damages to the musculoskeletal system are possible, attention should be paid to additional cardiological, angiological and also gastro-intestinal pathology in Ehlers-Danlos syndrome (Sobey 2014).

37.8.3　Diagnosis

The precise descriptive clinical examination is flanked by sonographic diagnostics, furthermore molecular analyses of structure genes of the connective tissue.

37.8.4　Therapy

The therapy aims at strengthening the muscles, possibly also the connective tissue through regular sports exercises, supported by physiotherapeutic exercise treatment.

37.8.5　Diagnosis

The diagnosis is primarily based on the clinical picture of the disease, possibly in combination with a skin biopsy and genetic diagnostics.

37.8.6　Prophylaxis

Strictly speaking, there is no prophylaxis to prevent the disease.

Conclusion

Patients with benign hypermobility and pain sensations should be managed from a clinical point of view, overdiagnosis through laboratory chemistry and imaging should be avoided. Significant pronounced connective tissue weakness syndromes can be assessed molecular genetically also with regard to risk factors. In the latter, multidisciplinary care from rheumatology, cardiology, dermatology, human genetics, flanked by intensive physiotherapy with promotion of musculoskeletal fitness has proven successful.

References

Beighton P (1972) Articular manifestations of the Ehlers-Danlos syndrome. Semin Arthritis Rheum 1:246–261

Beighton P, De Paepe A, Steinmann B, Tsipouras P, Wenstrup RJ (1998) Ehlers-Danlos syndromes: revised nosology, Villefranche, 1997. Ehlers-Danlos National Foundation (USA) and Ehlers-Danlos Support Group (UK). Am J Med Genet 77:31–37

Cattalini M, Khubchandani R, Cimaz R (2015) When flexibility is not necessarily a virtue: a review of hypermobility syndromes and chronic or recurrent musculoskeletal pain in children. Pediatr Rheumatol Online J 13:40. ► https://doi.org/10.1186/s12969-015-0039-3

De Paepe A, Malfait F (2012) The Ehlers-Danlos syndrome, a disorder with many faces. Clin Genet 82:1–11. ► https://doi.org/10.1111/j.1399-0004.2012.01858.x

Gedalia A, Brewer EJ Jr (1993) Joint hypermobility in pediatric practice – a review. J Rheumatol 20:371–374

Girschick HJ, Schneider P, Haubitz I, Hiort O, Collmann H, Beer M, Shin YS, Seyberth HW (2006) Effective NSAID treatment indicates that hyperprostaglandinism is affecting the clinical severity of childhood hypophosphatasia. Orphanet J Rare Dis 1:24. ► https://doi.org/10.1186/1750-1172-1-24

Girschick HJ, Mornet E, Beer M, Warmuth-Metz M, Schneider P (2007) Chronic multifocal non-bacterial osteomyelitis in hypophosphatasia mimicking malignancy. BMC Pediatr 7:3. ► https://doi.org/10.1186/1471-2431-7-3

Mayer K, Kennerknecht I, Steinmann B (2013) Clinical utility gene card for: Ehlers-Danlos syndrome types I-VII and variants – update 2012. Eur J Hum Genet 21. ► https://doi.org/10.1038/ejhg.2012.162

Silence DO, Rimoin DL (1978) Classification of osteogenesis imperfect. Lancet 1:1041–1042

Sobey G (2014) Ehlers-Danlos syndrome – a commonly misunderstood group of conditions. Clin Med (Lond) 14:432–436. ► https://doi.org/10.7861/clinmedicine.14-4-432

Sobey G (2015) Ehlers-Danlos syndrome: how to diagnose and when to perform genetic tests. Arch Dis Child 100:57–61. ► https://doi.org/10.1136/archdischild-2013-304822

A 3-Year-Old Toddler with Recurrent Fever Spikes, Maculopapular Exanthema, Polyarthritis, and Acute Neurological Symptoms Since Infancy

Christian Huemer

Contents

38.1 Medical History

A girl was referred to the rheumatology clinic by her pediatrician at the age of 3 years with a long-standing history of recurrent fever episodes. The child had started showing symptoms towards the end of her first year of life, with recurrent fever episodes up to 40 °C (evening fever increases), associated with rashes, which were described as maculopapular "exanthema" mainly in the area of the lower extremities. Initially, viral infections or allergic reactions to food were suspected, but a change in diet did not bring about any improvement, and symptomatic therapy during manifest temperature increase could only temporarily improve the course of the fever episodes. In the months before presentation in our rheumatology clinic, there was finally additional symptomatology of symmetrical polyarthritis, particularly affecting the finger joints as well as elbow joints and now a neurological symptomatology in the form of a questionable ataxia of the child (increased gait insecurity).

Further medical history unremarkable. Family history unremarkable, the parents are not consanguineous. The pediatrician suspected Still's disease and requested further clarification.

38.2 Examination Findings

Eutrophic toddler with slightly reduced general condition, temperature 39.4°C at first examination. Unremarkable cardiopulmonary examination, abdomen soft, indolent, no hepatosplenomegaly, no lymphadenopathy. ENT findings unremarkable. There is a trunk-accentuated, small-spotted, maculopapular exanthema, in the area of the lower extremities there is a clear livedo pattern (◘ Fig. 38.1). In the developmental neurological examination, developmental delay with gait insecurity, slightly atactic gait pattern and latent left-accentuated tetraspasticity.

In the musculoskeletal status, polyarthritis is impressive with involvement of the hands (wrist joints, MCP II–V and BIP II–V on both hands). There is a restriction of movement with loss of extension of 5° at both elbow joints.

38.3 Laboratory Values, Further Findings and Imaging

38.3.1 Laboratory Values and Further Findings

The first laboratory tests show a significant increase in inflammation parameters (ESR 70 mm/h, CRP 12 mg/dl) and leukocytosis (18.0 G/L). Autoimmunological findings (ANA, ENA C3, C4 complement, ANCA, rheumatoid factor) negative. Immunoglobulins unremarkable.

Further findings obtained: CSF findings unremarkable, blood and stool cultures, direct pathogen detection (PCR) and infection serological findings remained unremarkable. **Urine** findings unremarkable. **Cardiological examination** (ECG, heart echo) unremarkable.

Molecular genetic panel to exclude common periodic fever syndromes (FMF, HIDS, CAPS, TRAPS) showed no abnormal findings.

38.3.2 Imaging

Chest X-ray and abdominal ultrasound show no abnormalities.

38.4 Educational Questions

1. What differential diagnoses should be considered in this episodically occurring highly inflammatory process?

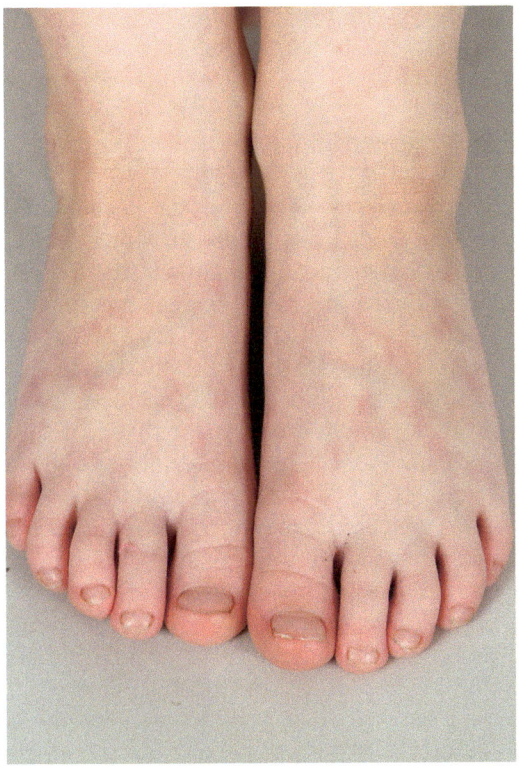 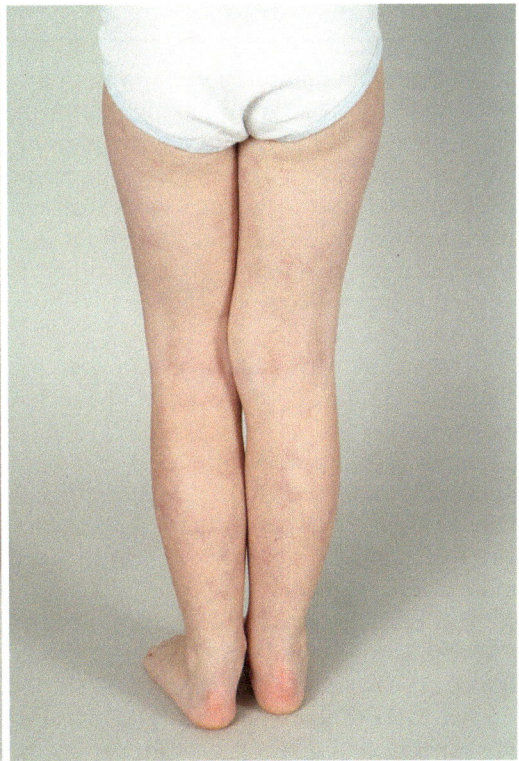

❏ **Fig. 38.1** Livedo reticularis in DADA-2 disease

2. What further findings would you suggest?
3. What acute therapy and further therapy should be discussed?

38.5 Differential Diagnostic Considerations and Educational Answers

A seriously ill child with clear indications of an episodically occurring, multisystemic and inflammatory process requires rapid and systematic clarification for *differentiation* between an infectious, malignant or autoinflammatory process. It is generally to be considered whether such a patient should not be presented in any case at a tertiary medical center. The possibilities of a rapid collection of important immunological and infectious diagnostic steps are to be exhausted.

The child with these symptoms quickly needs an infectious work-up (culture findings, infection serological findings, CSF diagnostics, measurement of inflammation activity and detection of possible organ systems by means of chest X-ray, abdominal sonography, heart echocardiogram, possibly MRI of suspected organs, PET scan) and an assessment by the specialists of hemato-oncology, neuropediatrics and rheumatology. By excluding an infectious process and a neoplasm, the suspected diagnosis of an autoinflammatory or autoimmunological process is to be specified.

38.6 Further Course

After the initial examination, the young patient was first given symptomatic treatment with ibuprofen (30 mg/kg body weight/day p.o.) after a 1-week i.v. antibiotic therapy (Cefotaxime) due to an unclear infectious work-up, which initially led to a slight improvement in symptoms. After another 6 days, there was a complication in the form of a renewed significant fever spike > 39.5 °C associated with sudden vision loss on the left and an acute paralysis of the lower extremities.

In the immediately initiated imaging diagnostics (**cranial MRI**), a signal disturbance of the optic nerve was found. In the MRI of the orbit, an optic sheath process with contrast medium uptake was seen. In the visually evoked potentials (VEP), a severe visual impairment on the left was found due to papilledema on the left.

An MRI of the spinal canal showed a myelopathy of unclear origin at the tip of the conus medullaris.

Due to these additional clinical symptoms, the diagnostics were expanded and finally a determination of the enzyme adenosine deaminase 2 (ADA2) was initiated. This showed a significant reduction (0.2 mU/g): The diagnosis of an **ADA2 deficiency** could thus be confirmed. A molecular genetic examination (**CECR1 gene**) remained inconspicuous. The patient initially received a systemic steroid therapy (intravenous methylprednisolone pulse therapy 30 mg/kg body weight/day) for 3 days and subsequently a multi-week oral steroid therapy.

At the same time, treatment with a TNF-α blocker (Adalimumab 1-time 20 mg s.c. every 2 weeks) was started. Already in the first weeks after the start of therapy, a significant reduction in inflammation parameters was observed, there were no further fever spikes or clinical complications. In a follow-up observation of 1 year, there was a partial clinical remission of the disease. The child still requires intensive physiotherapy and occupational therapy.

38.7 Summary

The **deficiency of adenosine deaminase 2 (DADA2)** is caused by homozygous or compound heterozygous variants in the CECR1 gene. There is a **wide clinical spectrum** of this disease (Wittkowski 2022). On the one hand, inflammatory manifestations such as recurrent fever, acute phase reaction, athromyalgias, livedo reticularis, polyarteritis nodosa and vasculitic manifestations (Navon Elkan et al. 2014; Zhou et al. 2014) occur. Particularly characteristic is the occurrence of lacunar **strokess** in childhood, i.e., strokes caused by occlusion of the small penetrating arteries in the area of the brainstem, internal capsule, or basal ganglia. The disease is confirmed by demonstrating a reduced ADA2 enzyme activity and/or the detection of pathogenic variants in the CECR1 gene. 25% of patients with DADA2 show a humoral immune deficiency similar to variable immune defect syndrome with hypogammaglobulinemia and increased susceptibility to infection (Schepp et al. 2017; Meyts and Aksentijevich 2018). Therapeutically, TNF blockade has proven to be particularly promising (Ombrello et al. 2019).

> **Conclusion**
>
> In the assessment of episodic multisystemic and inflammatory diseases, the important differential diagnoses of autoinflammatory diseases should always be included.
>
> ADA2 deficiency is one of the most exciting entities in this regard. The possibility of a rapid diagnosis through enzyme diagnostics and molecular genetics is important, as this opens up the chance of a specific therapy, e.g., with TNF-α-blocking drugs.

38

References

Meyts I, Aksentijevich I (2018) Deficiency of adenosine deaminase 2 (DADA 2): updates on the phenotype, genetics, pathogenesis, and treatment. J Clin Immunol 38(5):569–578

Navon Elkan P, Pierce SB, Segel R, Walsch T, Barash J, Padeh S, Zlotogorski A, Berkun Y, Press JJ, Mukamel M, Voth I, Hashkes PJ, Harel L, Hoffer V, Ling E, Yalcinkaya F, Kasapcopur O, Lee MK, Klevit RE, Renbaum P, Weinberg-Shukron A, Sener EF, Schormari B, Zeligson S, Marek-Yagel D, Strom TM, Shohat M, Singer A, Rubinow A, Pras E, Winkelmann J, Tekin M, Anikster Y, King MC, Levy-Lahad E (2014) Mutant adenosine deaminase 2 in a polyarteritis nodosa vasculopathy. N Engl J Med 370(10):921–931

Ombrello AK, Qin J, Hoffmann PM, Kumar P, Stone D, Jones A, Romeo T, Barham B, Pinto-Patarroyo G, Toro C, Soldatos A, Zhou Q, Deuitch N, Aksentijevich I, Sheldon SL, Kelly S, Man A, Barron K, Hershfield M, Flegel WA, Kastner DL (2019) Treatment strategies for deficiency of adenosine deaminase 2. N Engl J Med 380(16):1582–1584

Schepp J, Proietti M, Frede N, Buchta M, Hubscher K, Rojas Restrepo J, Goldacker S, Warnatz K, Pachlopnik- Schmid J, Duppenthaler A, Lougaris V, Uriarte I, Kelly S, Hershfield M, Grimbacher B (2017) Screening of 181 patients with antibody deficiency for deficiency of adenosine deaminase 2 sheds new light on the disease in adulthood. Arthritis Rheum 69(8):1689–1700

Wittkowski H (2022) Autoinflammatorische Syndrome bei Kindern und Jugendlichen. In: Wagner N, Dannecker G, Kallinich T (Hrsg) Pädiatrische Rheumatologie. Springer, Berlin/Heidelberg, S 783–791

Zhou et al (2014) Early-onset stroke and vasculopathy associated with mutations in ADA 2. N Engl J Med 370(10):911–920

A 2-Year-Old Boy with Severe Nocturnal Leg Pain

Christian Huemer

Contents

39.1 Medical History

A 2-year-old boy is presented via the emergency outpatient clinic. The parents are worried because for about 2 weeks the child has been complaining of extremely severe pain in his legs, especially towards the end of the day. The child regularly wakes up late in the evening, crying in pain. The parents are alarmed, they are not sure where the pain is located, but they have the impression that the pain is mainly in the legs of the child, where they notice no external abnormalities. Temperature was regularly measured and showed no elevated readings. No other symptoms in the child. Surprisingly for the parents, after administering a paracetamol suppository, the child falls asleep again and is completely symptom-free the next morning. Family history is unremarkable, however, the child's father believes he remembers having similar nocturnal pains as a toddler.

39.2 Examination Findings

Toddler in excellent general and nutritional condition. Musculoskeletal status without palpable synovitis or enthesopathy, functionally unremarkable findings. The child's gait is without abnormalities. No focal signs of inflammation. Internal status completely unremarkable.

39.3 Laboratory Values and Imaging

39.3.1 Laboratory Values

CRP, sedimentation rate and autoimmune findings are unremarkable. All other laboratory findings including complete blood count, differential blood count, liver and kidney function parameters are also unremarkable.

39.3.2 Imaging

Plain X-ray of the lower extremities without abnormalities.

39.4 Educational Questions

1. What important differential diagnosis should be discussed in these pronounced pain conditions?
2. Are there any suggestions for extended additional diagnostics?
3. How would you advise the parents of this child?

39.5 Differential Diagnostic Considerations and Educational Answers

The differential diagnosis for the above symptoms requires the exclusion of infectious and non-infectious (malignant, possibly also post-traumatic) diseases. The indication for a plain radiological examination is often given, a malignant process or a post-traumatic process can then be quickly "excluded". In any indication of systemic symptoms such as fever, cardiopulmonary or gastrointestinal symptoms, an infectious "work-up" is to be indicated, possibly also an extended imaging diagnosis using MRI to safely exclude an Osteomyelitis. The advice to the parents should be very deescalating and reassuring, as in principle, in the absence of the aforementioned further symptoms, a very benign diagnosis can be assumed.

39.6 Further Course

In the medical history and detailed clinical examination of our young patient, there was no indication of a systemic event, no indication of an infection prior to the onset of symptoms or during the pain symptoms. Already obtained laboratory findings showed no inflammatory activity, a plain X-ray of the lower extremities was unremarkable. Thus, after a detailed differential diagnosis, the **diagnosis of childhood growing pains** could be made.

39.7 Summary

39.7.1 Etiology

The term growing pains describes recurring, self-limiting pains in the lower extremities in children, which usually occur in the evening and at night and have no known cause. The medical term often used is "**nocturnal arthralgia**". The pains commonly referred to as "growing pains" in layman's terms usually occur in children between the ages of 2 and 12, with a prevalence between 4 and 35%, and about 10-20% of all school-age children complain of such pains at some point. The disease picture is not clearly characterized (Brandenberger et al. 2000), but it is important to note that childhood growing pains always have a benign course (Lehman and Carl 2017) and usually disappear within 1-2 years.

39.7.2 Clinic

The typical clinical symptoms usually consist of bilateral pain in the lower extremities, which cannot be clearly assigned to a structure (joint). Older children (> 6 years of age) also describe the pain as cramp-like creeping pain or as restlessness of the legs. The pain usually develops in the evening or overnight and can be so severe that children wake up from sleep and cry persistently.

Spontaneous improvement usually occurs in the morning hours. During the day, the children are symptom-free. Hypermobility is often associated and may contribute to the pain characteristics, often also physical/sporting activity throughout the day.

39.7.3 Therapy

Pain perception can be alleviated by massage, heat, or the use of analgesics. The family history often provides clues to similar complaints during childhood in parents or other relatives. An important part of therapy is educating the affected children and their families about the harmless nature of these symptoms. Parents can often anticipate their child's complaints after an active sports day. In this situation, a prophylactic NSAID in the evening may be helpful.

> **Conclusion**
>
> Childhood "growing pains" are very benign pain conditions, which cause no lasting impairment to the child. Prior to the diagnosis of childhood growing pains, it is important to have a detailed history and clinical examination, a comprehensive exclusion diagnosis, to securely rule out important differential diagnoses in this age group such as infectious and also neoplastic diseases.

References

Brandenberger G, Gronfier C, Chapotot F, Simon C, Piquard F (2000) Effect of sleep deprivation on overall 24 h growth-hormone secretion. Lancet 356:1408

Lehman PJ, Carl RL (2017) Growing pains. Sports. Health 9:132–138

A 9-Year-Old Girl with Elevated Body Temperature, Clear Protective Posture, and Pain in the Right Hip

Christian Huemer

Contents

© The Author(s), under exclusive license to Springer-Verlag GmbH, DE, part of Springer Nature 2024
C. Huemer and H. Girschick (eds.), *Clinical Examples in Pediatric Rheumatology*,
https://doi.org/10.1007/978-3-662-68732-1_40

40.1 Medical History

The 9-year-old girl was referred by the pediatrician to the pediatric emergency department. The girl had developed varicella 2 weeks ago, then after a week, she first started to adopt a protective posture and experienced pain in her right hip. The suspected diagnosis of a **Coxitis fugax** was made, initially symptomatic therapy with nonsteroidal anti-inflammatory drug and rest. Nevertheless, the complaints increased. Four days after the first appearance of joint symptoms, an increase in joint effusion was observed in the sonography at the pediatrician's office, along with an increased body temperature (maximum 38.0 °C) and rhinopharyngitis. On the day of referral to the emergency department of our clinic, the girl was presented again to the pediatrician due to the persistence of complaints. For the first time, the sonography showed clouding of the effusion.

40.2 Examination Findings

9-year-old girl in slightly reduced general condition, somewhat pale. Condition after **varicella** (older lesions visible, no fresh lesions). Musculoskeletal status shows restriction of external and internal rotation exclu-

sively in the area of the right hip joint, here end-stage significant pain symptoms, flexion of the right hip possible, end-stage also significant pain symptoms can be triggered. Heart sounds pure, rhythmic, normofrequent. Lungs ventilated equally on both sides, no rattling noises. Abdomen soft, no resistances, no pressure pain. No hepatosplenomegaly. ENT findings inconspicuous.

40.3 Laboratory Values and Imaging

40.3.1 Laboratory Values

CRP 1.1 mg/dl, **ESR 96 mm/h**, blood count leukocyte count 9.5/nl, Hb 9.9 g/dl, Hct 29%, platelets 631/nl. Differential blood count without left shift. Serum chemical findings: electrolytes inconspicuous, liver function parameters GOT, GPT inconspicuous. LDH inconspicuous.

40.3.2 Imaging

The hip sonography (◻ Fig. 40.1) showed an effusion around the right hip head, a capsule detachment of 9.7 mm, inhomogeneous,

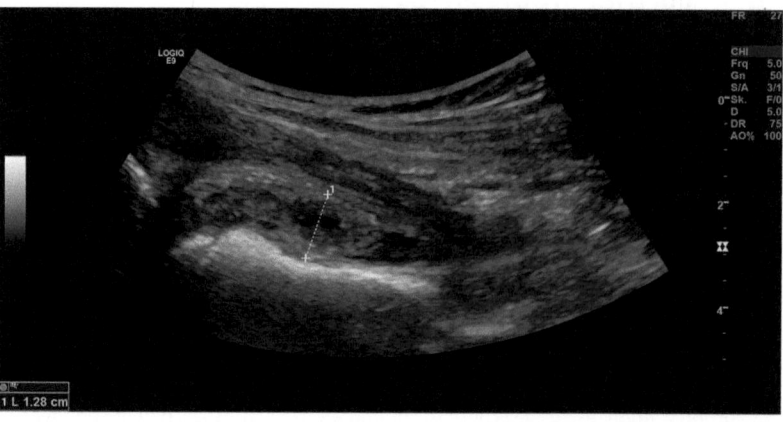

◻ **Fig. 40.1** Hip sonography of the patient. There is a significant echo-rich joint effusion and widened synovia of the right hip joint, capsule detachment, measured in the standard plane longitudinally on the femoral neck

40

echo-rich. A bony destruction sign was not sonographically presentable. Native X-ray (pelvic overview X-ray) without clear indications of osseous destructive changes or post-traumatic lesions.

40.4 Educational Questions

1. What differential diagnoses do you consider given the present clinical findings?
2. What next diagnostic steps would you suggest?
3. What therapeutic considerations need to be considered immediately and in the long term?

40.5 Differential Diagnostic Considerations and Educational Answers

The rapid *differential diagnostic* work-up in this child with pronounced protective posture and pain symptoms in the right hip as well as significantly increased inflammatory parameters (ESR dropped!), this after the onset of a **varicella infection**, makes the rapid evaluation of primarily an infectious or post-infectious process a priority. The child does not show high fever, but clearly increased inflammatory activity in the laboratory as well as an inhomogeneous echo-rich effusion in the hip joint sonography. In this constellation, an extended diagnosis to safely exclude an osteomyelitic process is urgently indicated. As *next diagnostic steps*, a diagnostic joint puncture in sedation and analgesia and an MRI must be planned quickly for this child. These steps are indispensable to *possibly initiate a rapid empirical antibiotic therapy*, possibly also a *joint lavage,* if necessary.

40.6 Further Progress

On the day of the initial presentation of the 9-year-old girl in the pediatric emergency department, an MRI and a joint puncture under sedoanalgesia were performed simultaneously. The joint puncture, which also appeared milky cloudy, showed 90,000 leukocytes/µl (5% mononuclear cells, 95% polynuclear cells). Thus, the **diagnosis of septic arthritis** was highly likely. The simultaneous MRI (◘ Fig. 40.2) already showed clear indications of **Coxitis** and **Osteomyelitis**, especially of the epiphysis and the adjacent femoral neck. There was also a significantly increased contrast uptake of the synovia, but also of the periarticular soft tissue including the adductor muscles. There was bone marrow edema and significant contrast uptake in the epiphysis (already with medial structural disorder), in the femoral neck and opposite in the acetabulum of the pelvis. As a secondary finding, a reactive inguinal lymphadenopathy was shown. MRI thus showed pronounced coxitis and osteomyelitis. Based on this finding, a joint irrigation was performed by pediatric orthopedics during the same sedoanalgesia, and empirical antibiotic therapy with a cephalosporin (Cefazolin 100 mg/kg body weight/day) was started intravenously. No growth of a pathological germ was found in the joint puncture (Gram stain negative, aerobic and anaerobic culture sterile after 48 h, panbacterial PCR and culture after long-term incubation [10 days] negative). The intravenous antibiotic therapy with cephalosporin was carried out for 3 weeks, the clinical condition improved increasingly, also the initially significantly increased blood sedimentation was significantly regressive (day 10: 35 mm/h, day 20: 12 mm/h, day 30: 7 mm/h). A control sonography and MRI after 20 days of antibiotic therapy still showed pronounced coxitis and

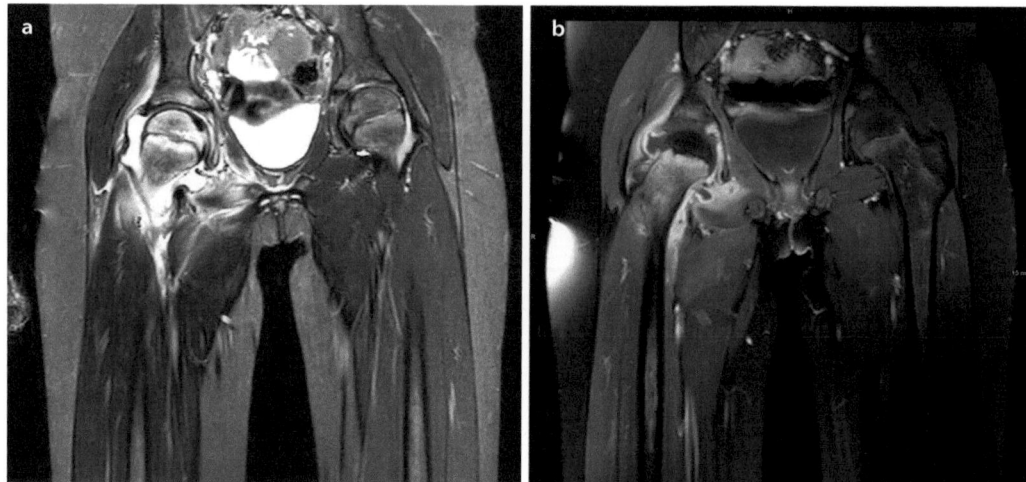

□ Fig. 40.2   a, b MRI of the hip joints with suspicion of septic infection. Clear T2-hyperintense effusion in the right hip joint with linear thickening of the synovia on the right to 3 mm. Significantly increased contrast uptake of the synovia and the periarticular soft tissue including adductors. Bone marrow edema and significant contrast uptake in the acetabulum and femoral neck on the right up to intertrochanteric. In summary, MRI shows pronounced bacterial coxitis on the right

progressive structural changes of the epiphysis, therefore, after consultation with pediatric orthopedics, an arthrotomy of the hip with open joint irrigation was performed again. The switch to oral antibiotic therapy took place after 4 weeks, this therapy was continued for another 4 weeks, until the complete normalization of all sonographic and laboratory inflammatory signs with a continued significant improvement of the child's clinical condition. The unusually long duration of antibiotic therapy in this child (a total of 8 weeks) was decided in this case, as early structural changes were already visible in the epiphysis, a second intervention was indicated on day 20 and completely negative pathogen findings did not allow a targeted change from the initially empirical antibiotic therapy to a targeted therapy. A normalization of all inflammatory parameters and a significant improvement of the clinical findings (not the sonographic findings) were already present when switching to oral antibiotic therapy (day 20).

Unfortunately, the follow-up examinations of the hip joint (□ Fig. 40.3) after

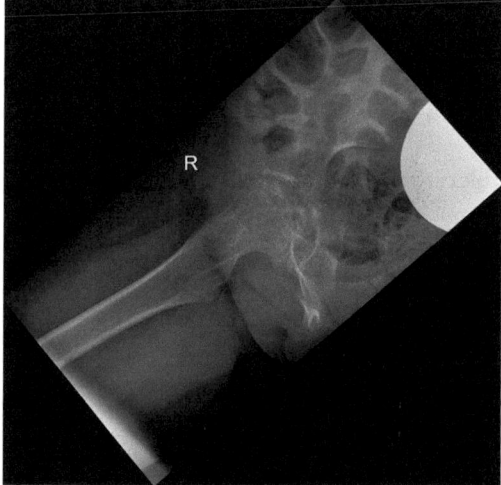

□ Fig. 40.3 X-ray of the right hip joint 1 year after diagnosis. The femoroacetabular joint space on the right is still narrowed. High-grade destruction of the femoral head, especially the epiphysis, widening of the femoral neck

6 and 12 months showed a significant destruction of the femoral head/epiphysis. The child has since been in regular check-ups by

pediatric orthopedics, requires supportive measures such as intensive physiotherapy and muscle-relaxing measures by means of Botox injection. The prognosis is currently reservedly unfavorable, the child may need an early joint endoprosthesis operation.

40.7 Summary

40.7.1 Etiology

The **septic (purulent) arthritis** and infectious **acute osteomyelitis** represent pediatric rheumatological emergency diagnoses, which require rapid diagnostic management as well as aggressive therapeutic approaches in both conservative and surgical forms. Joint pain or pain in the extremities with protective posture can be an important indication of an infection in the bone or surrounding soft tissues. Basically, isolated infections of the bone structures (Osteomyelitis), of the entire bone (**Osteitis**) are distinguished from infections of the bone and adjacent joint structures (septic arthritis in combination with osteomyelitis). The development of osteomyelitis or septic arthritis is due to different blood circulation conditions in children at different ages. Another cause can be external injuries, foreign bodies after an accident, or a local invasion of infectious agents, either per continuitatem in superficially located joints or through secondary spread via the bloodstream. Hematogenous osteomyelitis represents a bone and bone marrow inflammation that occurs via the bloodstream after bacterial invasion, with an acute or less commonly chronic course extending beyond 3-4 weeks.

Osteomyelitis often forms in the metaphyses of long tubular bones and is difficult to diagnose due to often obscured symptoms. The diagnosis is particularly difficult in the area of the pelvic bones or vertebral bodies.

Non-hematogenous osteomyelitis can occur through an external injury with the entry of bacteria through the skin and subsequent spread into the tissue. Infections of the skin (skin abscesses) and soft tissue (phlegmon, erysipelas), which manifest near large or small joints, are also possible causes of a per continuitatem inflammation of a joint capsule (septic arthritis). Hematogenous osteomyelitis or septic arthritis is more common in boys than in girls, overall it is a relatively rare but important infection for childhood, for which no reliable regional incidence figures are available (Schnabel et al. 2016).

40.7.2 Clinic

The clinical symptoms of osteomyelitis in the sense of classic inflammatory symptoms with pain, redness, heat, swelling, and functional restriction should be clearly documented (Wirth 2022). These symptoms are very pronounced in osteomyelitis of older children, especially when the extremities are affected, while the symptoms often appear less characteristic when the pelvic bones or spine are affected.

Particularly risky is the often only mildly pronounced symptomatology in osteomyelitis and septic arthritis of infants and newborns, in whom the most important clinical sign in addition to increased inflammatory activity is the sparing of a limb or painful restriction when testing passive mobility.

The manifestation of a bacterial infection on the vertebral bodies as spondylitis or in the case of joint-crossing image as spondylodiscitis often goes unnoticed for days or weeks and is initially attributed to other causes. The main symptom here is the affected and painful spinal region, which the patients manifest as a protective posture.

40.7.3 Diagnosis

The diagnosis of osteomyelitis or septic arthritis is based on typical changes in the laboratory with increased inflammatory activity (leukocytosis, left shift, increased ESR and CRP), but these parameters are not specific laboratory values for a bacterial infection, but are also found significantly increased in other inflammatory diseases such as the systemic forms of JIA or other chronic inflammations.

In any suspicion of osteomyelitis, taking a blood culture and microbiological pathogen detection is essential. Since the blood culture only succeeds in detecting the pathogen in a maximum of 50% of cases, cultures from joint aspirates are indicated as long-term cultures of 10 days. Currently, molecular biological detection methods, e.g. eubacterial 16S-rRNA amplification, or NGS-based detection methods are also available. The diagnostic joint puncture in suspected septic arthritis is mandatory to perform, in septic arthritis the granulocytes in the joint effusion are present in high numbers > 50,000/ul. Imaging diagnostics are crucial for the diagnosis of osteomyelitis, it is important to remember that conventional X-rays in the early phase of acute osteomyelitis do not yet allow the detection of the beginning bone changes, here an ultrasonographic finding with early detection of a soft tissue edema and in further course the rapid indication for an MRI examination is to be indicated. The MRI examination can effectively supplement the initial sonography, especially in the case of bone inflammations, the MRI finding is diagnostically decisive.

40.7.4 Therapy

The antibiotic therapy for osteomyelitis should be administered intravenously over a period of at least 3 weeks, with Clindamycin or Cephalosporins (Group 1 or 2) recommended. Once the culture result is available, a targeted antibiotic therapy can be indicated (Saavedra-Lozano et al. 2017). As soon as a diagnosis of septic arthritis is made, surgical relief of the joint must be carried out, either arthroscopically or by open **arthrotomy** (Fernandez et al. 2015). Except for septic arthritis of the infant hip, alternative therapy methods are propagated through repetitive aspirations with good therapeutic success (Pääkkönen et al. 2010). Delaying surgical therapy leads to progressive destruction and growth disturbance of the femoral head with serious implications for future life.

Conclusion

The diagnosis of septic arthritis and/or acute osteomyelitis in childhood represents a pediatric emergency. Only through rapid diagnosis and subsequent swift therapy can long-term damage be prevented. The diagnostic joint puncture is important for obtaining clear culture findings and for planning a swift antibiotic therapy.

References

Fernandez FF, Langendörfer M, Wirth T, Eberhardt O (2015) Die arthroskopische Therapie septischer Hüftgelenkentzündungen in der Kindheit. Oper Orthop Traumatol 27:262–269

Pääkkönen M, Kallio MJ, Peltola H, Kallio PE (2010) Pediatric septic hip with or without arthrotomy: retrospective analysis of 62 consecutive non-neonatoal culture-positive cases. J Pediatr Orthop B 19:264–269

Saavedra-Lozano J, Falup-Pecurariu O, Faust SN, Girschick H, Hartwig N, Kaplan S, Lorrot M, Mantadakis E, Peltola H, Rojo P, Zaoutis T, Le-Mair A (2017) Bone and joint infections. Pediatr Infect Dis J 36(8):788–799. ▶ https://doi.org/10.1097/INF.0000000000001635

Schnabel A, Range U, Hahn G, Siepmann T, Berner R, Hedrich CM (2016) Unexpectedly high incidences of chronic non-bacterial as compared to bacterial osteomyelitis in children. Rheumatol Int

36(12):1737–1745. ▶ https://doi.org/10.1007/s00296-016-3572-6 . Epub 2016 Oct 11.PMID: 27730289

Wirth T (2022) Orthopädische Differenzialdiagnosen und häufige Krankheitsbilder in der pädiatrischen Rheumatologie. In: Wagner N, Dannecker G, Kallinich T (Hrsg) Pädiatrische Rheumatologie. Springer, Berlin/Heidelberg, S 811–839

From Nail Bed Inflammation Straight to the Wheelchair— and When the Newborn No Longer Moves Its Leg

Moritz Klaas and Hermann Girschick

Contents

41.1 Medical History

Two cases are presented to outline various facets of bacterial osteomyelitis in children and adolescents.

▪▪ Ali

A 5-week-old infant had been favoring his left leg for 3 days, which was no longer actively moved. He had always been in good condition, without the presence of fever or other complaints. The peri- and postnatal course of the full-term newborn had been uncomplicated.

▪▪ Leo

The boy had repeatedly presented to the trauma surgeon due to acute pain in his left foot in the previous days. After an unremarkable X-ray, immobilization was recommended under the working diagnosis of an ankle sprain, even though the boy consistently denied any significant trauma. In addition, he had now had **fever up to 39 °C** for 3 days. Leo had been healthy so far, no previous illnesses were reported.

41.2 Examination Findings

▪▪ Ali

Upon examination, favoring of the left leg and slight thickening along the left knee joint were noticeable. The passive mobility of the joints was unremarkable. Furthermore, there was no overheating, no redness, and a regular pediatric-internal examination finding in a persistently fever-free child.

▪▪ Leo

13-year-old boy in significantly reduced general condition with swelling, overheating, limited mobility, and extreme sensitivity to touch in the area of the left upper ankle joint, which extended to the left lower leg up to halfway. The load on the left leg

was not tolerated. In addition, a **parony-chia** of the left big toe was noticeable. The remaining joint status as well as the pediatric-internal status were also unremarkable here.

41.3 Laboratory Values and Imaging

41.3.1 Laboratory Values

▪▪ Ali

The analysis of blood count, C-reactive protein (CRP), creatine kinase, and alkaline phosphatase showed no abnormalities.

▪▪ Leo

The laboratory analysis showed significantly increased inflammation parameters (**CRP 249 mg/l**, normal range < 5; **Erythrocyte sedimentation rate (ESR) 72 mm/h**, normal range <20; **Leukocytes 15/nl**, normal range 4–11.4) and mild **hyponatremia** (**130 mmol/l**, normal range 136–145).

41.3.2 Imaging

▪▪ Ali

In the musculoskeletal sonography, a round, approximately 7 mm in diameter **osteolysis** with hypoechoic to anechoic content could be demonstrated at the level of the distal lateral femoral epiphyseal plate on the left (◘ Fig. 41.1b, c) as well as surrounding echogenic soft tissue thickening (◘ Fig. 41.1a) along the distal femoral metaphysis (which ultimately corresponded to a subperiosteal abscess). Gonarthritis could be ruled out. The X-ray in 2 planes showed no discernible osteolysis or erosions and a regular representation of the epiphyseal nuclei (◘ Fig. 41.1d). Magnetic resonance imaging (MRI) confirmed the assessment of an abscessing osteomyelitis of the

41

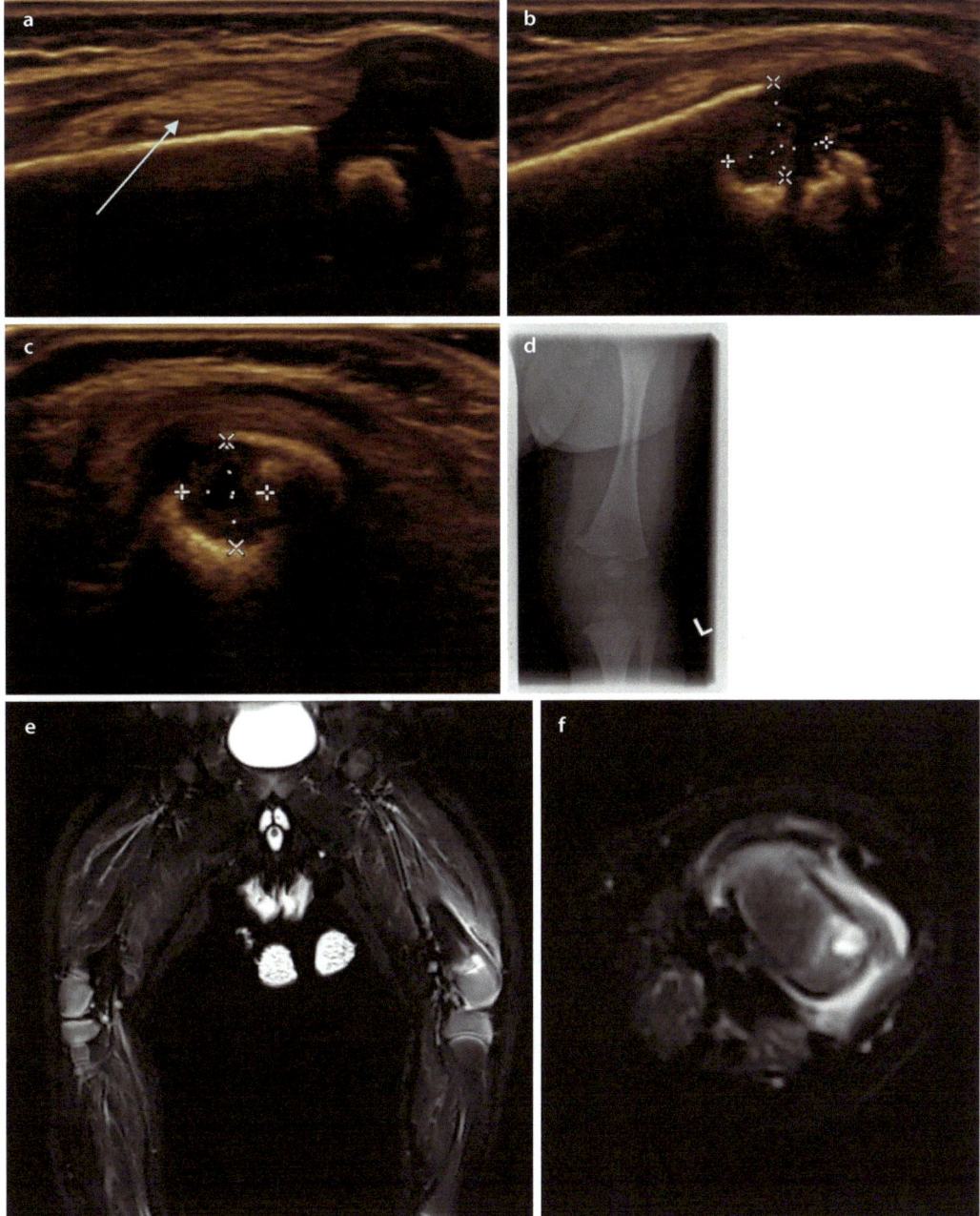

☐ **Fig. 41.1** **a–c** Sonography of the distal femur on the left, **d** conventional X-ray a.p., e,f MRI TIRM of Ali. **a–c** show along the epiphyseal plate a round erosion with hypoechoic content (**b,c**), a joint effusion in the area of the upper recessus is not demonstrable, however, an echogenic soft tissue inhibition along the distal femoral metaphysis, which we interpreted as a subperiosteal abscess (**a**, *arrow*). The X-ray showed a regular finding (**d**). In the strongly T2-weighted TIRM sequence with fat suppression, a signal intense round structure along the lateral epiphyseal plate with accompanying edema was shown transversely and frontally (**e,f**). (With kind permission from Prof. Dr. J. Wagner, Institute for Radiology and Interventional Therapy, Vivantes Klinikum im Friedrichshain, Berlin)

distal femur on the left, with a T1-hypointense and T2-hyperintense lesion along the lateral epiphyseal plate, faint marginal enhancement after contrast agent application and additional extension to the metaphysis (◘ Fig. 41.1e, f). In addition, there was intra- and intermuscular fluid accumulation of the lateral M. quadriceps femoris on the left as well as periosteal. The echocardiography and sonography of the skull were without pathological findings.

▪▪ Leo

The joint sonography was able to show arthritis with significant effusion and capsular distension in the area of the left upper ankle joint (◘ Fig. 41.2c). The conventional X-ray of the upper ankle joint showed no abnormalities (◘ Fig. 41.2a, b). In the transthoracic echocardiography, there was no evidence of valvular or endocardial vegetations.

41.4 Educational Questions

1. What are typical signs of a bacterial osteoarticular infection?
2. Which pathogens should empirical antibiotic therapy cover?
3. What should be considered in a musculoskeletal infection caused by *Kingella kingae*?
4. How long should bacterial osteomyelitis be treated with antibiotics?

41.5 Differential Diagnostic Considerations

In both cases, the working diagnosis of a bacterial infection of the musculoskeletal system was quickly established. Classically, the **Kocher criteria** (Kocher et al. 1999) are used to differentiate bacterial arthritis/osteomyelitis from reactive forms (e.g.,

Coxitis fugax). These include the inability to load the affected body part, the presence of fever (> 38.5 °C), leukocytosis (> 12/nl) in the blood count, and an acceleration of the ESR (> 40 mm/h). Here, a sensitivity of 93% or 99% is shown when 3 or 4 criteria are present, respectively.

In the second case, the classic picture of an **osteoarticular infection of the musculoskeletal system** was present, with all 4 Kocher criteria present. In the first case, however, only the pseudoparalysis of the left leg and a slight increase in the size of the knee joint were clinically and laboratory-chemically noticeable. The short duration of the disease and the age alone argued against the presence of a **chronic non-bacterial osteomyelitis** or a disease from the rheumatological spectrum. There were also no indications of a central nervous or traumatic origin of the movement restriction.

Possible further differential diagnoses could include trauma/abuse, a bone metabolism disorder or bone dysplasia for Ali, and malignancy, benign tumors, trauma, autoinflammation, and rare metabolic disorders such as hypophosphatasia for Leo.

41.6 Further Course Including Therapy

▪▪ Ali

Sonography-guided aspiration of the abscess content was performed and empirical therapy with ampicillin and gentamicin was started. In the bone punctate, *Streptococcus agalactiae* could be detected both culturally and molecular biologically, but not in the blood culture. During pregnancy care, the mother was found to have vaginal colonization with B streptococci and was given antibiotic prophylaxis in case of premature rupture of membranes. Even retrospectively, no signs of an early-onset neonatal infection could be identified from

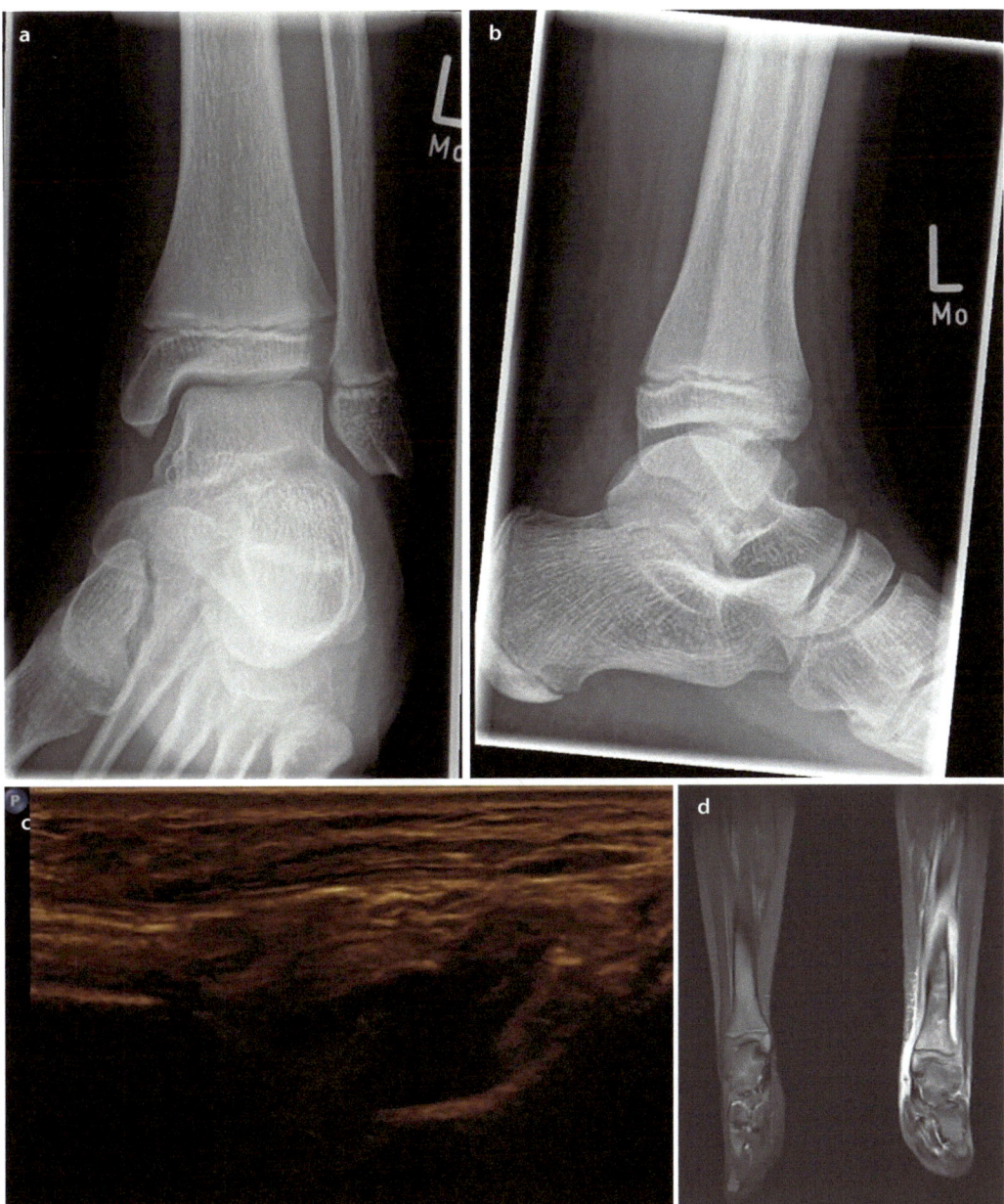

◨ **Fig. 41.2** **a,b** X-ray of Leo conventionally initial, **c** Sonography of the upper ankle joint initial, **d** MRI TIRM after 1 week of therapy, **e,f** X-ray conventionally after 6 months. Initially regular representation conventionally (**a,b**), however, sonographically significant effusion and capsular distension of the upper ankle joint (**c**). One week after the start of therapy, the strongly T2-weighted fat-suppressed TIRM sequence showed a signal intense inhomogeneous bone marrow signal of the distal half of the tibia with significant periosteal soft tissue edema (**d**). Radiologically, after 6 months, inhomogeneous bony structures could be shown without clear destructive changes or sequestration formation (**e, f**). (With kind permission from Prof. Dr. J. Wagner, Institute for Radiology and Interventional Therapy, Vivantes Klinikum im Friedrichshain, Berlin)

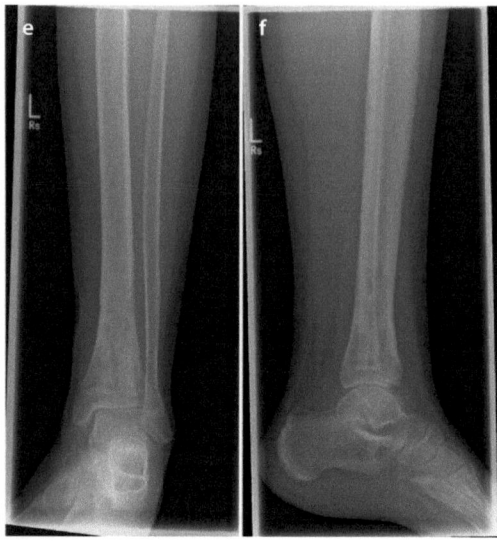

◘ Fig. 41.2 (continued)

the history. Due to the still quite young age and the present abscess formation, a total of 3 weeks of intravenous and subsequent 1 week of oral therapy with ampicillin or amoxicillin was carried out, with initial use of gentamicin for 3 days and clindamycin for 18 days i.v. In summary, the young infant had a **hematogenous osteomyelitis** in the area of the distal lateral femoral epiphyseal plate on the left, with a **subperiosteal abscess** and **accompanying myositis**, caused by *Streptococcus agalactiae* due to a late-onset neonatal infection. In the outpatient follow-up, there was a complete recovery, accompanied by age-appropriate development and percentile-appropriate and above all equal leg growth. The immunological immune defect diagnosis in the case of early major infection (lymphocyte subtyping, examination for granulocyte antibodies in case of transient neutropenia as well as the formation of general and specific antibodies and complement factors) gave no indication of the presence of a primary immune defect.

▪▪ Leo

An empirical intravenous therapy with Cefuroxim and Clindamycin was carried out, along with repeated arthroscopies and irrigations of the upper ankle joint. The MRI examination first performed on day 7 (◘ Fig. 41.2d) showed an increased inhomogeneous bone marrow signal of the lower half of the tibia extending into the distal epiphysis, with significant periosteal and soft tissue edema of the foot, indicative of a **diffuse osteomyelitis of the left tibia**. The arthritis of the upper ankle joint was fortunately no longer detectable on day 7. Due to persistent severe pain symptoms and persistent fever, further surgical cleanings were carried out, which included an anterograde marrow cavity drilling of the tibia, repeated lavages and Sulmycin inserts, as well as the treatment of the panaritium using Emmert plastic. From the samples of the upper ankle joint, tibia marrow cavity, big toe nail bed and blood culture, a **methicillin-sensitive Staphylococcus aureus (MSSA)** could be detected. This proved to be well sensitive to the antibiotics used in the test, but showed the **virulence factor Panton-Valentin-Leukocidin (PVL)**. PVL-producing staphylococci cause particularly invasive infections. By forming a pore-forming toxin, macrophages are lysed and human defense functions are significantly impaired (Shallcross et al. 2013). The very extensive findings of osteomyelitis and septic arthritis were certainly also due to this property. Therefore, we decided on a 6-week intravenous therapy (2 weeks Cefuroxim and Clindamycin, followed by 4 weeks Flucloxacillin). After 9 days of treatment, no bacterial growth could be detected for the first time from the samples taken and the inflammation parameters in the blood were well decreasing (CRP 71 mg/l, leukocytes 19/nl). The boy was fever-free from the 10th day of treatment. To eradicate the PVL-positive *Staphylococcus* *aureus*/MSSA, antiseptic washings were carried out, similar to colonization with a methicillin-resistant *Staphylococcus aureus* (**MRSA**). Due to the particularly protracted course of healing, we decided on a subsequent 4-week oral therapy with Cefuroxim.

On the basis of the considerable psychological stress, Leo developed a **pain amplification syndrome** with a **complex regional pain syndrome** (CRPS), with diffuse swelling, severe movement restriction, neuropathic pain, and anxiety. This required a multimodal pain therapy by the disciplines of pediatrics, trauma surgery, anesthesia, pain therapists, child and adolescent psychiatry, and physiotherapy, the use of epidural anesthesia, Metamizol, Ibuprofen, Morphine, Ketamine, Gabapentin, Risperidone and Tilidine, repeated dressing changes under analgosedation, and a 6-week follow-up treatment. Mobilization was not possible for a long time. In summary, there was a severe multifocal bacterial infection of the upper ankle joint in the form of a **septic arthritis** and the tibia as **osteomyelitis with periostitis** on the left, originating from a panaritium on the left big toe. The cause was a PVL-forming *Staphylococcus aureus*. The severe pain amplification problem with complex regional pain syndrome could be overcome. Over the next year, there was a steady improvement and achievement of remission. An X-ray control after 6 months (◘ Fig. 41.2e, f) still showed inhomogeneous bony structures in the area of the distal tibia without clearly destructive changes or sequestration. In the immunological diagnosis, there was **no indication** of an immunological defect (blood count, general and specific antibodies, immunoglobulin G subclasses, lymphocyte subpopulations and complement factors, leukocyte burst age-appropriate).

41.7 Educational Answers

- ### 1. What are typical signs of a bacterial osteoarticular infection?

Classically, children and adolescents with bacterial osteomyelitis develop a local painful restriction of movement/protective posture and also have fever, but not always. Laboratory chemistry shows leukocytosis as well as an increase in ESR and CRP.

- ### 2. Which pathogens should empirical antibiotic therapy cover?

The empirical antibiotic therapy for bacterial osteomyelitis depends on the age of the patient. In general, the therapy should be effective against staphylococci. The younger the children are, the more gram-negative germs must also be considered.

- ### 3. What should be considered in a musculoskeletal infection caused by *Kingella kingae*?

This gram-negative rod is increasingly detected in osteoarticular infections of toddlers thanks to improved detection methods. The clinical symptoms are considered milder compared to an infection with a *Staphylococcus aureus*. It is difficult to cultivate, which is why this bacterial species should always be considered in case of initially unsuccessful pathogen search. Long-term incubation of the punctate in aerobic blood culture bottles over 10 days or direct nucleic acid detection using PCR simplifies detection. *Kingella kingae* is sensitive to penicillins, 2nd and 3rd generation cephalosporins, but not to clindamycin.

- ### 4. How long should bacterial osteomyelitis be treated with antibiotics?

An uncomplicated bacterial osteomyelitis is usually treated for (2–)**3**(–4) weeks. The switch from the initial parenteral to oral therapy often occurs after a few days, given a good clinical and laboratory response (CRP, leukocytes). In very young infants, complicated or septic course, unusual pathogens (e.g., salmonella, tuberculosis) or locations (e.g., spine), an individual determination is made regarding the duration of the overall therapy and the intravenous portion (Saavedra-Lozano et al. 2017).

41.8 Summary

41.8.1 Etiology/Pathogenesis

Bacterial arthritis/osteomyelitis in children and adolescents predominantly occurs as a result of **hematogenous spread**. Occasionally, direct infection can occur due to foreign bodies, surgery, and trauma, or from the spread of an adjacent infection. The long tubular bones of the lower extremity are most commonly affected, followed by the humerus and less frequently the pelvis, spine, or tarsal bones. Multifocal involvement of several bones is rare. The further spread of the bone infection into the surrounding tissue or joint depends particularly on age, closure of the epiphyseal plate, and thickness of the compacta. Thus, in children under 2 years of age, due to the shared blood supply of the epiphysis from the metaphyseal arteries and the still quite thin compacta, osteomyelitis can spread both into the joint and continuously into the soft tissues, while with increasing age, after closure of the epiphyseal plate and separate vascular supply with still quite thin compacta, transfers into the soft tissue predominate (rarely also from there into the joint in intracapsular position). In adults, due to the thick bone cortex, a preferred spread through the epiphysis into the joint can result, whereas a subperiosteal abscess is rather unlikely.

The spectrum of pathogens differs particularly according to age and the presence of underlying diseases (◘ Table 41.1). Across all age groups, *Staphylococcus aureus* is most frequently detected, followed by *Streptococcus pyogenes*. Infections by *Streptococcus pneumoniae* and *Haemophilus influenzae* type B have receded due to specific vaccinations. In infants and toddlers, *Kingella kingae* is increasingly detected, whose diagnosis, although complicated by

◘ Table 41.1 Spectrum of pathogens in osteoarticular infections according to age and underlying disease (Saavedra-Lozano et al. 2017; Hospach et al. 2018a). The list of pathogens by possible frequencies has also been sorted for orientation within the individual age groups

Age	Pathogen
Infants (< 3 months)	*Staphylococcus aureus* Group B Streptococci *Escherichia coli* *Pseudomonas spp.* *Candida spp.* *Neisseria gonorrhoeae*
Infants and Toddlers	*Staphylococcus aureus* *Kingella kingae* Group A Streptococci Pneumococci *Haemophilus influenzae* Type B *Salmonella spp.*
Schoolchildren	*Staphylococcus aureus* Group A Streptococci *Neisseria gonorrhoeae*
Underlying Disease	
Leukemia/ Neutropenia	*Staphylococcus aureus* Gram-negative pathogens *Candida spp.*
Sickle Cell Disease	Mainly: *Salmonella spp.* *Escherichia coli*
Cellular Immune Defects	Among others: *Mycobacterium tuberculosis* Non-tuberculous mycobacteria

often mild laboratory inflammation and demanding cultivation, is reliably possible using molecular biological methods from the punctate. In newborns, group B streptococci and *Escherichia coli* are also found.

41.8.2 Clinic

Typically, an acute or subacute painful protective posture of the affected body part occurs. In addition, local (swelling, redness, and warmth) and systemic signs of inflammation (fever, impaired general condition) may be present. In infants and infections caused by *Kingella kingae*, the symptoms are often more subtle, making detection difficult. Therefore, the above-mentioned Kocher criteria are only indicative for the diagnosis of classic pus pathogens such as *Staphylococcus aureus*. An inadequately or too late treated osteomyelitis can cause **a bone necrosis**, **sequestrum**formation or destruction of the epiphyseal plate and joint cartilage (in arthritis) with subsequent growth disturbance and osteoarthritis.

41.8.3 Diagnosis

The focus is on the protective posture or pseudoparalysis and significant pain in the affected body region. In case of suspected bacterial osteomyelitis, differential blood count, CRP, and ESR are determined. Especially with classic pathogens, elevated inflammation parameters and a leukocytosis with left shift are detected. In addition, one or more **aerobic and anaerobic blood cultures**, in case of bacterial arthritis a **joint puncture**, and in case of osteomyelitis with abscess formation a **bone puncture** should be performed before starting therapy. Here, a minimally invasive procedure, a **mini arthrotomy**, and short-term drainage may be helpful (Saavedra-Lozano et al. 2017). Microbiological diagnosis is made by microscopy of the Gram stain and cultural cultivation. The diagnosis of difficult-to-cultivate pathogens (especially *Kingella kingae*), but also in case of already started antibiotic therapy, can be achieved by long-term incubation (up to 10 days) in blood culture bottles and nucleic acid analysis, e.g., by pathogen-specific polymerase chain reaction (PCR), from the punctate. Newer microbiological diagnostics based on **Next generation sequencing** can further increase the probability of detection. Furthermore, the analysis of cell count and differentiation of the joint punctate can indicate a bacterial infection.

Magnetic resonance imaging is the gold standard for the representation of a musculoskeletal infection and should be performed within the first week after the start of therapy. Sonography is quickly available and can quickly detect arthritis, subperiosteal and intramuscular abscesses, and periosteal soft tissue swelling, and can also be used for puncture. However, it is highly dependent on the examiner's experience and, unlike MRI, can only detect intraosseous changes to a very limited extent. Conventional X-rays cannot rule out osteomyelitis and are often inconspicuous in the acute course. Together with computed tomography, they are used to rule out other pathologies (such as bone tumors and fractures) or in the event of complications of osteomyelitis in the course (e.g., osteolysis and sequestrum). If there is suspicion of multifocal involvement, a whole-body MRI in TIRM technique is initially performed with gadolinium administration.

In case of complicated course or atypical germs, further **immunological and hematological diagnostics** should be carried out to rule out an immune defect. This should consider immune defects such as granulocytopenia, septic granulomatosis, an antibody deficiency, or sickle cell disease.

41.8.4 Therapy

Intravenous antibiotic therapy should be initiated immediately after sample collection and should not be delayed, for example, due to the unavailability of an MRI examination. This is initially done empirically, taking into account sufficient staphylococcal efficacy. Regional resistance patterns, e.g., origin from high-risk countries for MRSA and an underlying disease, should be considered. A proposal for empirical antibiotic therapy according to age, underlying disease, and MRSA prevalence in the population is listed in ◘ Table 41.2. It should be noted that particularly at the beginning of therapy, higher dosages are usually used.

After receiving the microbiological diagnosis with pathogen detection, targeted therapy is carried out. Classic applications are Flucloxacillin for *Staphylococcus aureus*/MSSA, Amoxicillin/Clavulanic acid or Cefuroxime for *Kingella kingae*. The total

◘ **Table 41.2** Empirical antibiotic therapy of osteoarticular infections according to age until the pathogen is identified (suggestion) (Saavedra-Lozano et al. 2017; Hospach et al. 2018). Higher dosages are usually used at the beginning of therapy

Age	Calculated Therapy	Intravenous Dosage
Infants (< 3 months)	Ampicillin + Gentamicin or Ampicillin + Cefotaxime	Ampicillin: 100–200 mg/kg BW in 3 single doses (SD) Gentamicin: 5 mg/kg BW in 1 SD Cefotaxime: 100–200 mg/kg BW in 3 SD
Infants (> 3 months) and toddlers	Cefuroxime + Clindamycin or Ampicillin/Sulbactam	Cefuroxime: 100–150 mg/kg BW in 3 SD Clindamycin: 20–40 mg/kg BW in 3 SD Ampicillin/Sulbactam: 100–150 mg/kg BW in 3 SD
School children	Cefuroxime + Clindamycin or Ampicillin/Sulbactam or Cefazolin	Cefazolin: 50–100 mg/kg BW in 2–3 SD **Dosage Adolescents:** Ampicillin/Sulbactam: 2.25–6.75 g in 3 SD Cefazolin: 2–6(–8) g in 2–3 SD Cefotaxime: 3–6 g in 3 SD Cefuroxime: 3–4.5(–6) g in 3 SD Clindamycin: 1.8–2.7 g in 3 SD Cotrimoxazole (p.o.): 320 mg Trimethoprim component in 2 SD Rifampicin (p.o.): 450–600 mg in 1–2 SD Vancomycin: 2(–3) g in 2–3 SD
MRSA prevalence > 10–15 %	Vancomycin (critically ill) or Clindamycin or Rifampicin or Cotrimoxazole (Consider combinations with a gram-negative effective antibiotic)	Vancomycin: 40–60 mg/kg BW in 2–3 SD Rifampicin (p.o.): 10–20 mg/kg BW in 1–2 SD Cotrimoxazole (p.o.): 6 mg Trimethoprim component/kg BW in 2 SD
Sickle cell disease	Cefotaxime + Clindamycin	Cefotaxime: 100–200 mg/kg BW in 3 SD

41

duration of therapy for bacterial osteomyelitis is (2–)3(–4) weeks. The switch to oral therapy can usually occur after a few days, given a good clinical response with stable defervescence, significant reduction of CRP (usually <20 mg/l), confirmed medication intake, and the possibility of follow-up checks (Saavedra-Lozano et al. 2017; Howard-Jones and Isaacs 2013; Hospach et al. 2018a, b). In Central Europe, this switch is usually possible after about 7 days. On the other hand, a lack of initial therapy response or a septic disease pattern may require therapy escalation and longer intravenous therapy. In the presence of pus, in addition to puncture, irrigation, osteotomy, abscess clearance, and possibly arthroscopy should be pursued.

A consistent therapy with nonsteroidal anti-rheumatic drugs has an analgesic effect and promotes recovery due to its anti-inflammatory effect. With the exception of vertebral body affection, long-term immobilization is usually not necessary. It is discussed whether adjuvant dexamethasone therapy (0.6 mg/kg body weight/day in 3–4 doses in the first 4 days) in the presence of bacterial arthritis can accelerate the healing of acute symptoms. However, there is no general recommendation for this (Saavedra-Lozano et al. 2017; Hospach et al. 2018a, b; Odio et al. 2003). The therapy should be coordinated interdisciplinary with the specialties of pediatrics, infectious diseases, microbiology, orthopedics, physiotherapy, etc.

41.8.5 Diagnosis

The wide clinical and laboratory chemical spectrum of bacterial osteomyelitis in children and adolescents is impressively demonstrated by both children, especially with regard to pathogens, age, laboratory chemical and systemic inflammation.

41.8.6 Prophylaxis

With adequate therapy, a complete recovery is to be expected. Regular follow-up checks should be ensured, especially in the first year, to detect defect healing (Hospach et al. 2018a; Odio et al. 2003). If *Staphylococcus aureus*/MRSA or a PVL-producing *Staphylococcus aureus* is detected, decolonization measures are carried out to reduce the germ load and the risk of a new invasive infection. If an underlying immune defect is relevant, then infection prophylaxis with antibiotics, immunoglobulin substitution, and possibly other measures in interdisciplinary care should also be considered.

> **Conclusion**
> Bacterial musculoskeletal infections can present differently depending on age and pathogen. Especially young children often develop only a few symptoms, such as pseudoparalysis, while classic signs (e.g., fever, fatigue, and increased inflammation values) are missing.

References

Hospach T, Hedrich C, Fernandez F, Girschick H, Borte M, Günther A, Martin L, Hahn G, von Kalle T, Horneff G, Kallinich T, Huppertz HI (2018a) Bakterielle Arthritis bei Kindern und Jugendlichen, Schwerpunkt Diagnostik. Monatsschr Kinderheilkd 166:141–147

Hospach T, Hedrich C, Fernandez F, Girschick H, Borte M, Günther A, Martin L, Hahn G, von Kalle T, Horneff G, Kallinich T, Huppertz HI (2018b) Bakterielle Arthritis bei Kindern und Jugendlichen, Schwerpunkt Therapie. Monatsschrift Kinderheilkunde. 166:239–248

Howard-Jones AR, Isaacs D (2013) Systematic review of duration and choice of systemic antibiotic therapy for acute haematogenous bacterial osteomyelitis in children. J Paediatr Child Health 49(9):760–768. ▶ https://doi.org/10.1111/jpc.12251

Kocher MS, Zurakowski D, Kasser JR (1999) Differentiating between septic arthritis and transient synovitis of the hip in children: an evidence-based clinical prediction algorithm. J Bone Joint Surg 81(12):1662–1670. ► https://doi.org/10.2106/00004623-199912000-00002

Odio CM, Ramirez T, Arias G, Abdelnour A, Hidalgo I, Herrera ML, Bolaños W, Alpízar J, Alvarez P (2003) Double blind, randomized, placebo-controlled study of dexamethasone therapy for hematogenous septic arthritis in children. Pediatr Infect Dis J 22(10):883–888. ► https://doi.org/10.1097/01.inf.0000091293.32187.7b

Saavedra-Lozano J, Falup-Pecurariu O, Faust SN, Girschick H, Hartwig N, Kaplan S, Lorrot M, Mantadakis E, Peltola H, Rojo P, Zaoutis T, Le-Mair A (2017) Bone and joint infections. Pediatr Infect Dis J 36(8):788–799. ► https://doi.org/10.1097/INF.0000000000001635

Shallcross LJ, Fragaszy E, Johnson AM, Hayward AC (2013) The role of the Panton-Valentine leucocidin toxin in staphylococcal disease: a systematic review and meta-analysis. Lancet Infect Dis 13:43–54. ► https://doi.org/10.1016/S1473-3099(12)70238-4

Bone Pain, Suspicion of Leukemia—And Yet the Blood Count is Unremarkable

Henner Morbach

Contents

42.1 Medical History

An 8-year-old boy suddenly developed a limping gait due to pain in both feet and lower legs. The complaints were mainly in the afternoon and intensified towards the evening. About a week after the onset of symptoms, swelling and discrete redness appeared in the area of both mid-feet, with emphasis on the left side. Due to increasing pain intensity, walking was no longer possible and the boy moved only by crawling. An X-ray of both feet taken during an orthopedic examination showed no abnormal findings. Analgesic/anti-inflammatory therapy with ibuprofen and local zinc paste bandage did not improve the symptoms. In addition, the attending pediatrician prescribed antibiotic therapy with amoxicillin-clavulanic acid for a possible bacterial infection. Due to the persistence of the symptoms, the boy was referred to the hospital for further investigation and treatment.

42.2 Examination Findings

Upon hospital admission, there was significant tenderness to pressure in the area of the metatarsals of both feet and slight swelling in the area of the tendon sheaths of the toe extensors. The rest of the joint status was unremarkable. The rest of the pediatric-internal examination findings were also unremarkable. There were no elevated body temperatures.

42.3 Laboratory Values and Imaging

42.3.1 Laboratory Values

The blood count showed a discrete **leukopenia** with **3100 leukocytes/μl** (55% neutrophils, 42% lymphocytes, 3% monocytes) with normal Hb (12.5 g/dl) and age-appropriate platelet count (282,000/μl). The **inflammatory parameters** were slightly **elevated (CRP 1.6 mg/dl; ESR 35 mm/h; ferritin 174 μg/l)**. The overview values of clinical chemistry (electrolytes, renal retention parameters, transaminases, cell decay parameters) were unremarkable.

42.3.2 Imaging

An MRI of both feet (◘ Fig. 42.1a–d) showed multiple lesions with hyperintense signal in the TIRM sequence (◘ Fig. 42.1a, c), hypointense signal in the T1 sequence, and increased contrast uptake in the inflammatory regions, but also inhomogeneous fat distribution e.g. in the calcaneus and in the distal tibia (◘ Fig. 42.1b, d).

42.4 Educational Questions

1. How do you interpret the current laboratory diagnostics and imaging diagnostics in terms of possible differential diagnoses?
2. Would you initiate further diagnostic measures?

42.5 Differential Diagnostic Considerations

The clinical symptoms (**bone pain**) and imaging diagnostics (bone edema with contrast uptake) first suggest an osteomyelitis. Despite normal body temperatures and only slightly elevated inflammatory parameters, an infectious cause cannot be ruled out. In addition to an infection by *Staphylococcus aureus* or *Kingella kingae*, tuberculosis should also be included in the differential diagnostic considerations. As a non-infectious cause of inflammatory bone changes, chronic non-bacterial osteomyelitis (CNO) is certainly a consideration. Rarer

TIRM   **T1 + contrast agent**

left

right

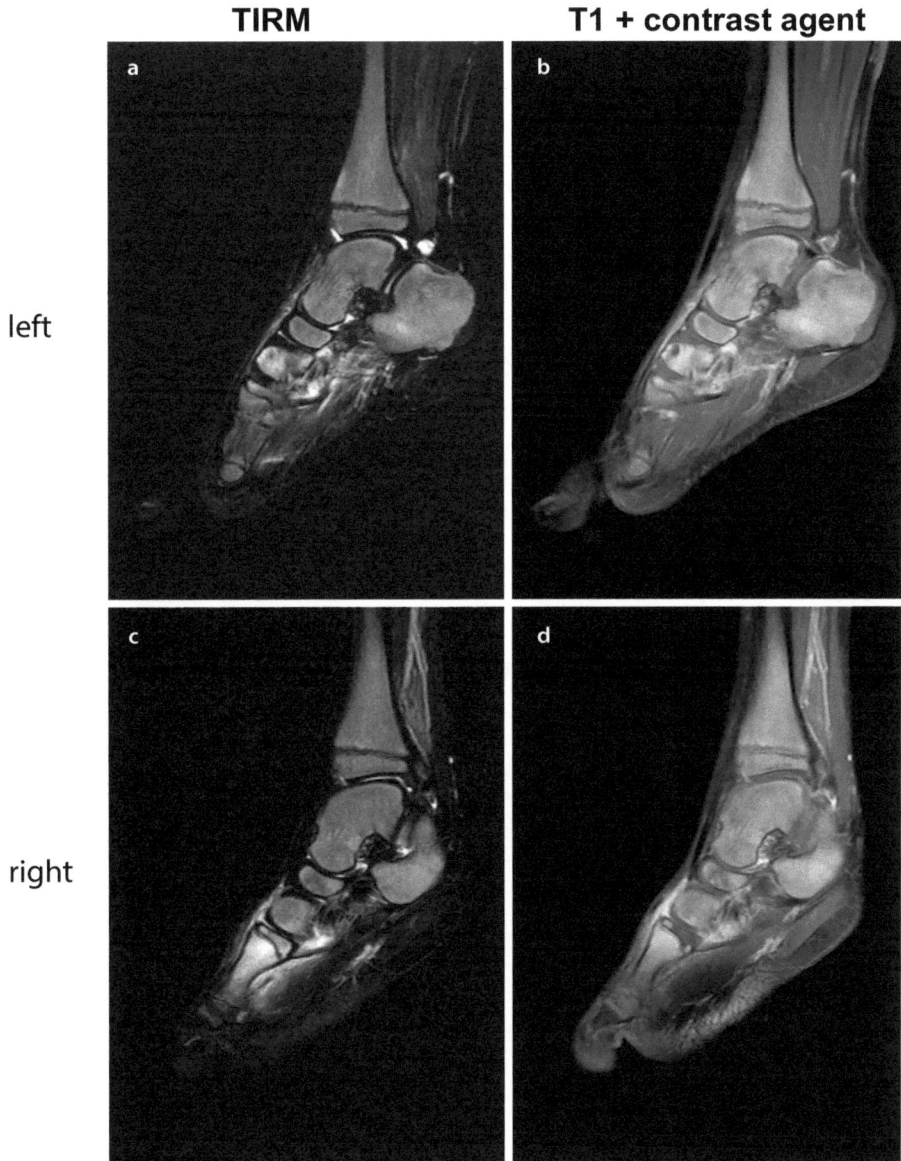

◘ **Fig. 42.1** **a–d** MRI diagnostics for unclear joint and bone pain. **a,c** show fat-saturated, strongly T2-weighted MRI sequences (TIRM) of both feet with noticeable bone edema in the midfoot on both sides, furthermore some effusion in the left ankle joint, mild periostitis in the right midfoot. **b,d** show the corresponding T1-weighted sequences after contrast agent uptake

differential diagnoses that can resemble osteomyelitis in MRI imaging are e.g. bone metabolism disorders (e.g. hypophosphatasia), although the late manifestation and acute onset are atypical for this. In the case of load-related changes, bone edema can also be depicted in MRI. Malignant hematological diseases and bone tumors are another important differential diagnosis for unclear bone and joint pain.

42.6 Further Progress

Due to a bacterial genesis of osteomyelitis that could not be definitively ruled out, the antibiotic therapy was initially continued intravenously. The anti-inflammatory therapy with ibuprofen was also continued. A bone biopsy was not performed due to prior antibiotic treatment. The blood cultures remained sterile. On the 3rd day of treatment, the boy developed arthritis in both elbow joints with pronounced effusion and limited mobility (◘ Fig. 42.2). The MRI of the elbow joints showed effusion without evidence of bone involvement. The puncture of the left elbow joint showed a granulocytic cell image, the cultural and molecular biological microbiological diagnostics could not detect any pathogens.

In the course of further follow-up checks of the laboratory values, a decrease in CRP was observed, but with persistent **leukopenia** (minimal 2100/μl). No morphological abnormalities could be detected in the microscopic examination of the blood smear. A bone marrow puncture was performed for differential diagnostic clarification of the leukopenia. Here, the microscopic examination of the smear showed a high proportion of lymphoblastic cells (about 40%), so the suspected diagnosis of acute lymphoblastic leukemia (ALL) was made. The flow cytometric analysis confirmed the suspected diagnosis and assigned

TIRM   **T1 + contrast agent**

◘ Fig. 42.2   **a, b** MRI diagnostics for unclear joint and bone pain. **a** shows a fat-saturated, strongly T2-weighted MRI sequence (TIRM) of the left elbow with effusion. **b** shows the corresponding T1-weighted sequence with increased contrast agent uptake in the area of the synovia the leukemia to a pre-B-cell ALL. In the retrospective examination of 3 smears of peripheral blood made up to the time of diagnosis, at least one suspect lymphatic cell could be identified in one smear with "complete" review, but ultimately there was still a state of **aleukemic leukemia**, which had not been washed out into the peripheral blood.

42.7 Educational Answers

■ **1. How do you interpret the previous laboratory diagnostics and imaging diagnostics with regard to possible differential diagnoses?**

Bacterial osteomyelitis can rarely manifest with multifocal lesions. However, the symmetrical pattern of involvement in the patient with multiple lesions in the area of the distal lower legs and feet is rather atypical for an infectious origin. Here, a CNO would be more likely to be considered (Girschick et al. 2018). The slightly elevated inflammation values are consistent with a CNO. Load-related changes in the bone can also be noticeable in MRI due to bone marrow edema. However, the sometimes very focal accentuated lesions in the patient ultimately appeared atypical for this differential diagnosis.

Due to the noticeable divergence between elevated humoral inflammation parameters (CRP) and simultaneous leukopenia in the laboratory tests, disorders of hematopoiesis should also be included in the differential diagnostic considerations. The **Majeed syndrome** is a very rare, monogenetically caused disease with the occurrence of non-bacterial osteomyelitis and disturbed hematopoiesis, with dyserythropoietic anemia being predominant (Morbach et al. 2013). Malignant hematological diseases are far more common causes of unclear bone and joint pain. In addition to nonspecific bone pain, manifest rheumatic symptoms can also occur as a symptom of a **leu-**

kemia and initially lead to the diagnosis of an inflammatory rheumatic disease, such as reactive arthritis, juvenile idiopathic arthritis or osteomyelitis (Brix et al. 2022; Brix et al. 2020; Louvigne et al. 2020; Marwaha et al. 2010; Tsujioka et al. 2018). In some of these patients, signs of arthritis and/or osteomyelitis can be detected in imaging (�‍ Fig. 42.3) (Tsujioka et al. 2018). In addition to hepatosplenomegaly, cytopenia of

T1

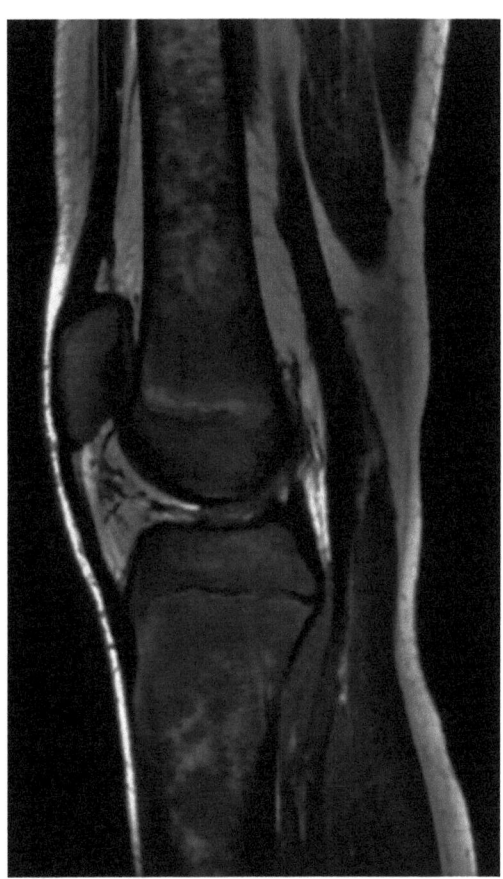

◘ **Fig. 42.3** MRI diagnostics for unclear joint and bone pain. The image shows a T1-weighted MRI sequence of the distal femur and the proximal tibia with band-like to diffusely speckled changes in the epiphyseal metaphyses in a child with leukemia

one or more cell lines is particularly suspicious of the presence of a malignant hematological disease, with cases of inconspicuous blood count in the sense of aleukemic leukemia as described in our patient (Brix et al. 2022; Louvigne et al. 2020; Tsujioka et al. 2018).

- **2. Would you initiate further diagnostic measures?**

To clarify an infectious origin in suspected osteomyelitis, identification of the pathogen should be sought. Blood cultures should always be taken here, in addition, a biopsy with cultural and molecular biological pathogen search should be considered. Since the patient had already received antibiotic pretreatment, a biopsy in the foot area was waived considering the expected information gain and possible risks and side effects. Since this also did not result in a histological examination of the T2 signal conspicuous lesions detected in the MRI, their origin ultimately remains unclear. It would be discussed whether these are inflammatory lesions in the sense of a paraneoplastic symptom or a bone marrow infiltration of the leukemia. In leukemia, MRI typically shows T1-hypointense and T2-hyperintense band-like to diffusely speckled changes in the epiphyseal metaphyses (◘ Fig. 42.3). In the case of bone and/or joint pain of unclear origin, a malignant hematological disease should always be considered as the cause and the examination of a differential blood count should be indicated. The differential blood count does not always have to show pancytopenia in the presence of leukemia and can even show only discrete or even no abnormalities in the white row in aleukemic forms. Especially in the case of bone pain that cannot be assigned to a joint, unclear bone (marrow) lesions in MRI and/or cytopenias, a bone marrow puncture should be carried out for differential diagnostic clarification (Fordham et al. 2022). Ultimately,

however, a leukemia could also remain undetected here, should the spread of the malignant disease in absolutely rare cases not yet have covered all areas of the bone marrow.

42.8 Summary

42.8.1 Etiology

ALL is a malignant disease that originates from immature precursors of lymphocytes. It is the most common form of leukemia in childhood.

42.8.2 Pathogenesis/Clinic

Bone pain is a common symptom of leukemia and occurs in about 30–40% of children. About 10% develop arthritis and/or osteomyelitis prior to diagnosis, initially suggesting the diagnosis of a rheumatic disease.

42.8.3 Therapy

The initial treatment of ALL is carried out using glucocorticoids and chemotherapy, in cases of central nervous system involvement also in combination with radiation therapy. Depending on the presence of molecular risk factors and the response to therapy, an allogeneic stem cell transplantation is carried out during the course to intensify the therapy.

42.8.4 Diagnosis

An abnormal differential blood count can indicate leukemia, the diagnosis is confirmed by an examination of the bone marrow.

Conclusion

Leukemia can manifest itself not only through nonspecific bone pain but also through arthritis and/or osteomyelitis. The differential blood count is an important diagnostic tool, but despite existing "leukemia", it can sometimes only show nonspecific, not yet indicative changes.

References

Brix N, Rosthoj S, Glerup M, Hasle H, Herlin T (2020) Identifying acute lymphoblastic leukemia mimicking juvenile idiopathic arthritis in children. PLoS One 15(8):e0237530. ▶ https://doi.org/10.1371/journal.pone.0237530

Brix N, Amstrup J, Norgaard M, Hagstrom S, Hasle H, Herlin T (2022) Musculoskeletal diagnoses before cancer in children: a Danish registry-based cohort study. J Pediatr 242:32–38 e32. ▶ https://doi.org/10.1016/j.jpeds.2021.11.024

Fordham NJ, Bartram J, Ghorashian S, O'Connor D, Taylor A, Sibson K, Rao A, Pavasovic V, Cheng D, Ancliff P, Vora A, Samarasinghe S (2022) What is the diagnostic yield of bone marrow aspiration to exclude leukaemia prior to systemic treatment in juvenile idiopathic arthritis? Br J Haematol 199(3):447–451. ▶ https://doi.org/10.1111/bjh.18413

Girschick H, Finetti M, Orlando F, Schalm S, Insalaco A, Ganser G, Nielsen S, Herlin T, Kone-Paut I, Martino S, Cattalini M, Anton J, Mohammed Al-Mayouf S, Hofer M, Quartier P, Boros C, Kuemmerle-Deschner J, Pires Marafon D, Alessio M, Schwarz T, Ruperto N, Martini A, Jansson A, Gattorno M, Paediatric Rheumatology International Trials O, the Eurofever r (2018) The multifaceted presentation of chronic recurrent multifocal osteomyelitis: a series of 486 cases from the Eurofever international registry. Rheumatology (Oxford) 57(8):1504. ▶ https://doi.org/10.1093/rheumatology/key143

Louvigne M, Rakotonjanahary J, Goumy L, Tavenard A, Brasme JF, Rialland F, Baruchel A, Auclerc MF, Despert V, Desgranges M, Jean S, Faye A, Meinzer U, Lorrot M, Job-Deslandre C, Bader-Meunier B, Gandemer V, Pellier I, Group G (2020) Persistent osteoarticular pain in children: early clinical and laboratory findings suggestive of acute lymphoblastic leukemia (a multicenter case-control study of 147 patients). Pediatr Rheumatol Online J 18(1):1. ▶ https://doi.org/10.1186/s12969-019-0376-8

Marwaha RK, Kulkarni KP, Bansal D, Trehan A (2010) Acute lymphoblastic leukemia masquerading as juvenile rheumatoid arthritis: diagnostic pitfall and association with survival. Ann Hematol 89(3):249–254. ▶ https://doi.org/10.1007/s00277-009-0826-3

Morbach H, Hedrich CM, Beer M, Girschick HJ (2013) Autoinflammatory bone disorders. Clin Immunol 147(3):185–196. ▶ https://doi.org/10.1016/j.clim.2012.12.012

Tsujioka T, Sugiyama M, Ueki M, Tozawa Y, Takezaki S, Ohshima J, Cho Y, Yamada M, Iguchi A, Kobayashi I, Ariga T (2018) Difficulty in the diagnosis of bone and joint pain associated with pediatric acute leukemia; comparison with juvenile idiopathic arthritis. Mod Rheumatol 28(1):108–113. ▶ https://doi.org/10.1080/14397595.2017.1332474

Severe Bone Pain and Subfebrile Temperatures— Osteomyelitis?

Henner Morbach

Contents

43.1 Medical History

A 12-year-old girl with known homozygous sickle cell disease presents to the emergency room due to severe pain in her right upper arm, which has been present for 3 days. The pain has not been well controlled with ibuprofen analgesic therapy. Since the morning of admission, she has had subfebrile temperatures. No trauma is remembered. A few days ago, she had exerted her arm more while bowling.

The patient is connected to a hematological outpatient clinic due to her sickle cell disease. In the past, there were repeated episodes of severe pain in the musculoskeletal system. For about 3 years, the patient has been taking a continuous therapy with hydroxycarbamide. In addition, a continuous antibiotic prophylaxis with penicillin is taken.

43.2 Examination Findings

The joint status is unremarkable and without signs of active arthritis. There is general pain in the area of the right upper arm, which intensifies under local pressure. There is no swelling and/or redness in this area. The spleen can be felt about 2 cm below the rib arch. A slight **scleral icterus** is noticeable. The body temperature is 38.8 °C.

43.3 Laboratory Values and Imaging

43.3.1 Laboratory Values

The blood count shows a **normochromic-normocytic anemia** with an **Hb of 8.8 g/dl**. The **inflammatory parameters** are initially slightly elevated (CRP 2.8 mg/dl; ESR 25 mm/h) and significantly increased the day after next **(CRP 16.2 mg/dl)**. There is a hyperbilirubinemia (total bilirubin 3.9 mg/dl, direct bilirubin 0.5 mg/dl) and an **increased activity of LDH** (589 U/l, reference 110–330). Transaminases, ALP and GGT were unremarkable. The **ferritin** was slightly elevated at **209 μg/l** (reference 9–59).

43.3.2 Imaging

In the MRI of the right arm, an extensive **medullary bone marrow edema** in the **diaphysis of the humerus** throughout its course, in addition to a **periosteal edema with contrast uptake** in the sense of periostitis (❏ Fig. 43.1). After contrast administration, the **proximal third of the diaphysis shows no contrast uptake** with preserved cortex. The middle and distal diaphysis shows contrast uptake. The other surrounding soft tissues and bones were unremarkable. An X-ray of the right upper arm showed no localized osteolysis or cortical destruction in the area of the humerus.

43.4 Educational Questions

1. How do you interpret the clinical symptoms and imaging findings, also considering the underlying disease?
2. What therapy would you initiate?

43.5 Differential Diagnostic Considerations

Localized bone pain and fever with simultaneously elevated inflammatory parameters are highly suspicious of a **bacterial osteomyelitis**. The detection of bone marrow edema in the MRI supports this suspected diagnosis. However, the lack of contrast uptake in part of the lesion is noticeable. This could be a bone sequestration or abscess formation in the context of bacterial

TIRM   T1 + contrast agent   X-ray

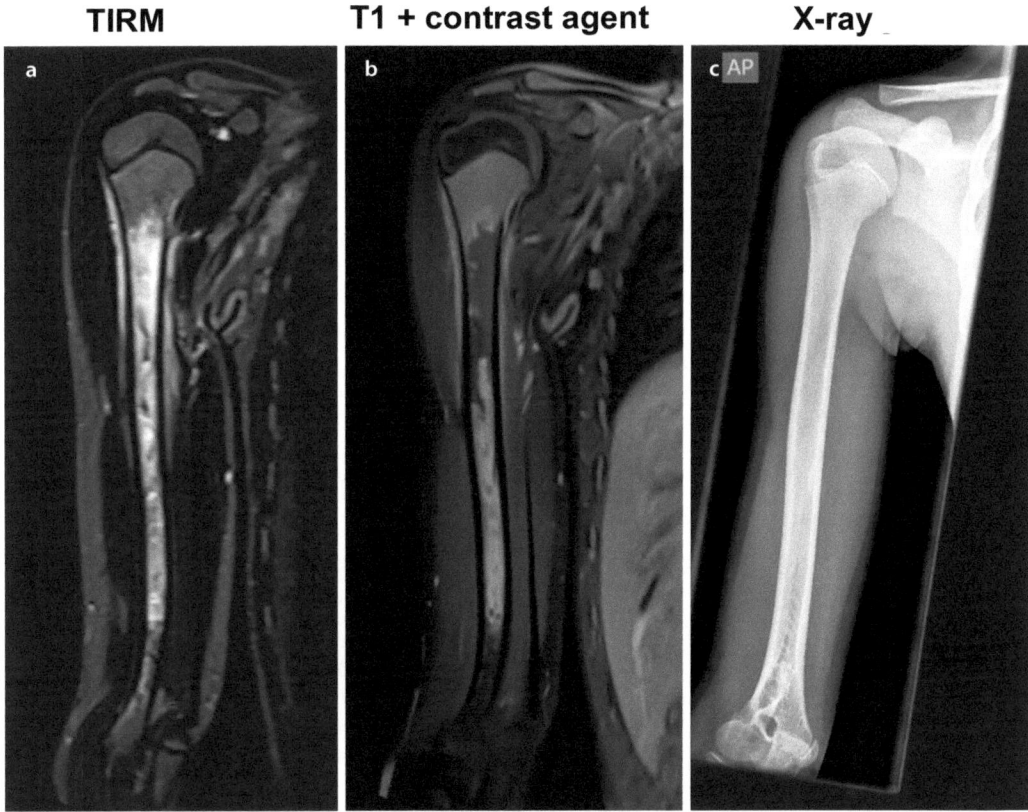

☐ **Fig. 43.1   a, b** MRI and X-ray diagnostics for bone pain. **a** shows a fat-saturated, strongly T2-weighted MRI sequence (TIRM) of the right humerus with noticeable diaphyseal bone edema. **b** shows corresponding T1 sequences after application of contrast medium with increased contrast uptake in the distal two thirds of the lesion and lack of contrast uptake in the proximal third of the lesion. **c** showed an X-ray of the right humerus with at most slight increase in transparency at the transition from the proximal to the middle third of the humerus diaphysis without localized osteolysis or cortical destruction

osteomyelitis. On the other hand, a **bone infarction** in the context of a **microcirculation disorder** in sickle cell disease could also produce this image.

43.6 Further Course

Under the initial suspicion of bacterial osteomyelitis, intravenous antibiotic therapy with cefotaxime was started. In the initially taken blood culture, **Salmonella** of group B (*Salmonella Typhimurium*) were detected, which were subsequently also detectable in a stool sample. With the continuation of the antibiotic therapy, the inflammation parameters decreased, and the fever subsided. Parallel to the antibiotic therapy, infusion therapy was started to improve rheological conditions. In addition, analgesic therapy was carried out, initially with piritramide and later solely with ibuprofen. The intravenous antibiotic therapy with cefotaxime was administered for a total of 2 weeks and was converted into an oral sequence therapy with ciprofloxacin for another 4 weeks.

15 months after this episode, the patient presented again with severe pain, this time localized in the lumbar spine area and the right shoulder. There was no fever. The inflammation parameters were elevated (CRP max. 6.9 mg/dl). In the whole-body MRI, disseminated osseous signal alterations with corresponding contrast enhancement and partly periosteal reaction zones were noticeable. Lesions were found in the spinous and transverse processes of several vertebral bodies, in the manubrium sterni, in the lateral clavicle on the right, in individual ribs, the proximal humeri on both sides, and in the right ilium (◘ Fig. 43.2). Due to the multiple lesions and sterile blood culture, these lesions were most likely interpreted in the context of microcirculation disorders/incipient bone infarctions, and infusion therapy to improve rheology and pain therapy was started. However, since bacterial osteomyelitis could not be ruled out based on imaging, additional antibiotic therapy was administered.

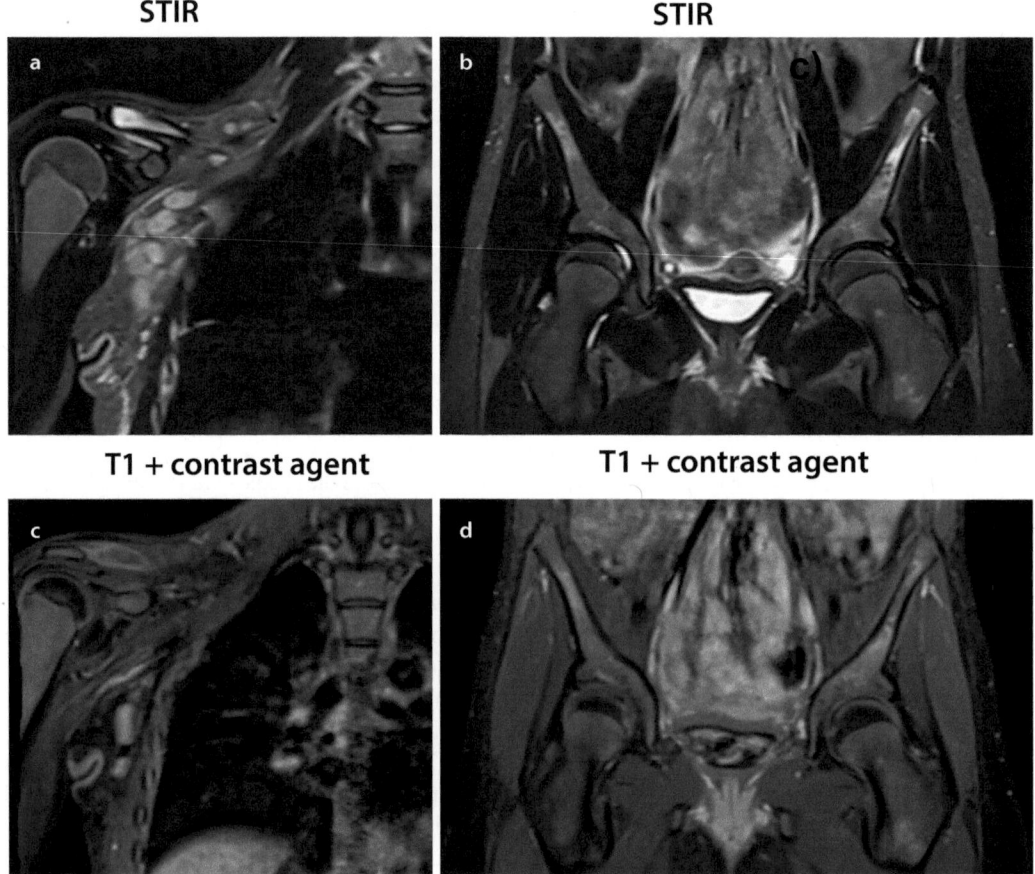

◘ **Fig. 43.2**   **a–d** MRI diagnostics for bone pain. **a** and **b** show a fat-saturated MRI sequence (STIR) of the right shoulder girdle and the pelvis with edema formation in the area of the clavicle as well as the ilium and the proximal femur. **c** and **d** show the corresponding T1-weighted sequence with increased contrast agent uptake in the area of the lesions

43

43.7 Educational Responses

■ **1. How do you interpret the clinical symptoms and imaging findings, also considering the underlying disease?**

The patient has sickle cell disease as an underlying condition. This is an autosomal recessive blood disorder characterized by altered hemoglobin (Kavanagh et al. 2022). This is particularly prone to polymerization in erythrocytes in the deoxygenated state, which restricts their deformability. A shortening of the lifespan of erythrocytes with chronic hemolysis and microcirculatory disorders in the capillary bed with resulting infarcts are the consequence. Inflammatory processes are also involved in the vascular occlusions, mediated by substances released by hemolysis, among other things (Ofori-Acquah 2020). Infarcts can occur in all organs, especially bone marrow infarcts manifest with severe pain (**"pain crises"**). Frequently affected are bones containing a lot of bone marrow, such as the long tubular bones, the vertebral bodies, and the sternum. In infants and toddlers, dactylitis (**hand-foot syndrome**) is a common manifestation of the osseous microcirculatory disorder (Kavanagh et al. 2022). As a complication of circulatory disorders, **avascular bone necrosis** can develop. The hip joint (femoral head necrosis) and shoulder joint (femoral head necrosis) are particularly predisposed to this.

Patients with sickle cell disease have a **significantly increased risk of severe bacterial infections**, which is explained, among other things, by a progressive dysfunction of the spleen during the course of the disease (Kavanagh et al. 2022). Pneumococci, meningococci, but also salmonella, *Haemophilus influenzae*, and staphylococci are common infectious agents in these patients (Narang et al. 2012; Ochocinski et al. 2020). The bones are a common site of bacterial infections. Salmonella is a typical infectious

agent and is more common than *Staphylococcus aureus* (Kaplan et al. 2019). However, distinguishing between a microcirculatory disorder with an incipient bone marrow infarct and osteomyelitis can often be difficult, as in the case of the patient described here. Pain crises due to microcirculatory disorders are much more common in sickle cell disease than bacterial osteomyelitis. However, the reduced blood flow in the bone caused by the microcirculatory disorder can also pave the way for bacterial osteomyelitis. Similarly, iatrogenic iron overload in patients with sickle cell disease can promote increased susceptibility to infection with siderophilic bacteria, with some bacteria also able to utilize the host's ferritin-stored iron for their own use (Nairz et al. 2010)

■ **2. What therapy would you initiate?**

In the case of the patient described, the treatment goals are aimed at treating bacterial osteomyelitis, pain, and the bone's microcirculatory disorder (Brandow and Liem 2022). In suspected bacterial osteomyelitis in patients with sickle cell disease, the typical spectrum of pathogens for the disease with susceptibility to salmonella must be considered. Cefotaxime or ciprofloxacin are suitable antibiotics. For adequate pain therapy in sickle cell disease pain crises, paracetamol and/or ibuprofen are usually not sufficient, so analgesic therapy with morphine should be initiated promptly. Intravenous fluid administration of about 1.5–2 l/ m^2 BSA/day is intended to improve the rheology of the blood and thus the microcirculatory disorders.

Transfusions of erythrocyte concentrates are an important part of treatment for certain acute complications with severe anemia as well as under defined indications in long-term treatment, e.g., in the prophylaxis of strokes (Han et al. 2021). Transfusions can lead to improved oxygen supply to the tissue, but also increase the viscosity of the blood. Transfusions are not generally indicated for the acute treatment of pain crises. Hydroxyurea is used as long-term therapy in sickle cell disease to reduce the occurrence of pain crises. Hydroxyurea increases the synthesis of fetal hemoglobin, which in turn prevents polymer formation in sickle hemoglobin. The prevention of local hypoxemia (e.g., due to cold) should be avoided. Allogeneic stem cell therapy is recommended/considered as a curative treatment option if there is an HLA-identical sibling as a stem cell donor.

43.8 Summary

43.8.1 Etiology

Recurrent pain crises, bone infarctions, and bacterial osteomyelitis in the context of sickle cell disease.

43.8.2 Pathogenesis/Clinic

Sickle-shaped erythrocytes lead to blockages in the smallest vessels, resulting in subsequent microcirculation disorders. Bones are particularly often affected by these vascular occlusions, which can lead to bone infarctions.

43.8.3 Therapy

Intravenous fluid therapy to improve the rheological situation. Adequate pain therapy, where ibuprofen usually does not have sufficient potency and opioid analgesics are used early. In case of suspected bacterial osteomyelitis, rapid and consistent antibiotic therapy is additionally required. There is often no general indication for erythrocyte concentrates for the primary treatment

of the pain crisis. However, if there are indications of a vaso-occlusion and subsequent local tissue ischemia, the indication for this should be checked. The aim is to improve the supply of oxygen in the tissue in order to avoid the irreversible sickling of the erythrocytes as much as possible. The vascular inflammation processes in the context of vaso-occlusion are increasingly being discussed as a therapeutic target in sickle cell disease.

43.8.4 Diagnosis

The diagnosis is based on clinical symptoms and imaging (MRI).

> **Conclusion**
> Microcirculation disorders with subsequent painful bone infarctions are typical symptoms of sickle cell disease. The differentiation from bacterial osteomyelitis is sometimes difficult.

References

Brandow AM, Liem RI (2022) Advances in the diagnosis and treatment of sickle cell disease. J Hematol Oncol 15(1):20. ▶ https://doi.org/10.1186/s13045-022-01237-z

Han H, Hensch L, Tubman VN (2021) Indications for transfusion in the management of sickle cell disease. Hematology Am Soc Hematol Educ Program 2021(1):696–703. ▶ https://doi.org/10.1182/hematology.2021000307

Kaplan J, Ikeda S, McNeil JC, Kaplan SL, Vallejo JG (2019) Microbiology of osteoarticular infections in patients with sickle hemoglobinopathies at Texas Children's Hospital, 2000–2018. Pediatr Infect Dis J 38(12):1251–1253. ▶ https://doi.org/10.1097/INF.0000000000002478

Kavanagh PL, Fasipe TA, Wun T (2022) Sickle cell disease: a review. JAMA 328(1):57–68. ▶ https://doi.org/10.1001/jama.2022.10233

Nairz M, Schroll A, Sonnweber T, Weiss G (2010) The struggle for iron – a metal at the host-pathogen interface. Cell Microbiol 12(12):1691–1702. ▶ https://doi.org/10.1111/j.1462-5822.2010.01529.x

Narang S, Fernandez ID, Chin N, Lerner N, Weinberg GA (2012) Bacteremia in children with sickle hemoglobinopathies. J Pediatr Hematol Oncol 34(1):13–16. ► https://doi.org/10.1097/MPH.0b013e318240d50d

Ochocinski D, Dalal M, Black LV, Carr S, Lew J, Sullivan K, Kissoon N (2020) Life-threatening infectious complications in sickle cell disease: a concise narrative review. Front Pediatr 8:38. ► https://doi.org/10.3389/fped.2020.00038

Ofori-Acquah SF (2020) Sickle cell disease as a vascular disorder. Expert Rev Hematol 13(6):645–653. ► https://doi.org/10.1080/17474086.2020.1758555

A 7-Year-Old Patient with Known Leukodystrophy and Skin Abnormalities

Christiane Reiser

Contents

© The Author(s), under exclusive license to Springer-Verlag GmbH, DE, part of Springer Nature 2024
C. Huemer and H. Girschick (eds.), *Clinical Examples in Pediatric Rheumatology*,
https://doi.org/10.1007/978-3-662-68732-1_44

44.1 Medical History

A 7-year-old severely developmentally de-layed patient with a rare infantile, usually fatal in early childhood form of leukodys-trophy is admitted to the hospital due to in-creasing restlessness. The following addi-tional points are asked in the medical history:

Skin/Joints: The parents reported that for several months after an antibiotic ther-apy for urinary tract infection, non-itchy "spots" existed on the arms, which were in-terpreted as "allergy". Two weeks before admission, the rash spread to the entire body except for the feet, hands, and back. The presentation in the emergency depart-ment of a children's hospital suggested a vi-ral **exanthem** (◘ Fig. 44.1). In addition, a swelling of both dorsum of the feet had oc-curred a few days ago, which was referred to as "edema". A swelling of the right knee has been present for about 2 months.

Bleeding tendency: Furthermore, in-creased **gum bleeding** has been reported for a few days, no nosebleeds, no noticeable he-matoma formation. Fresh blood overlay has been detectable for years in known con-stipation.

Susceptibility to infection: The last uri-nary tract infection occurred 5 months ago and was treated with antibiotics. Since a tooth extraction surgery 6 weeks ago, recur-rent elevated temperature.

Neurology: No seizures for 4-5 years. The patient has "unlearned" many skills in the last year, e.g., crawling and sitting up independently. Spasticity has increased in recent months.

Current therapy: Ibuprofen as needed, Baclofen 5 mg due to increased spastic-ity for a week, Sultiam 50 mg twice a day, Movicol.

44.2 Examination Findings

7 ½-year-old girl in reduced general con-dition, very restless, reacts defensively to touches on the legs. Known spasticity and developmental delay. Weight 20.9 kg, length 103 cm, head circumference 51.2 cm. Blood pressure 110/75 mmHg, heart rate: 138/min, temperature: 37.5 °C. Skin: nu-merous **purpura**-like efflorescences, **perifolli-cular**, slightly swollen knee joints, edema on both dorsum of the feet. Cor/Pulmo/Abdo-men: unremarkable, large hematoma (5 cm) perianal, 2nd degree hemorrhoids. ENT: Gum hyperplasia, gum bleeding. Throat ring not reddened, oral mucosa moist.

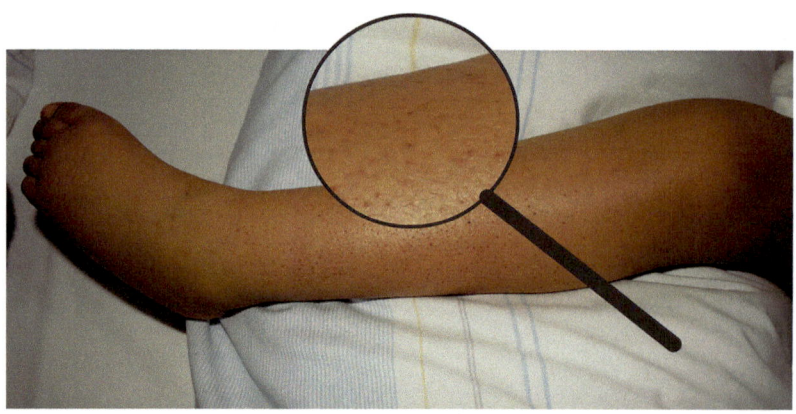

◘ **Fig. 44.1**   Cutaneous findings: Follicular petechiae clearly visible in the magnifying glass

Upon admission, **petechiae** (■ Fig. 44.1) and **gingival hyperplasia** of unclear etiology (■ Fig. 44.2a, b) were observed. The examination findings then additionally revealed knee and ankle arthritis with swelling and effusion (■ Fig. 44.3), the existing spasticity made it difficult to adequately assess the restriction of movement.

44.3 Labor Values

44.3.1 Labor Values at Admission

Hb 7.2 g/dl (normochromic, normocytic), leukocytes 7600/μl, platelets 170,000/μl, differential blood count unremarkable. CRP max. 3 mg/dl. **ESR 95 mm/h**. The remaining laboratory values (electrolytes, liver, kidney, muscles, bones) were unremarkable. Coagulation diagnostics: unremarkable, factor 13 reduced (34%). Immunology: The rheumatological diagnostics showed normal values for complement and no autoantibodies. No evidence of p- and c-ANCA. Nonspecific antibody stimulation. Neopterin: 6.8 ng/ml (max. 2.5). The urinalysis revealed the presence of a urinary tract infection caused by *E. coli*.

44.3.2 Educational Questions— Part 1

1. What is your suspected diagnosis?

44.4 Further Course

The patient was admitted to the hospital on suspicion of **Henoch-Schönlein purpura**. The symptoms and laboratory values were assessed as consistent with vasculitis, due to the reduced general condition and suspicion of **intestinal bleeding** with an intermittent Hb drop to 5.8 g/dl without evidence

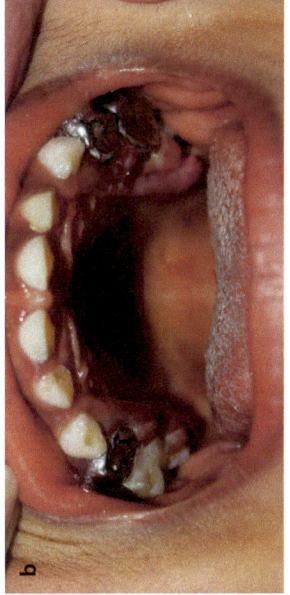
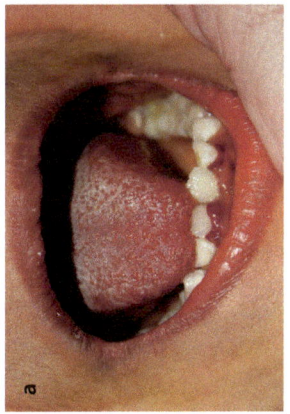

■ Fig. 44.2 a, b Enoral findings. Gingival hyperplasia with inflammatory component

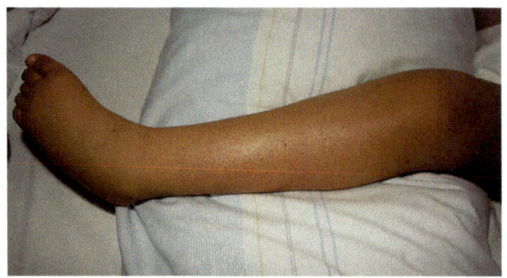

◘ Fig. 44.3 Musculoskeletal findings. Swelling of the knee and ankle

of a bleeding source, immunosuppressive therapy with prednisolone was started, under which no significant improvement initially occurred. After transfusion, good stabilization of Hb around 9.5 g/dl.

In the course of the disease, the pediatric rheumatological co-assessment was also carried out in the case of unclear disease events. Noteworthy in the examination findings were the **petechiae**, which in contrast to the classic bleeding efflorescences e.g. in vasculitis in the present case were strictly **follicular/perifollicular**. The **gingival hyperplasia**/gingivitis (◘ Fig. 44.2) was impressive and not to be considered as a typical symptom of Henoch-Schönlein purpura. The swelling of the knee and ankle joints in the sense of joint inflammation could be well reconciled with the original suspected diagnosis, but overall there were doubts about the diagnosis of vasculitis. The detailed history revealed that the patient had been receiving the same two types of baby food jars several times a day for at least 4 years. On some days she also received pudding. The manufacturer of the baby food confirmed that these 2 jars, as well as the dessert, did not contain **vitamin C**. Due to a diaper dermatitis developing from the consumption of fruit juices, the parents had also refrained from giving juices for years, the patient drank only water.

After detailed nutritional counseling, our patient received a balanced diet. After 3 months of balanced nutrition, there were no more gum bleeding, the restlessness was significantly improved. The parents felt that their daughter seemed more relaxed and interested again, even if the lost motor skills had not yet been completely relearned. There were no more skin symptoms, the joint swellings had subsided.

44.5 Educational Questions— Part 2

2. What further diagnostic steps should be initiated to make the differential diagnosis of scurvy more likely?
3. Is scurvy a disease relevant also in our latitudes or does it almost never exist outside of old sailor stories?
4. How is the disease treated? How can it be prevented?

44.6 Educational Answers

▪ 1. What is your suspected diagnosis?

In this patient, it was initially unclear what was causing the complaints. The petechiae and joint involvement seemingly fit with Henoch-Schönlein purpura. Atypical for Henoch-Schönlein purpura was the significantly reduced general condition, the regression of abilities, the course over months with ultimately aggravation of complaints and the manifestation of purpura sparing the dependent body parts. In a mostly lying patient, one would expect the purpura also on the back and legs. The elevated inflammatory markers also fit well with the urinary tract infection, which however could not explain the long-term changes. Therefore, an antibiotic therapy was initially carried out, in addition to symptomatic therapy with rehydration, balanced nutrition according to body weight, pain and anti-in-flammatory therapy.

- **2. What further diagnostic steps should be initiated to make the differential diagnosis scurvy more likely?**

Laboratory diagnostics: The diagnosis of vitamin C measurement in leukocytes is superior to the measurement in plasma, but it is subject to strong fluctuations. The medical history and clinical findings are decisive for the diagnosis. In our case, the determination of vitamin C was delayed. At the time of determination, the vitamin C level in the serum was 0.22 mg/dl (normal value from 0.5 mg/dl), symptoms of scurvy are generally expected from a level of < 0.2 mg/dl (Mertens and Gertner 2011).

Radiology: The X-ray examination of the knee joint then showed the classic conventional radiological signs of Möller-Barlow's disease, i.e., infantile scurvy (**osteopenia, Frankl line, metaphyseal extensions**) (◘ Fig. 44.4).

- **3. Is scurvy a disease relevant in our latitudes, or does it almost never exist outside of old seafarer stories?**

In the literature, one regularly finds reports of patients with scurvy. Particularly affected are severely developmentally delayed children, children with psychiatric diseases, e.g.,

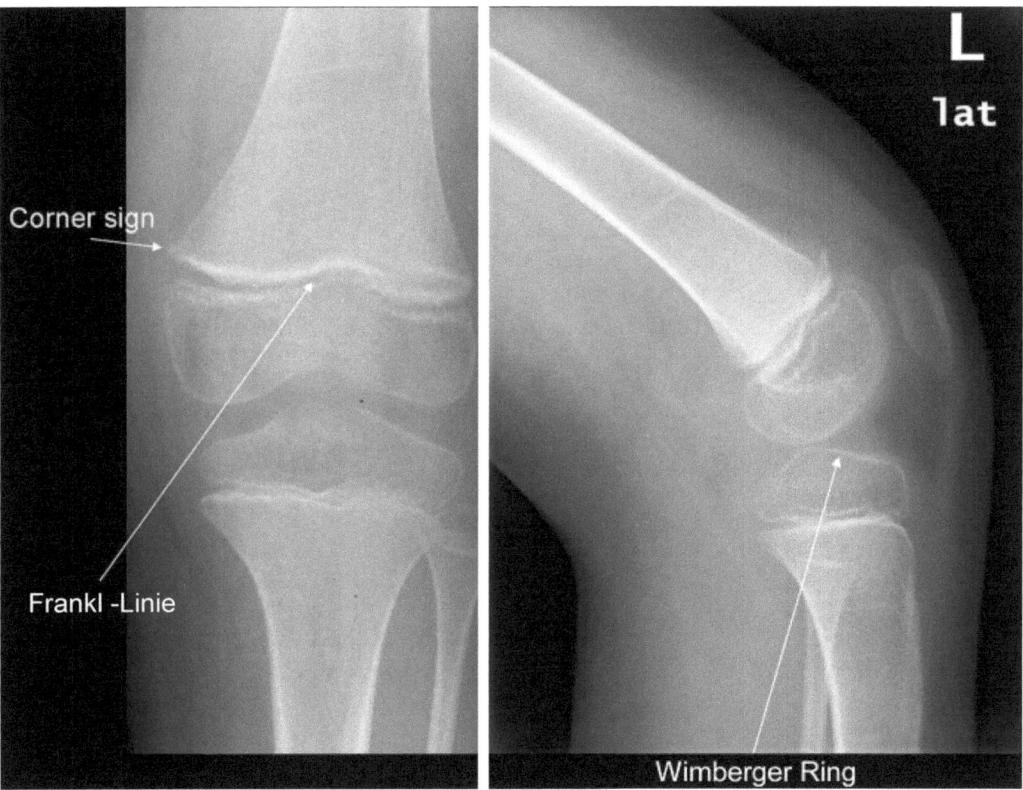

◘ **Fig. 44.4**　Radiological signs of the child consistent with scurvy. (With kind permission from Prof. Dr. J. F. Schäfer, Ped. Radiology, University Children's Hospital Tübingen)

anorexia nervosa, and occasionally (small) children with glaring nutritional errors (supposed refusal of the child to eat fruits and vegetables). The disease is also regularly reported in adulthood, here it is often psychiatric patients or patients with pronounced addictive behavior (e.g., alcohol).

- **4. How is the disease treated? How can it be prevented?**

The therapy is carried out with the substitution of vitamin C 100 mg, 3 times daily, ideally in the form of vitamin C-containing foods. To prevent vitamin C deficiency states, there are age-dependent recommendations for daily intake (◘ Table 44.1, German Society for Nutrition, Austrian Society for Nutrition, Swiss Society for Nutrition Research, Swiss Association for Nutrition 2015).

44.7 Differential diagnostic considerations

The presented symptoms initially resembled, for example, leukocytoclastic vasculitis, which is why therapy with steroids was also initiated. However, the strictly (peri-)follicular petechiae combined with gingival hyper-

◘ **Table 44.1** Age-dependent recommendations for vitamin C needs. (From: Reference values German Society for Nutrition e. V., Vitamin C, last revised 2015. ► www.dge.de . Downloaded on 27.01.2022)

Age	Vitamin C mg/day
1st year of life to end of 4th year of life	20
4th to end of 7th year of life	30
7th to end of 10th year of life	45
10th to end of 13th year of life	65
13th to end of 15th year of life	85
15 to 18 years	105 (m)/90 (w)

plasia/gingivitis were decisive for a detailed medical history, which then revealed the patient's severe malnutrition. These described symptoms should still make us think of the differential diagnosis of scurvy today, which still occurs in western countries and often presents with rheumatological symptoms.

44.8 Summary

44.8.1 Etiology

Unlike many animals, humans cannot produce ascorbic acid, so vitamin C is an **essential vitamin** (Levine 1986). Vitamin C is a powerful antioxidant and, in addition to its stabilizing function in **collagen biosynthesis**, it has a number of other important functions, such as increasing iron absorption or its role in the synthesis of neurotransmitters or neuroendocrine hormones (Schwetje et al. 2020).

44.8.2 Pathogenesis/Clinic

Depending on the severity and duration of the deficiency, different symptoms occur. These symptoms arise after 1–3 months of insufficient supplementation and are listed in ◘ Table 44.2 (Hamperl 1944; Hodges et al. 1969; Fain 2005; Biesalski et al. 2010):

44.8.3 Diagnosis

If one thinks of it, the diagnosis can be made clinically with the appropriate history, with the typical radiological signs being helpful in the assessment. These include generalized demineralization, Frankl line (also Fränkel line) (calcification zone at the end of the metaphysis), "corner sign" (also "Pelkin spur": lateral metaphyseal spur after infarction) and Wimberger ring (framing line

◘ **Table 44.2**   Possible sequelae of severe vitamin C deficiency

Skin/Mucous Membrane	Follicular petechiae, ecchymoses, corkscrew hairs, gingival hyperplasia with mucosal bleeding, tooth loss
Musculoskeletal System	Bone pain due to subperiosteal hemorrhages, arthritis, arthralgia, hemarthrosis
Hematology	Anemia (multifactorial: e.g., iron deficiency, other hypovitaminoses, bleeding)
Immune System	Susceptibility to infection, delayed wound healing Increased CRP and ESR
Neurology	Irritability

around the epiphyses) (see also ◘ Fig. 44.4) (Popovich et al. 2009; Miraj and Abdullah 2020).

It is important to highlight in the differential diagnosis that in malnourished children, a combination of rickets, scurvy, and other hypovitaminoses can occur, which can potentially complicate the diagnosis. This aspect was already highlighted in a paper on avitaminoses in 1941 (Eddy and Dalldorf 1941). Nowadays, other rheumatic diseases, such as vasculitis, but also physical abuse can present a similar picture at first glance (Clemetson 2002).

44.8.4 Therapy

High-dose substitution of vitamin C, dietary advice, possibly substitution of other vitamins in frequently associated malnutrition.

44.8.5 Prevention

The recommendations for vitamin C supplementation vary. The WHO recommends the multiple daily intake of unprocessed fruits and vegetables. The average daily intake of vitamin C in Europe and the USA is between 50 and 100 mg, which also corresponds to the recommendations of the German, Austrian and Swiss societies for nutrition 2000 (age-dependent from newborn to adolescence from 20–90 mg/day) (German Society for Nutrition, Austrian Soci-

ety for Nutrition, Swiss Society for Nutrition Research, Swiss Association for Nutrition 2015). However, it should be noted that the vitamin requirement shows large individual and disease-related fluctuations (German Society for Nutrition, Austrian Society for Nutrition, Swiss Society for Nutrition Research, Swiss Association for Nutrition 2015). In refugee camps, it has been observed that even significantly lower amounts (10 mg/day) of vitamin C can prevent the development of scurvy (Hodges et al. 1969; Hodges 1971).

> **Conclusion**
>
> Scurvy is a disease that is now rarely seen. However, it is occasionally reported in patients with low socioeconomic status and severe disabilities, or with malnutrition in the case of severe, e.g., oncological underlying diseases (Weinstein et al. 2001; Rosati et al. 2005; Ghedira Besbes et al. 2010; Schwetje et al. 2020).

References

Biesalski, Bischoff, Puchstein (2010) Ernährungsmedizin: Nach dem Curriculum Ernährungsmedizin der Bundesärztekammer und der DGE. Georg Thieme, Verlag, Stuttgart

Clemetson C a B (2002) Barlow's disease. Med Hypotheses 59:52–56.   ▶ https://doi.org/10.1016/s0306-9877(02)00114-7

Deutsche Gesellschaft für Ernährung, Österreichische Gesellschaft für Ernährung, Schweizerische Gesellschaft für Ernährungsforschung, Schweizerische

44

Vereinigung für Ernährung (2015) Referenzwerte für die Nährstoffzufuhr

Eddy WH, Dalldorf G (1941) The avitaminoses; the chemical, clinical and pathological aspects of the vitamin deficiency diseases. Williams & Wilkins, Baltimore

Fain O (2005) Musculoskeletal manifestations of scurvy. Joint Bone Spine 72:124–128. ▶ https://doi.org/10.1016/j.jbspin.2004.01.007

Ghedira Besbes L, Haddad S, Ben Meriem C et al (2010) Infantile scurvy: two case reports. Int J Pediatr 2010:717518. ▶ https://doi.org/10.1155/2010/717518

Hamperl (1944) Ribberts Lehrbuch der allgemeinen Pathologie und der Pathologischen Anatomie. Springer, Berlin

Hodges R (1971) Clinical manifestations of ascorbic acid deficiency in man. Am J Clin Nutr 24:432–443

Hodges RE, Baker EM, Hood J et al (1969) Experimental scurvy in man. Am J Clin Nutr 22:535–548. ▶ https://doi.org/10.1093/ajcn/22.5.535

Levine M (1986) New concepts in the biology and biochemistry of ascorbic acid. N Engl J Med 314:892–902. ▶ https://doi.org/10.1056/NEJM198604033141407

Mertens MT, Gertner E (2011) Rheumatic manifestations of scurvy: a report of three recent cases in a major urban center and a review. Semin Arthritis Rheum 41:286–290. ▶ https://doi.org/10.1016/j.semarthrit.2010.10.005

Miraj F, Abdullah A (2020) Scurvy: Forgotten diagnosis, but still exist. Int J Surg Case Rep 68:263–266. ▶ https://doi.org/10.1016/j.ijscr.2020.03.002

Popovich D, McAlhany A, Adewumi AO, Barnes MM (2009) Scurvy: forgotten but definitely not gone. J Pediatr Health Care 23:405–415. ▶ https://doi.org/10.1016/j.pedhc.2008.10.008

Rosati P, Boldrini R, Devito R et al (2005) A child with painful legs. Lancet Lond Engl 365:1438. ▶ https://doi.org/10.1016/S0140-6736(05)66381-7

Schwetje D, Zillekens A, Kieback J-D et al (2020) Infantile scurvy: still a relevant differential diagnosis in Western medicine. Nutrition 75–76:110726. ▶ https://doi.org/10.1016/j.nut.2020.110726

Weinstein M, Babyn P, Zlotkin S (2001) An orange a day keeps the doctor away: scurvy in the year 2000. Pediatrics 108:E55. ▶ https://doi.org/10.1542/peds.108.3.e55

Supplementary Information

Abbreviations

AAV - ANCA-associated vasculitis

ACE - Angiotensin converting enzyme

ACPA/Anti-CCP - Antibodies against citrullinated proteins

ACR/VF - American College of Rheumatology/Vasculitis Foundation

ADA-2 - Adenosine Deaminase- 2

ADB - Anti-Deoxyribonucleotidase B

AB - Antibody

ALL - acute lymphatic leukemia

ALT - Alanine Aminotransferase

ANA - antinuclear antibodies

ANCA - antineutrophil cytoplasmic antibodies

Anti-dsDNA-AB - Antibodies against double-stranded DNA

AOSD - Adult-onset Still's Disease

AP - alkaline phosphatase

APLAID - Autoinflammation with PLCG2-associated antibody deficiency and immune dysregulation

ARA - American Rheumatism Association

ARDS - Acute Respiratory Distress Syndrome

ARF - acute rheumatic fever

ASL - Antistreptolysin Test/Titer

aSLE - adult systemic lupus erythematosus

ASS - Acetylsalicylic acid

AST - Aspartate Aminotransferase

AZ - General condition

BE - Base Excess

BGA - Blood gas analysis

BLyS - B-Lymphocyte Stimulator

BMI - Body Mass Index

BMP - Bone morphogenetic protein

BSG - Erythrocyte sedimentation rate

BWK - Thoracic vertebrae

CAPS - Cryopyrin-associated periodic syndrome (OMIM191900, 120100, 607115)

CARD - Caspase recruitment domain-containing protein

CARRA - Childhood Arthritis and Rheumatology Research Alliance

CED - chronic inflammatory bowel disease

CES - Camuratti-Engelmann Syndrome

CINCA - Chronic Infantile Neurologic Cutaneous and Articular Syndrome

CK - Creatine kinase

CMAS - Childhood Myositis Assessment Scale

CMV - Cytomegalovirus

CMV - Cytomegalovirus

CNO - chronic nonbacterial osteomyelitis

CREST Syndrome - Calcinosis, Raynaud's Syndrome, Esophageal Dysmotility, Sclerodactyly, and Telangiectasia

CRMO - chronic recurrent multifocal osteomyelitis

CRP - C-reactive Protein

CRPS - complex regional pain syndrome

csDMARD - conventional synthetic disease modifying antirheumatic drugs

CT - Computer Tomography

c-TA - Takayasu Arteritis in childhood

CTGF - Connective tissue growth factor

DADA2 - Deficiency of Adenosine Deaminase 2

DIC - disseminated intravascular coagulation

DIP - distal interphalangeal joints

dsDNA - Double-stranded DNA

EAA - Enthesitis-associated arthritis

EBV - Epstein-Barr Virus

ECF - Slipped capital femoral epiphysis

EDS - Ehlers-Danlos Syndrome

EGPA - eosinophilic granulomatosis with polyangiitis (formerly: Churg-Strauss syndrome)

ECG - Electrocardiogram

ELISA - Enzyme-linked immunosorbent assay

EMA - European Medicines Agency

ENA - extractable nuclear antigens

EOS - Early-Onset Sarcoidosis

ERA - European Dialysis and Transplant Association

EULAR - European League Against Rheumatism

EZ - Nutritional status

FCAS - familial cold-induced autoinflammatory syndrome

FEV - forced expiratory volume

FMF - familial Mediterranean fever (OMIM 249100)

GAS - Group A Streptococci

GFR - glomerular filtration rate

GGT - Gamma-Glutamyl-Transferase

GK - Glucocorticoids

GKJR - Society for Pediatric and Adolescent Rheumatology

GnRH - Gonadotropin-Releasing Hormone

GOT - Glutamate Oxaloacetate Transaminase

GPA - Granulomatosis with Polyangiitis (formerly: Wegener's Granulomatosis)

GPT - Glutamate-Pyruvate Transaminase

GvHD - Graft-versus-Host Disease

Hb - Hemoglobin

HIDS - Hyperimmunoglobulin D Periodic Fever Syndrome (OMIM 260920)

HIV - human immunodeficiency virus

Hk - Hematocrit

HLA - human leukocyte antigen

HLH - hemophagocytic lymphohistiocytosis

HPP - Hypophosphatasia

HSP - Henoch-Schönlein Purpura

HSV - Herpes simplex virus

HUS - hemolytic uremic syndrome

HWS - Cervical spine

IFN - Interferon

Ig - Immunoglobulin

IL - Interleukin

ILAR - International League of Associations for Rheumatology

IP-10 - Interferon-γ induced protein 10

IUIS - International Union of Immunological Societies

IVIG - intravenously administered immunoglobulins

JAK - Janus kinase

JIA - juvenile idiopathic arthritis

JPsA - juvenile Psoriasis Arthritis

KD - Kawasaki Syndrome

KG - Body weight

KM - Contrast agent

KOF - Body surface area

LDH - Lactate dehydrogenase

LWK - Lumbar vertebrae

MAA - Myositis-associated antibodies

MAS - Macrophage Activation Syndrome

MCH - mean corpuscular hemoglobin

MCP - Metacarpophalangeal joint

MCP-1 - Monocyte chemoattractant protein 1

MCV - mean corpuscular volume

MIS-C - Multisystem Inflammatory Syndrome in Children

MMF - Mycophenolate mofetil

MMP - Matrix Metalloproteinase

MPA - Microscopic Polyangiitis

MPO - Myeloperoxidase

MRA - Magnetic Resonance Angiography

MRSA - Methicillin-resistant *Staphylococcus aureus*

MRT - Magnetic Resonance Imaging

MSA - Myositis-specific antibodies

MSSA - Methicillin-sensitive *Staphylococcus aureus*

MTP - Metatarsophalangeal joint

MTX - Methotrexate

MVK - Mevalonate kinase

MWS - Muckle-Wells Syndrome

NET - Neutrophil extracellular traps

NF-κB - Nuclear factor kappa-light-chain-enhancer of activated B-cells (Nuclear factor kappa-light-chain-enhancer of activated B-cells)

NGS - Next generation sequencing

NLRP3 - NACHT, LRR and PYD domains-containing protein

NOD2 - Nucleotide-binding oligomerization domain containing 2

NOMID - Neonatal Onset Multisystemic Inflammatory Disease

NSAID - nonsteroidal anti-inflammatory drugs

NSAR - nonsteroidal anti-inflammatory drugs

NT-proBNP - N-terminal prohormone of brain natriuretic peptide

OI - Osteogenesis imperfecta

OMIM - Online Mendelian Inheritance in Man

OSG - upper ankle joint

PAAND - Pyrin-associated autoinflammation with neutrophilic dermatosis

PCR - Polymerase Chain Reaction

PET-CT - Positron Emission Tomography-Computed Tomography

PFAPA Syndrome - periodic fever, aphthous stomatitis, pharyngitis, and adenopathy

PID - primary immune deficiency

PIMS - Pediatric Inflammatory Multisystem Syndrome

PIP - proximal interphalangeal joints

PJP - Pneumocystis jiroveci pneumonia

PLCG2 - Phospholipase C Gamma 2; Phospholipase-C-Gamma-2

Pm-SCl - Polymyositis-Scleroderma

PR3 - Proteinase 3

PReS - Pediatric Rheumatology European Society

PRINTO - Pediatric Rheumatology International Trials Organization

PSRA - Post-Streptococcal Arthritis

PTT - partial thromboplastin time

PTX - Pentraxin

PVAS - Pediatric Vasculitis Activity Score

PVL - Panton-Valentine Leukocidin

RF - Rheumatoid Factor

RR - Riva-Rocci blood pressure measurement

SAA - Serum Amyloid A

SAA - Scleroderma-associated antibodies

SAMHD1 - SAM domain and HD domain-containing protein 1

SAP - Signaling lymphocytic activation molecule associated protein

SEA Syndrome - Seronegativity-Enthesiopathy-Arthropathy Syndrome

SHARE - Single Hub and Access Point for Paediatric Rheumatology in Europe

SIGLEC1 - Sialic acid-binding immunoglobulin-like lectin 1

sJIA - systemic juvenile idiopathic arthritis

SLE - systemic lupus erythematosus

SLEDAI - Systemic Lupus Erythematosus Disease Activity Index

SLICC (SDI) - Systemic Lupus International Collaborating Clinics/American College of Rheumatology Damage Index

SpA - Spondyloarthritis

ssDNA - single-stranded DNA antibodies

SSW - Weeks of pregnancy

STING - Stimulator of interferon genes

STIR - Short-tau inversion recovery

SURF - Syndrome of Undifferentiated Fever

SZT - Stem cell transplantation

T3 - Triiodothyronine

T4 - Tetraiodothyronine

TGF - Transforming growth factor

TH - Helper T cells

TIRM - Turbo inversion recovery magnitude

TLCO - Carbon monoxide transfer factor

TMEM173 - Transmembrane protein 173, corresponds to STING1

TMS - Trimethoprim-Sulfamethoxazole

TNF - Tumor necrosis factor

TNSALP - Tissue non-specific alkaline phosphatase

TPO - Thyroid peroxidase

TRAPS - Tumor necrosis factor receptor-associated periodic syndrome (OMIM 142680)

TREX - DNA 3'-repair exonuclease 1

TSH - Thyrotropin

USG - lower ankle joint

VCAM - Vascular cell adhesion protein

VUS - Variants of Uncertain Significance

VZV - Varicella-Zoster Virus

XIAP - X-linked inhibitor of apoptosis protein